RECENT ADVANCES IN CLINICAL PSYCHIATRY

Recent Advances in Clinical Psychiatry

By

KENNETH GRANVILLE-GROSSMAN

M.D. (Lond.), M.R.C.P., D.P.M.

Physician-in-Charge, Department of Psychiatry,
St. Mary's Hospital, London

J. & A. Churchill · London

1971

First Published 1971

International Standard Book Number
0 7000 1501 9

Printed in Great Britain

For Pat,
with respect to the onlookers,
Deborah, David and Helen

PREFACE

THE rate of progress in clinical psychiatry is steadily increasing and important advances now occur more frequently and are more varied than at any previous time. In this book my aim has been to give a discerning account of some of the more recent developments in this field particularly in relation to previous knowledge and current practice. My emphasis is on the clinical situation and I have tried to avoid an academic approach, but I have not hesitated to discuss theoretical aspects where an understanding of these seems essential for the proper handling of clinical problems.

The work involved in preparing this book has been much eased by the help of others. I am indebted to Mrs Ann Jackman and Mrs Isabel Vincent for their enthusiastic secretarial assistance, to Mr K. J. Wass for his careful preparation of the diagrams and to Mr J. A. Rivers and Mr A. S. Knightley of Messrs. J. & A. Churchill for their courteous guidance. For kind permission to reproduce illustrations, I am grateful to:

Professor Michael Shepherd and English Universities Press, for Figure 1.3.

Dr Maurice Victor and the Elsevier Publishing Company for Figure 4.1.

Dr Ian Oswald, Dr Robert Priest and the Editor, *British Medical Journal*, for Figure 4.4.

Dr Malcolm Lader and the Editor, *Journal of Neurology, Neurosurgery and Psychiatry*, for Figure 5.1

Dr Malcolm Lader and the Editor-in-Chief, *British Journal of Psychiatry*, for Figure 5.2.

Dr Colin Murray Parkes and the Editor, *British Medical Journal*, for Figure 6.1

The Editor, *The Lancet*, for Figure 7.1.

Lastly, I would like to express my gratitude to my colleagues for many very helpful discussions and to thank my wife and family for their patient encouragement and understanding.

London, 1970   K. L. G-G.

CONTENTS

CHAPTER 1

PHYSICAL TREATMENTS OF AFFECTIVE DISORDERS

Convulsive Therapy. Lithium Therapy. Monoamines and Affective Disorders. Hypertensive Reactions with Monoamine Oxidase Inhibitors

CONVULSIVE THERAPY

Preparation of the Patient

MOST psychiatrists now agree that patients receiving convulsive therapy should have atropine as premedication and should be anaesthetized and paralysed before the fit is induced. As with other procedures involving the administration of an anaesthetic, the patient should have been examined physically and his urine tested; the stomach must be empty and dentures removed.

Premedication

Electrical stimulation of the brain activates the autonomic nervous system and commonly causes transient cardiac irregularities. At the onset of the fit the pulse rate and blood pressure fall for several seconds and then increase to above normal values. Generally, these changes are of little importance clinically but sometimes they are associated with sudden cardiovascular failure (Perrin, 1961). Atropine, by its vagolytic action, prevents many of these adverse effects on the heart, but Cropper and Hughes (1964) point out that the conventional dose of 0·65 mg (1/100 gr) may be inadequate to prevent vagal overstimulation, and that the required dose may be of the order of 2 mg (1/35 gr). Intravenous administration (either immediately before, or in the same syringe as the anaesthetic) seems to be more effective than the more conventional subcutaneous injection some time before the treatment. Clement (1962) observed the arterial pulse of 200 patients immediately after the electrical stimulus; half had received atropine 1 mg intravenously at the same time as the anaesthetic and of these only one developed severe bradycardia, whereas there were 22 such instances among the 100 patients who had been premedicated subcutaneously half an hour before the anaesthetic. Hargreaves (1962) and Parry-Jones (1964) have also advocated the intravenous route. Bodley and Fenwick (1966) have reported findings similar to those of Clement in a smaller series. These authors also investigated the blood pressure responses to ECT with and without atropine premedication in hypertensive subjects. They noted a much greater increase in blood pressure in these patients when atropine was used than when it was omitted. A dilemma therefore arises in hypertensive subjects; if atropine is given, the heightened blood pressure response might increase the risk of a cerebrovascular accident, while if it is not given, the transient reduction in cardiac output due to excessive vagal stimulation might be dangerous. It seems better, however, to give atropine since ECT more commonly causes cardiac arrest than cerebral haemorrhage. A further reason for using atropine is that it lessens the increased salivary and bronchial secretion associated with convulsive therapy.

The Anaesthetic

Intravenous thiopentone sodium ("Pentothal") is the most widely used anaesthetic. The average dose is 150-250 mg and it is best given as a 2·5 per cent solution; at this concentration serious damage following accidental injection outside the vein or into an artery is unlikely. During the past few years, methohexitone sodium ("Brietal sodium"; "Brevital sodium") and propanidid ("Epontol") have been used as the anaesthetic agent. Methohexitone is an ultra-short acting barbiturate given intravenously usually as a 1 per cent solution in an average dose of 100-125 mg. Pitts, Desmarais, Stewart and Schaberg (1965) compared 500 electrical convulsive treatments in which methohexitone was given with 500 treatments using thiopentone. They found that thiopentone had the greater tendency to produce post-ictal ECG abnormalities, particularly atrial and ventricular ectopic beats, and that both induction and recovery were quicker using methohexitone. These findings have been confirmed in other studies (Woodruff, Pitts and Craig, 1969). In spite of these claims that methohexitone is the better anaesthetic, most psychiatrists seem to prefer thiopentone because it allows the patient to sleep during the period of post-ictal confusion whereas methohexitone does not. Further experience, however, may show methohexitone to be preferable when unilateral electrical stimulation or flurothyl is used (see below).

Propanidid is a non-barbiturate short-acting anaesthetic available as a 5 per cent oily solution which is administered intravenously at the rate of 1-2 ml per second; the average dose is about 7 mg per kilogramme body weight. Propanidid and thiopentone have been compared in a number of controlled studies on patients receiving ECT (Heifetz, Birkhan and Davidson, 1969; Naftalin, Haw and Bevans, 1969; Finlayson, Burnheim and Boots, 1970). Recovery of consciousness is much quicker when propanidid is used, but apnoea tends to be prolonged and occasionally patients may begin to recover consciousness before spontaneous respiration is satisfactorily re-established. Although Finlayson *et al.* (1970) noted that post-ictal confusion was more common among patients who had received thiopentone, there seems little or no advantage in using propanidid except rarely where barbiturates are contraindicated.

Muscle Relaxation

Suxamethonium chloride (succinylcholine chloride, "Scoline"), a depolarizing short-acting muscle relaxant, is now routinely given in convulsive therapy immediately before induction of the fit. Since it is hydrolysed by alkaline solutions it should not be given in the same syringe as thiopentone or methohexitone. The usual dose is 30-50 mg I.V.; it should not be so large that the convulsion cannot be detected. In patients with skeletal disease or with reduced cardiac or respiratory reserve, the technique described by Adderley and Hamilton (1953) may be useful. An arterial tourniquet is applied to one arm immediately before a full paralysing dose of the relaxant is given and the seizure is evident in the ischaemic arm if not elsewhere.

Suxamethonium markedly reduces muscular activity, especially that at the onset of the convulsion, when sudden muscular contractions may cause fractures and dislocations; a further advantage of its use is a reduction in cardiovascular disturbance, especially that due to the Valsalva effect (Perrin, 1961). The paralysis and associated apnoea usually last for about two minutes. Recovery is due to hydrolysis of the suxamethonium by serum pseudo-cholinesterase. (This enzyme is quite distinct from acetylcholinesterase, which is responsible for the degradation of acetylcholine liberated at neuromuscular junctions during normal nerve impulse transmission.) Rarely, normal pseudo-cholinesterase is replaced by an "atypical" enzyme which is very much less active in hydrolysing suxamethonium, and in these individuals the apnoea and paralysis may last two or three hours (Liddell, 1968). The abnormality is a genetically determined recessive characteristic; heterozygotes represent about 3·8 per cent of the general population, but only homozygotes (about 1:2800 of the population) show increased sensitivity to suxamethonium (Kattamis, Zannos-Mariolea, Franco et al., 1962).

Suxamethonium apnoea also arises in rare cases where the enzyme that is present is a third variant, different from both the normal and the common "atypical" forms (Lehmann, Liddell, Blackwell et al., 1963), and even more rarely where there is complete absence of plasma pseudocholinesterase activity (Liddell, Lehmann and Silk, 1962). Whittaker (1968) has described another variant and it seems likely that further phenotypes will be discovered.

Treatment of apnoea consists of intubation and continuing with intermittent positive pressure respiration until recovery. Anticholinesterase drugs such as neostigmine given early tend to potentiate the block and increase the paralysis, but they may accelerate recovery when given later; the critical point when these drugs change their effect seems to be about 90 minutes after the onset of the apnoea (Vickers, 1963). Reconstituted freeze-dried plasma contains active pseudocholinesterase and transfusion with it has been suggested as a specific treatment, but it needs to be given rapidly, and it may be ineffective when paralysis has persisted for one hour or more (Bush, 1968). Sensitivity to suxamethonium does not absolutely contraindicate its further use. Bidder, Sattin and Dowling (1963) described a patient who became apnoeic for three hours following the administration of a dose of 60 mg prior to ECT. Further convulsive treatments using 4 mg of suxamethonium were quite satisfactory, the apnoea and paralysis lasting only 10 minutes on these occasions.

REFERENCES

ADDERLEY, D. J. and HAMILTON, M. (1953). Use of succinylcholine in E.C.T. with particular reference to its effect on blood pressure. *Brit. med. J.* **1**, 195-197.

BIDDER, T. G., SATTIN, A. and DOWLING, A. S. (1963). Sensitivity to succinyl-choline. *Arch. gen. Psychiat.* **9**, 96-101.

BODLEY, P. O. and FENWICK, P. B. C. (1966). The effects of electroconvulsive therapy on patients with essential hypertension. *Brit. J. Psychiat.* **112**, 1241-1249.

BUSH, G. H. (1968). Pharmacogenetics and anaesthesia. *Proc. roy. Soc. Med.* **61**, 171-174.

CLEMENT, A. J. (1962). Atropine premedication for electric convulsion therapy. *Brit. med. J.* **1**, 228-229.

CROPPER, C. F. J. and HUGHES, M. (1964). Cardiac arrest (with apnoea) after E.C.T. *Brit. J. Psychiat.* **110**, 222-225.

FINLAYSON, P., BURNHEIM, R. B. and BOOTS, U. J. (1970). A comparison of propanidid (Epontol) and thiopentone anaesthesia in ECT. *Brit. J. Psychiat.* **116**, 79-83.

HARGREAVES, M. A. (1962). Intravenous atropine premedication before electro-convulsion therapy. *Lancet*, **1**, 243.

HEIFETZ, M. J., BIRKHAN, H. J. and DAVIDSON, L. J. (1969). Clinical evaluation of propanidid in electroconvulsive therapy. *Anesth. Analg. Curr. Res.* **48**, 293-296.

KATTAMIS, C., ZANNOS-MARIOLEA, L., FRANCO, A. P., LIDDELL, J., LEHMANN, H. and DAVIES, D. (1962). Frequency of atypical pseudocholinesterase in British and Mediterranean populations. *Nature (Lond.)*, **196**, 599-600.

LEHMANN, H., LIDDELL, J., BLACKWELL, B., O'CONNOR, D. C. and DAWS, A. V. (1963). Two further serum pseudocholinesterase phenotypes as causes of suxamethonium apnoea. *Brit. med. J.* **1**, 1116-1118.

LIDDELL, J. (1968). Cholinesterase variants and suxamethonium apnoea. *Proc. roy. Soc. Med.* **61**, 168-170.

LIDDELL, J., LEHMANN, H. and SILK, E. (1962). A "silent" pseudocholinesterase gene. *Nature (Lond.)*, **193**, 561-562.

NAFTALIN, A. L., HAW, M. E. and BEVANS, H. G. (1969). A comparison of propanidid and thiopentone as induction agents for electroconvulsive therapy. *Brit. J. Anaesth.* **41**, 506-515.

PARRY-JONES, W. LL. (1964). Oral atropine in premedication for electroconvulsive therapy. *Lancet*, **1**, 1067-1068.

PERRIN, G. M. (1961). Cardiovascular aspects of electric shock therapy. *Acta psychiat. scand.* Supplement 152.

PITTS, F. N., DESMARAIS, G. M., STEWART, W. and SCHABERG, K. (1965). Induction of anaesthesia with methohexital and thiopental in electroconvulsive therapy. *New Engl. J. Med.* **273**, 353-360.

VICKERS, M. D. A. (1963). The mismanagement of suxamethonium apnoea. *Brit. J. Anaesth.* **35**, 260-268.

WHITTAKER, M. (1968). An additional pseudocholinesterase phenotype occurring in suxamethonium apnoea. *Brit. J. Anaesth.* **40**, 579-582.

WOODRUFF, R. A., PITTS, F. N. and CRAIG, A. (1969). Electrotherapy: the effects of barbiturate anesthesia, succinylcholine and pre-oxygenation on EKG. *Dis. nerv. Syst.* **30**, 180-185.

Electrical Stimulation

Position of the Electrodes

The two electrodes are usually placed one on each side in the temporo-frontal regions so that the current passes between them across the anterior part of both cerebral hemispheres. In 1958, Lancaster, Steinert and Frost introduced a unilateral technique in which both electrodes are placed on the right (i.e. non-dominant) side of the head. One electrode is put in the temporal region 3-4 cm above the midpoint of a line joining the lateral angle of the orbit and the external auditory meatus, and the other is placed above the ear in the parietal region 7-10 cm from the first (Figure 1.1). Lancaster *et al.* observed that unilateral stimulation was associated with much less post-ictal disorientation and impairment of memory than the bilateral technique, although the therapeutic effect of the two methods was approximately equivalent. Most other investigators have reported similar findings (Cannicott

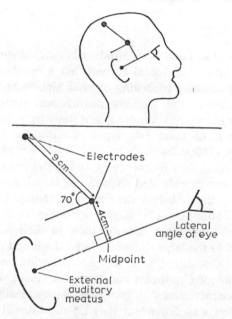

Figure 1.1 Placement of electrodes using
unilateral clcctrical stimulation

and Waggoner, 1967; Valentine, Keddie and Dunne, 1968; Zinkin and Birtchnell, 1968; Halliday, Davison, Browne and Kreeger, 1968; Strain, Brunschwig, Duffy *et al.*, 1968; Abrams and de Vito, 1969; Sutherland, Oliver and Knight, 1969; Costello, Belton, Abra and Dunn, 1970). Some studies, however, have failed to show that unilateral stimulation of the non-dominant hemisphere lessens the adverse effects of the treatment (McAndrew, Berkey and Matthews, 1967; Levy, 1968). There is some evidence that the unilateral technique is advantageous only when the stimulus is applied to the non-dominant hemisphere, and that placing the electrodes on the dominant side, though therapeutically as effective, may produce more mental disturbance than the bilateral method (Gottlieb and Wilson, 1965; Zamora and Kaelbling, 1965; Halliday *et al.*, 1968). Hence unilateral stimulation should only be used in patients who are clearly right-handed, and it should then be applied to the right side of the head. With left-handed and ambidextrous patients, where cerebral dominance cannot be located with certainty, the bilateral technique should be employed.

Inglis (1969) has pointed out that interference with the function of the dominant temporal lobe leads to disruption of learning. He suggests that it is the passage of the electric current through the dominant temporal lobe that is responsible for the memory impairment after ECT and that this accounts for the variation in intensity of the memory loss with the different techniques. If his hypothesis is correct he predicts that extreme anterior placement of the electrodes would cause the least mental disturbance.

Type of Stimulus

Originally when Cerletti and Bini introduced electrical stimulation in 1938, they used an alternating sinusoidal current, but a number of studies have since shown that a stimulus consisting of brief high-voltage pulses leads to less post-ictal confusion and memory disturbance. (Ottosson, 1960, has reviewed the earlier literature.) A more recent study by Valentine et al. (1968) compared the effects of these two types of stimulus. Patients receiving bidirectional pulses (750 volts peak to peak, each lasting about one two-thousandth of a second, at a frequency of 21·5 cycles per second) recovered their orientation more quickly and showed less impairment of memory for material learnt immediately before the treatment, than patients receiving the diphasic sinusoidal stimulus. The therapeutic effect of both methods was comparable, and the difference between them in their adverse effects can probably be related to the large difference in total amount of current passing through the brain. Consistent with this interpretation are the findings of Ottosson (1960) and of Cronholm and Ottosson (1960), who showed that memory disturbance increased with increasing electrical stimulation, but that the therapeutic effect was dependent only on the intensity of the epileptic activity.

REFERENCES

ABRAMS, R. and DE VITO, R. A. (1969). Clinical efficacy of unilateral ECT. Dis. nerv. Syst. 30, 262-263.
CANNICOTT, S. M. and WAGGONER, R. W. (1967). Unilateral and bilateral electro-convulsive therapy. Arch. gen. Psychiat. 16, 229-232.
COSTELLO, C. G., BELTON, G. P., ABRA, J. C. and DUNN, B. E. (1970). The amnesic and therapeutic effects of bilateral and unilateral ECT. Brit. J. Psychiat. 116, 69-78.
CRONHOLM, B. and OTTOSSON, J-O. (1960). Experimental studies of the therapeutic action of electroconvulsive therapy in endogenous depression. The role of the electrical stimulation and of the seizure studied by variation of the stimulus intensity and modification by lidocaine of seizure discharge. Acta psychiat. scand. Supplement 145, pp. 69-102.

GOTTLIEB, G. and WILSON, I. (1965). Cerebral dominance: temporary disruption of verbal memory by unilateral electroconvulsive shock treatment. *J. comp. physiol. Psychol.* **60**, 368-372.

HALLIDAY, A. M., DAVISON, K., BROWNE, M. W. and KREEGER, L. C. (1968). A comparison of the effects on depression and memory of bilateral ECT and unilateral ECT to the dominant and non-dominant hemispheres. *Brit. J. Psychiat.* **114**, 997-1012.

INGLIS, J. (1969). Electrode placement and the effect of ECT on mood and memory in depression. *Canad. psychiat. Ass. J.* **14**, 463-471.

LANCASTER, N. P., STEINERT, R. R. and FROST, I. (1958). Unilateral electro-convulsive therapy. *J. ment. Sci.* **104**, 221-227.

LEVY, R. (1968). The clinical evaluation of unilateral electroconvulsive therapy. *Brit. J. Psychiat.* **114**, 459-463.

MCANDREW, J., BERKEY, B. and MATTHEWS, C. (1967). The effects of dominant and non-dominant ECT as compared to bilateral ECT. *Amer. J. Psychiat.* **124**, 483-490.

OTTOSSON, J-O. (1960). Experimental studies of memory impairment after electro-convulsive therapy. *Acta psychiat. scand.* Supplement 145, pp. 103-132.

STRAIN, J. J., BRUNSCHWIG, L., DUFFY, J. P., AGLE, D. P., ROSENBAUM, A. L. and BIDDER, T. G. (1968). Comparison of therapeutic effects and memory changes with bilateral and unilateral ECT. *Amer. J. Psychiat.* **125**, 294-304.

SUTHERLAND, E. M., OLIVER, J. E. and KNIGHT, D. R. (1969). E.E.G., memory and confusion in dominant, non-dominant and bitemporal E.C.T. *Brit. J. Psychiat.* **115**, 1059-1064.

VALENTINE, M., KEDDIE, K. M. G. and DUNNE, D. (1968). A comparison of techniques in electro-convulsive therapy. *Brit. J. Psychiat.* **114**, 989-996.

ZAMORA, E. N. and KAELBLING, R. (1965). Memory and electroconvulsive therapy. *Amer. J. Psychiat.* **122**, 546-554.

ZINKIN, S. and BIRTCHNELL, J. (1968). Unilateral electro-convulsive therapy: its effects on memory and its therapeutic efficacy. *Brit. J. Psychiat.* **114**, 973-988.

Flurothyl Induction of Convulsions

The use of chemicals such as camphor and leptazol ("Cardiazol", "Metrazol") to induce convulsions became obsolete with the introduction of electrical stimulation. A new chemical convulsant with some possible advantage over electrical stimulation is flurothyl (hexafluorodiethyl ether, "Indoklon") a colourless, volatile, non-inflammable liquid first used by Krantz, Esquibel, Truitt *et al.* in 1958.

Administration

Flurothyl is most commonly administered by inhalation when the patient is anaesthetized and relaxed. Rose and Watson (1967*b*), Gander, Bennett and Kelly (1967), and Small, Small, Sharpley and Moore (1968) have described their experiences with the drug and have reviewed the literature. Since salivation seems to be greater with flurothyl than with electrical stimulation, Rose and Watson (1967*b*) advise premedication with larger than usual doses of atropine; they give 1·2 mg I.M. 30 minutes before treatment. Thiopentone blocks the convulsant action of the drug and methohexitone may be preferable. The apparatus for administering the flurothyl consists of a vaporizer attached to a face mask and to a double-ended bag filled with oxygen. About 0·5 ml flurothyl is injected into the vaporizer and an oxygen-flurothyl mixture is blown into the lungs by gently squeezing the bag once every five seconds. The response usually occurs after 40-60 sec, a period of myoclonus (irregular movements of the hands and feet) preceding the tonic and clonic phases. If no response is obtained (and this is particularly likely if the patient has been taking anticonvulsant drugs, or if thiopentone has been used) more flurothyl must be injected into the vaporizer.

Flurothyl has also been administered intravenously as a 10 per cent solution in polyethylene glycol (Nussbaum and Kurland, 1962). The initial injection of 5 ml is followed 30 seconds later by further injections of 0·5-1 ml every 10 seconds until signs appear of a fit developing; the average dose required is 6-8 ml. The solvent currently available is however not satisfactory, since it may cause renal damage (Rose and Watson, 1967b).

Comparison with ECT

All investigations (including the double-blind study on 100 patients by Small et al., 1968) report that flurothyl and electrical convulsive therapies are equally effective in treating psychiatric disorders. Side-effects, particularly confusion and memory disturbances, are generally much less severe with flurothyl, although the fits last longer. Flurothyl is significantly associated with headache, and other adverse effects seen with this treatment but not with ECT are nausea, vomiting and recurrence of the convulsion. Contrary to the reports of most investigators, Gander et al. (1967) found a much higher incidence of side-effects (including confusion and memory disturbance) with flurothyl than with ECT, but they used larger doses of the drug than most other workers have found necessary. At present, flurothyl should not be used in pregnancy as its teratogenic activity has not been investigated, but there does not seem to be any other contraindication to its use. It can be used, however, in circumstances where ECT is contraindicated (e.g. where the patient has an implanted electronic device such as a cardiac pacemaker) or where electrical stimulation has repeatedly failed to cause a convulsion (Rose and Watson, 1967a).

REFERENCES

GANDER, D. R., BENNETT, P. J. and KELLY, D. H. W. (1967). Hexafluorodiethyl ether (Indoklon) convulsive therapy; a pilot study. Brit. J. Psychiat. 113, 1413-1418.

KRANTZ, J. C., ESQUIBEL, A., TRUITT, E. B., LING, A. S. C. and KURLAND, A. A. (1958). Hexafluorodiethyl ether (Indoklon)—an inhalant anaesthetic. Its use in psychiatric treatment. J. Amer. med. Ass. 166, 1555-1562.

NUSSBAUM, K. and KURLAND, A. A. (1962). Intravenous hexafluorodiethyl ether (Indoklon) modified by succinylcholine chloride. Clinical studies in convulsive psychiatric treatment. Curr. ther. Res. 4, 44-56.

Rose, L. and Watson, A. (1967a). Flurothyl-induced convulsions. Two specific indications. *Clin. Trials J.* 4, 749-751.
Rose, L. and Watson, A. (1967b). Flurothyl (Indoklon). Experience with an inhalational convulsant agent. *Anaesthesia*, 22, 425-434.
Small, J. G., Small, I. F., Sharpley, P. and Moore, D. F. (1968). A double blind comparative evaluation of flurothyl and ECT. *Arch. gen. Psychiat.* 19, 79-86.

Indications for Convulsive Therapy in Affective Disorders

Depression

Convulsive therapy is the most effective treatment of depression. Given twice weekly, the mental state reverts to normal in responsive cases commonly after four to six treatments, though sometimes as many as ten or twelve are necessary. Improvement occurs with each treatment with some regression during the two or three days between them. The Medical Research Council (1965) carried out a trial of four different treatments of depression, namely electroconvulsive therapy (four to eight applications), imipramine 200 mg daily, phenelzine 60 mg daily and placebo. Most of the patients in the trial would probably be regarded as having an endogenous type of illness, because the main criteria for inclusion were that the depression was the primary manifestation of the illness and that it was accompanied by one or more of the five following symptoms: self-depreciation with a morbid sense of guilt, sleep disturbance, hypochondriasis, retardation of thought and action, agitated behaviour. In addition only patients aged 40-69 years were included, their illnesses were less than 18 months duration and they had had no adequate treatment during the six months prior to the trial. The 250 patients in the investigation were allocated randomly to the four regimes and assessments of the mental state were made before treatment and at various later times. After four weeks, 71 per cent of patients treated by ECT had recovered compared with only 39 per cent of those on placebo, and on this short-term basis ECT was undoubtedly the best treatment. Hutchinson and Smedberg (1963) reported an 86·7 per cent recovery rate in their series of depressed patients treated with ECT, better than the results in comparable patients treated with various drugs. Bratfos and Haug (1965) treated 315 patients suffering from manic-depressive disorder; with ECT recovery was more than twice as common as with drugs and the length of stay in hospital was significantly shorter.

Estimates of the relapse rate after successful electroconvulsive therapy vary. Recurrence within three months occurred in 8 per cent of Perris and D'elia's (1966) series, and in 38 per cent of similar patients studied by Bratfos and Haug (1965). When depression recurs, further ECT is likely to be successful.

The response to convulsive therapy varies. The best results are obtained in cases of severe depression with retardation, arising suddenly in patients with good premorbid personalities, where guilt feelings and delusions of a depressive nature are prominent, where the symptoms are much worse in the mornings and where there is early wakening. (This clinical picture corresponds to that of classical "endogenous" depression.) In these patients convulsive therapy is the treatment of choice, especially if there has been a similar previous illness with a good response. The majority of depressed patients have illnesses not typical of "endogenous" depression and here the response to ECT is less certain, but various studies have attempted to define the features of the illness which have value in predicting the response. In an early, but still useful, investigation Hobson (1953) constructed a check list based on an analysis of the history and clinical state of 127 depressives treated by ECT. Six items were associated with a favourable response to ECT and nine with a poor response (Table 1.1). To predict the response, one is scored for the *absence* of each favourable item, and one for the *presence* of each unfavourable feature; the higher the total score the less likely is the patient to respond. In Hobson's series a score of 7 or less was associated with a good result, but this criterion misclassified 27 of his 127 cases.

Table 1.1

PREDICTION OF RESPONSE TO ECT
(Hobson, 1953)

Favourable features (Score 1 for each feature *absent*)

1. Sudden onset
2. Good insight
3. Obsessional previous personality
4. Self-reproach
5. Duration of illness less than one year
6. Pronounced retardation

Unfavourable features (Score 1 for each feature *present*)

1. Hypochondriasis
2. Depersonalization
3. Emotional lability
4. Neurotic traits in childhood
5. Neurotic traits in adult life
6. Hysterical attitude to illness
7. Above average intelligence
8. Fluctuating course since onset
9. Ill-adjusted or hysterical previous personality

More recently, Carney, Roth and Garside (1965) assessed 35 aspects of the illness of 108 depressed patients treated by ECT. Ten items correlated significantly with the mental state six months after completion of the treatment. The items and their weightings are given in Table 1.2. On this scale a total score of 1 or more suggests a good response (i.e. full social recovery with or without residual symptoms) and one of zero or less, a poor result (i.e. incomplete social recovery, slight improvement only, or no change or worse). Use of this criterion does, however, predict wrongly in a proportion of cases. Thus, of 44 of Carney *et al.*'s patients who had a good response to ECT, nine would have been predicted as responding poorly, while of 64 patients with a poor result, eight had scores of 1 or more and would have therefore been predicted as responding well.

Other recent studies which reach conclusions similar to those of Carney *et al.* have been reported by Mendels (1965) and Nyström (1965).

Table 1.2

PREDICTION OF RESPONSE TO ECT
(Carney *et al.*, 1965)

Feature	Score[1]
Weight loss	+3
Pyknic body build	+3
Early wakening	+2
Somatic delusions[2]	+2
Paranoid delusions	+1
Self pity	−1
Anxiety	−2
Worse in evenings	−3
Hysterical features or attitude	−3
Hypochondriasis[3]	−3

[1] Score only if feature present. Ignore features which are absent.
[2] Delusions of body change or disease, usually of a bizarre nature.
[3] Excessive or morbid preoccupation with bodily sensations which have little or no organic basis.

Depersonalization is sometimes considered to contraindicate convulsive therapy; Roth (1959) found that ECT often aggravated it, and Sargant and Slater (1963) advised caution in using ECT in its presence. Ackner and Grant (1960) compared the effects of ECT on 50 depressed depersonalized patients with 50 matched subjects without depersonalization. They found that depersonalization responded favourably to ECT in patients whose depression was clearly endogenous, while in those with neurotic or reactive features, the depersonalization was often unchanged. Hence, if the depression merits ECT it should be given even if depersonalization is present.

Mania

Convulsive therapy is sometimes used in mania, but to be effective it may have to be given very frequently, two or three shocks per day, when remission may occur within two or three days (Kalinowsky and Hoch, 1961; Paterson, 1963). Schiele and Schneider (1949) summarized 16 statistical reports of the use of ECT in a total of 466 manic patients. Overall, the recovery rate was 62 per cent and a further 18 per cent were considered improved by the treatment. In their own experience, Schiele and Schneider found ECT to be most useful in extremely excited patients but that relapse was common when treatment was stopped.

REFERENCES

ACKNER, B. and GRANT, Q. A. F. R. (1960). The prognostic significance of depersonalization in depressive illnesses treated with electroconvulsive therapy. *J. Neurol. Neurosurg. Psychiat.* **23**, 242-246.

BRATFOS, O. and HAUG, J. O. (1965). Electroconvulsive therapy and antidepressant drugs in manic-depressive disease. Treatment results at discharge and 3 months later. *Acta psychiat. scand.* **41**, 588-596.

CARNEY, M. W. P., ROTH, M. and GARSIDE, R. F. (1965). The diagnosis of depressive syndromes and the prediction of ECT response. *Brit. J. Psychiat.* **111**, 659-674.

HOBSON, R. F. (1953). Prognostic factors in electric convulsive therapy. *J. Neurol. Neurosurg. Psychiat.* **16**, 275-281.

HUTCHINSON, J. T. and SMEDBERG, D. (1963). Treatment of depression: A comparative study of ECT and six drugs. *Brit. J. Psychiat.* **109**, 536-538.

KALINOWSKY, L. B. and HOCH, P. H. (1961). *Somatic Treatments in Psychiatry.* New York.

MEDICAL RESEARCH COUNCIL (1965). Clinical trial of the treatment of depressive illness. *Brit. med. J.* **1**, 881-886.

MENDELS, J. (1965). Electroconvulsive therapy and depression. III. A method for prognosis. *Brit. J. Psychiat.* **111**, 687-690.

NYSTRÖM, S. (1965). On relation between clinical factors and efficacy of E.C.T. in depression. *Acta psychiat. scand.* Supplement 181.

PATERSON, A. S. (1963). *Electrical and Drug Treatments in Psychiatry.* Amsterdam.

PERRIS, C. and D'ELIA, G. (1966). A study of bipolar (manic-depressive) and unipolar recurrent depressive psychosis. IX. Therapy and prognosis. *Acta psychiat. scand.* Supplement 194, pp. 153-171.

ROTH, M. (1959). The phobic anxiety-depersonalization syndrome. *Proc. roy. Soc. Med.* **52**, 587-595.

SARGANT, W. and SLATER, E. (1963). *An Introduction to Physical Methods of Treatment in Psychiatry*, 4th edition. Edinburgh.

SCHIELE, B. C. and SCHNEIDER, R. A. (1949). The selective use of electroconvulsive therapy in manic patients. *Dis. nerv. Syst.* **10**, 291-297.

Adverse Effects and Contraindications

Physical Complications

Convulsive therapy carries a definite though small mortality risk. Perrin (1961) has summarized a number of mainly American studies involving a total of more than 40,000 patients. He found overall that one patient in 950 died, that one treatment in 12,500 was fatal, and that 50 per cent of the deaths were due to adverse effects on the cardiovascular system. Estimates of the mortality rate in Great Britain have been somewhat lower. Tewfik and Wells (1957) calculated that during the years 1949-53 in England and Wales one patient in 2300 died, while Barker and Baker (1959) estimated the risk as one fatality per 28,000 treatments during the years 1956-57. There is some suggestion that the mortality rate has fallen during the past twenty years. Table 1.3 shows how the absolute numbers of deaths due to convulsive therapy has declined substantially during this time. Unfortunately the number of patients treated and the number of treatments given each year are not known so that it is not possible to demonstrate that there has been a fall in mortality rate, but this seems likely since it is improbable that there has been as rapid a decrease in the use of ECT over the years as there has been in the number of deaths.

Fatalities occur most commonly during or shortly after treatment, and at autopsy the lesions found are usually only secondary to cardiac failure. Forty-nine cases in Tewfik and Wells series of 90 cases and six of Barker and Baker's nine cases, fell into this category. Some of these deaths were due to cardiac arrest consequent on vagal inhibition, and cases of cardiac arrest have since been reported by Arneson and Butler (1961), Cropper and Hughes (1964) and Barron and Sullivan (1967), who advocate premedication with larger than customary doses of atropine to prevent this complication.

Table 1.3

DEATHS ASSOCIATED WITH ELECTROCONVULSIVE
THERAPY (England and Wales, 1947-66)

Year	Source	Number of deaths	Deaths per year
1947		4	4
1948		3	3
1949	Maclay (1953)	13	13
1950		14	14
1951		19	19
1952-53	Tewfik and Wells (1957)	21*	10·5*
1954-56	Registrar-General (1958)	34	11·3
1957-58		11	5·5
1959		8	8
1960		1	1
1961		3	3
1962	Registrar-General (1970)	3	3
1963		6	6
1964		0	0
1965		3	3
1966		1	1

* Estimated.

The second most common cause of death reported by Tewfik and Wells (1957) and by Barker and Baker (1959) was coronary thrombosis (17 and 2 cases respectively). Coronary thrombosis has also been reported by Heggtveit (1963), by Matthew and Constan (1964) and by Hussar and Pachter (1968). Other causes of death include pneumonia, cerebral haemorrhage and pulmonary embolism.

Perrin (1961) has reviewed some of the non-fatal complications. These include fractures, dislocations and fat embolism (practically non-existent when muscle relaxants are used), pulmonary disorders, bleeding from peptic ulcers, and perforation of abdominal viscera. On the basis of his review Perrin lists a number of contraindications to convulsive therapy (Table 1.4).

Adverse Mental Effects

Convulsive therapy sometimes precipitates mania in manic-depressive subjects, but this is rare and the commonest psychological disturbances are confusion and memory impairment. Williams (1966) has reviewed the disturbances of memory which have been shown objectively to occur with ECT. First, there is some retrograde amnesia immediately preceding the convulsion, similar to that seen in concussional head injuries, and which lessens with time. Secondly, there is a period of amnesia following the shock similar to post-traumatic amnesia, during which the patient is disorientated, confused, unable to respond to questions in a coherent manner, and sometimes so disturbed in his behaviour that he needs to be restrained; and thirdly, after return to full consciousness there are often some gaps in the patient's past memories and a difficulty in retaining newly learnt material. It is this last type of memory defect which is clinically the most important, but it improves with time and rarely lasts longer than a few weeks after the last treatment. Cronholm and Molander (1964) examined 28 patients and found no evidence of memory impairment one month after the completion of a course of ECT.

Table 1.4

CONTRAINDICATIONS TO CONVULSIVE THERAPY
(Perrin, 1961)

1. *Cardiovascular*

(a) Myocardial infarction within previous three months
(b) Angina pectoris
(c) Congestive heart failure
(d) Aneurysm of major vessel
(e) Thrombophlebitis

2. *Orthopaedic*

(a) Severe osteoporosis
(b) Major fracture

3. *Pulmonary*

(a) Acute respiratory infection
(b) Severe chronic pulmonary disease, including tuberculosis

4. *Neurological*

(a) Cerebrovascular accident in previous three months
(b) Brain tumour

5. *Other*

(a) Peptic ulcer
(b) Remediable conditions such as pernicious anaemia, thyrotoxicosis, pregnancy, etc., if immediate psychiatric treatment is not imperative

In contrast to objectively determined evidence of memory disturbance which appears to be related only to the treatment, complaints by patients may be symptomatic of depression. Cronholm and Ottosson (1963) found that patients treated by ECT were often unable to judge their memory accurately, and that a favourable response was associated with fewer complaints, even where there was objective evidence of impairment.

Of the variables which affect memory, intensity and type of electrical stimulus and position of the electrodes have already been mentioned. The impression of most psychiatrists is that the impairment increases with the number of treatments given and that it is most marked when they are given very frequently, but there have been no studies to substantiate or refute this (Williams, 1966).

REFERENCES

ARNESON, G. A. and BUTLER, T. (1961). Cardiac arrest and electroshock therapy. *Amer. J. Psychiat.* **117**, 1020-1022.

BARKER, J. C. and BAKER, A. A. (1959). Deaths associated with electroplexy. *J. ment. Sci.* **105**, 339-348.

BARRON, S. P. and SULLIVAN, T. M. (1967). The use of the cardiac pacemaker in an ECT-induced cardiac arrest. *Amer. J. Psychiat.* **124**, 395-396.

CRONHOLM, B. and MOLANDER, L. (1964). Memory disturbances after electro-convulsive therapy. 5. Conditions one month after a series of treatments. *Acta psychiat. scand.* **40**, 212-216.

CRONHOLM, B. and OTTOSSON, J-O. (1963). The experience of memory function after electroconvulsive therapy. *Brit. J. Psychiat.* **109**, 251-258.

CROPPER, C. F. J. and HUGHES, M. (1964). Cardiac arrest (with apnoea) after E.C.T. *Brit. J. Psychiat.* **110**, 222-225.

HEGGTVEIT, H. A. (1963). Coronary occlusion during EST. *Amer. J. Psychiat.* **120**, 78-79.

HUSSAR, A. E. and PACHTER, M. (1968). Myocardial infarction and fatal coronary insufficiency during electroconvulsive therapy. *J. Amer. med. Ass.* **204**, 1004-1007.

MACLAY, W. S. (1953). Death due to treatment. *Proc. roy. Soc. Med.* **46**, 13-20.

MATTHEW, J. R. and CONSTAN, E. (1964). Complications following ECT over a three-year period in a state institution. *Amer. J. Psychiat.* **120**, 1119-1120.

PERRIN, G. M. (1961). Cardiovascular aspects of electric shock therapy. *Acta psychiat. scand.* Supplement 152.

REGISTRAR-GENERAL (1958). *Statistical Review of England and Wales for the year 1956 Part III Commentary*, p. 232. London: H.M.S.O.

REGISTRAR-GENERAL (1970). *Statistical Review of England and Wales for the year 1966 Part III Commentary*, p. 126. H.M.S.O. London.

TEWFIK, G. I. and WELLS, B. G. (1957). The use of Arfonad for the alleviation of cardio-vascular stress following electro-convulsive therapy. *J. ment. Sci.* **103**, 636-644.

WILLIAMS, M. (1966). Memory disorders associated with electroconvulsive therapy. In *Amnesia* (Editors Whitty, C. W. M. and Zangwill, O. L.). London.

Mode of Action of Convulsive Therapy

The mechanism by which convulsive therapy exerts its beneficial effects is not known. Various psychological theories have been proposed postulating that it is the patient's emotional attitude to the treatment which determines its efficacy and these have been reviewed by Miller (1967). First, it has been suggested that fear induced by the treatment is the effective agent; secondly, that if the patient regards the shock as a punishment, his conscience will be assuaged and his guilt and depression relieved; and thirdly, that the stresses involved in the treatment cause regression of behaviour to infantile levels allowing the patient to resolve early conflicts. These theories, as Miller points out, are inconsistent with the fact that it is the induction of a fit (and not the other circumstances) which is of therapeutic value. Indeed, Cronholm and Ottosson (1960) showed that artificially shortening the duration of the epileptic discharge by means of lidocaine makes the treatment less effective.

Other theories (also reviewed by Miller, 1967) attribute the therapeutic effect to the confusion and amnesia, but there is good evidence that the therapeutic effect and the mental side-effects can be dissociated, as when the stimulus is unilateral. Furthermore, Ottosson (1960) has shown convincingly that the memory impairment is related to the degree of electrical stimulation; the therapeutic effect is independent of this but varies with the duration of epileptic discharge.

There is some evidence from animal studies that convulsive therapy leads to biochemical changes within the brain, and it may be these changes that are beneficial. Garattini, Kato and Valzelli (1960) found that electroconvulsive stimulation increases the 5-hydroxytryptamine (serotonin) level in the brain in a number of different species of animals, peak concentrations, especially in the midbrain, occurring 10 minutes and 36 hours after the shock. Breitner, Picchioni, Chin and Burton (1961) also found that stimulation sufficient to produce a convulsion increased the level of 5-hydroxytryptamine, particularly in the brain stem, but that localized stimulation of the brain stem alone did not. Schildkraut, Schanberg, Breese and Kopin (1967) gave electroconvulsive shocks to animals that had received a prior intracisternal injection of tritiated noradrenaline; their results suggest that the shock increases the neuronal discharge of noradrenaline in the brain. Hinesley, Norton and Aprison (1968) have reported that electroconvulsive shock is followed, in rats, by increased concentrations in the brain of serotonin, noradrenaline and dopamine, while Cooper, Moir and Guldberg (1968) have found that, after a series of experimentally produced convulsions in dogs, there is a rise in the CSF concentration of serotonin and catecholamine metabolites.

These findings, if applicable to humans, are consistent with the monoamine theory of depression and suggest that the beneficial effect of ECT, like that of the monoamine oxidase inhibitors and of the tricyclic antidepressants, is due to an increase in the amount of monoamines available to central adrenergic receptors.

REFERENCES

BREITNER, C., PICCHIONI, A., CHIN, L. and BURTON, L. E. (1961). Effect of electrostimulation on brain 5-hydroxytryptamine concentration. *Dis. nerv. Syst.* **22**, Supplement (April), pp. 93-96.
COOPER, A. J., MOIR, A. T. B. and GULDBERG, H. C. (1968). The effect of electroconvulsive shock on the cerebral metabolism of dopamine and 5-hydroxytryptamine. *J. Pharm. Pharmacol.* **20**, 729-730.
CRONHOLM, B. and OTTOSSON, J-O. (1960). Experimental studies of the therapeutic action of electroconvulsive therapy in endogenous depression. The role of the electrical stimulation and of the seizure studied by variation of stimulus intensity and modification by lidocaine of seizure discharge. *Acta psychiat. scand.* Supplement 145, pp. 69-102.

GARATTINI, S., KATO, R. and VALZELLI, L. (1960). Biochemical and pharmacological effects induced by electroshock. *Psychiat. et Neurol. (Basel)*, **140**, 190-206.

HINESLEY, R. K., NORTON, J. A. and APRISON, M. H. (1968). Serotonin, norepinephrine and 3,4-dihydroxyphenylethylamine in rat brain parts following electroconvulsive shock. *J. psychiat. Res.* **6**, 143-152.

MILLER, E. (1967). Psychological theories of E.C.T: A review. *Brit. J. Psychiat.* **113**, 301-311.

OTTOSSON, J-O. (1960). Experimental studies of memory impairment after electroconvulsive therapy. *Acta psychiat. scand.* Supplement 145, pp. 103-132.

SCHILDKRAUT, J. J., SCHANBERG, S. M., BREESE, G. R. and KOPIN, I. J. (1967). Norepinephrine metabolism and drugs used in the affective disorders. A possible mechanism of action. *Amer. J. Psychiat.* **124**, 600-608.

LITHIUM THERAPY

Lithium salts are now commonly used in the treatment of mania and to prevent recurrence of psychosis in manic-depressive subjects. The most widely used preparation is the carbonate ("Camcolit", "Lithane", "Lithonate", "Priadel") although the citrate and acetate are as effective. The advantage of the carbonate is that it is much more potent than the other two preparations, since its lithium content is very much greater. Comprehensive reviews on the use of the drug have been prepared by Gershon (1970), Christodoulou (1968), Schou (1968) and Noyes (1969).

Metabolism

Lithium carbonate is absorbed completely from the gastro-intestinal tract. The plasma concentration reaches its maximum about two hours after ingestion, thereafter declining so that the drug has to be given every few hours and wide fluctuations in plasma level occur during the day (Amdisen, 1969). With slow release preparations (e.g. "Priadel"), the plasma concentration remains fairly constant throughout the 24 hours after a single morning dose (Coppen, Bailey and White, 1969). After absorption the lithium ion is distributed throughout the body water, but in an irregular fashion. It readily crosses the blood-brain barrier (Baker and Winokur, 1966; Platman, Rohrlich and Fieve, 1968) and its administration causes a slowing of EEG rhythms (Platman and Fieve, 1969b). It is also concentrated intracellularly in kidney, muscle, bone and thyroid (Schou, 1968).

Lithium is excreted almost entirely in the urine and accumulation leading to toxic effects is likely where renal function is impaired. Renal clearance varies widely between individuals, decreasing with advancing age (Schou, 1969). It also depends on sodium intake; restriction of dietary sodium leads to lithium retention and conversely urinary loss is promoted by the administration of sodium salts (Platman and Fieve, 1969a). Most diuretics including water, frusemide, ethacrynic acid and mercurial and thiazide preparations do not influence lithium excretion, but sodium bicarbonate, acetazolamide, urea and aminophylline all increase the urinary loss (Thomsen, 1969).

Administration

The therapeutic dose of lithium carbonate varies between individuals and must be determined in each case by serial estimation of the plasma or serum lithium concentration. Since these levels vary widely throughout the day when the usual type of preparation is administered the concentration is best determined on a morning sample of blood taken before the first dose of the day. At that time levels of less than 0·6 mEq/l suggest that the dose is too low, while concentrations above 1·6 mEq/l are usually associated with untoward effects and indicate impending toxicity (Schou and Baastrup, 1967). With sustained release preparations the serum level remains constant throughout the day and can be determined at any convenient time (Coppen et al., 1969). The most commonly used method of determining the blood concentration employs a flame photometer (Amdisen, 1967) although atomic absorption spectroscopy (Blijenberg and Leijnse, 1968) also gives reliable results. Emission by sodium, potassium and calcium may interfere with the flame photometric estimation of lithium and it is important to use lithium standard solutions containing these cations in concentrations of the same order as in the serum sample. (Lithium in therapeutic levels does not, however, interfere significantly with the flame photometric estimation of sodium, potassium or calcium.)

Since the dose is dependent on the rate at which the drug is eliminated in the urine, impairment of renal function increases the risk of intoxication; hence the need for routine examination of the urine and estimation of the blood urea before treatment is started. Moreover, since renal clearance declines with advancing age, elderly patients should be given low doses at first. Body weight and dietary intake of sodium are other factors which must be considered in determining the initial dose, as is the type of preparation of lithium carbonate that is administered. Somewhat larger daily amounts of sustained release preparations are required to maintain the blood level at a given value (Coppen et al., 1969).

Where as rapid a response as possible is required (for example where mania is being treated) therapy may be started with lithium carbonate 500 mg three times daily (less if the patient is elderly or of low body weight) reducing to 250 mg three times daily after about six days or before then if early morning plasma lithium levels are above 1·6 mEq/l or if symptoms of overdosage appear (Schou and Baastrup, 1967). Even at high dosage manic patients do not usually show any worthwhile improvement for six to ten days and this delay may necessitate the concurrent administration of other drugs such as chlorpromazine or haloperidol which can be withdrawn as the lithium takes effect. The dose of lithium is then adjusted so as to maintain the plasma level within the therapeutic range (on average about 250 mg three times daily) and thereafter plasma estimations need be carried out every few weeks only, unless symptoms suggesting intoxication appear. During the initial period of treatment side-effects including nausea, vomiting, slight abdominal discomfort, diarrhoea, fine tremor of the hands and transient tiredness and sleepiness may occur, usually intermittently and coinciding with peak plasma lithium levels after each dose (Amdisen, 1969). Their appearance does not usually necessitate reducing the dose unless the plasma level is rising. These early side-effects may be avoided by using a slow release compound, given as one dose every morning (Coppen *et al.*, 1969).

If the drug is administered to a symptom-free person to prevent relapse there is less urgency, and the early absorptive side-effects may be avoided by initially giving a small daily dose, increasing gradually over the course of one week or so until the plasma level is in the therapeutic range (Schou and Baastrup, 1967). The average prophylactic dose is 750-1000 mg daily.

Efficacy of Lithium Treatment

Mania

Lithium has been used increasingly in the treatment of mania since Cade (1949) described 10 manic patients (including two who had been continuously ill for five years) who all responded dramatically to lithium therapy. Schou, Juel-Nielsen, Strömgren and Voldby (1954), Maggs (1963) and Goodwin, Murphy and Bunney (1969) have conducted double-blind cross-over studies comparing the effects of lithium and placebo on mania and have obtained markedly better results with the drug. Johnson, Gershon and Hekimian (1968) have reported a double-blind study on 28 manic patients comparing chlorpromazine (250-400 mg daily) with lithium carbonate (in doses sufficient to maintain the serum lithium concentration above $1 \cdot 0$ mEq/l). They noted that complete control of symptoms was obtained in 78 per cent of patients treated with lithium compared with only 36 per cent of patients treated with chlorpromazine. Moreover, they observed (as have other investigators, e.g. Schou, 1968) that lithium leaves the patient alert whereas chlorpromazine induces unpleasant feelings of sluggishness and drowsiness. Schou (1968), summarizing the literature up to 1967, concludes that 70 to 80 per cent of all manic patients show distinct improvement within one to two weeks but that 20 to 30 per cent do not respond satisfactorily. More recently, Fann, Asher and Luton (1969) obtained a good response in 27 of 29 manic patients; Wolpert and Mueller (1969) noted that 11 of 13 cases benefited markedly, while 12 of 14 patients treated by Hullin, Swinscoe, McDonald and Dransfield (1968) were free of symptoms within six or seven days of starting lithium therapy.

The beneficial effect of lithium in mania is independent of age, sex, or duration of illness but depends to some extent on the clinical picture. The best response is seen in typical cases of mania, that is where the predominant symptoms are either mood elevation, garrulousness and jocularity or irritability and restlessness, where any delusions are consistent with the mood, where hallucinations are inconspicuous, and where it is easy to establish contact with the patient (Schou, 1968).

The response to lithium has been correlated with biochemical findings.

Serry (1969) measured the four-hour urinary excretion of lithium after administering a single loading dose of 1200 mg lithium carbonate to 30 manic patients and noted that a good response to lithium therapy was associated with low urinary lithium output (less than 20 mg in the four-hour period). Baer, Durell, Bunney *et al.* (1970) have observed that the response tends to be better in those patients where administration of the drug leads to an increase in the 24-hour exchangeable body sodium.

Depression

The consensus of opinion is that lithium is of little or no value in the treatment of depression, but there are a few reports suggesting that it may have some antidepressant action. Dyson and Mendels (1968) treated 31 depressed patients in an uncontrolled investigation and observed an apparently favourable response in 19 cases; improvement was particularly noticeable in those patients whose depression had "endogenous" features. Goodwin *et al.* (1969) have reported a double-blind cross-over study of lithium and placebo therapies in 18 depressed patients and noted that the drug appeared to be effective in five cases, all of whom had a history of recurrent depressive episodes. The possible antidepressant effect is not very great, however, and in a double-blind study comparing lithium with imipramine on 29 acutely depressed patients, imipramine gave the better results (Fieve, Platman and Plutchik, 1968).

Other Conditions

Lithium salts appear to have no therapeutic effect in schizophrenia, schizo-affective psychosis, paranoid psychosis or delirium (Schou, 1968). Johnson *et al.* (1968) observed a deterioration in the condition of most patients with schizo-affective disorder when treated with lithium and Rimón and Räkköläinen (1968) found that lithium was without effect in confusional states.

Prophylaxis in Manic-depressive Disorder

Lithium is now widely used to prevent recurrences in manic-depressive psychosis. Baastrup and Schou (1967, 1968) have described their experiences with 88 female manic-depressive patients treated with lithium carbonate, 300 mg three times daily, continuously for at least one year. Each patient had had previous episodes of mania or depression so that it was possible to compare the frequency and duration of the psychotic episodes before and after the start of the lithium therapy. Lithium administration was associated with a striking decline in relapse rate. Before lithium, relapses occurred on average at intervals of about eight months; during lithium therapy the average interval was five years. Another indication of lithium's efficacy was that before lithium the patients each spent on average 13 weeks per year in a psychotic state; with lithium it was less than two weeks per year. Patients with a history of manic episodes appeared to benefit more than patients with recurrent depression. Melia (1967) in a similar study compared the course of the illness before and after starting lithium in 23 patients and found that 16 were better during the period of lithium administration. Angst, Dittrich and Grof (1969) studied 91 patients with recurrent affective psychoses and also noted a very obvious decrease in the frequency of relapses after starting lithium treatment, particularly in patients with bipolar illnesses (i.e. those with a history of both manic and depressive episodes) but also, to a lesser extent, in patients with recurrent depression. From an analysis of the intervals between relapses among 979 patients with recurrent affective psychosis who were not receiving prophylactic drugs, these authors concluded that relapses tend to increase in frequency as time goes by and that lithium reverses this tendency. They contrast this action of lithium with another study in which they showed that long-term administration of imipramine (150-200 mg daily) was without effect on the relapse rate.

Blackwell and Shepherd (1968) have criticized Baastrup and Schou's study, and their criticisms are also relevant to the other investigations. They suggest that the evidence for a supposed prophylactic effect may be due to faulty selection of patients and evaluation and to observer bias. Saran (1969) has also challenged the interpretation of these studies. Using an experimental design similar to them, he investigated 51 comparable patients with recurrent affective psychosis who had not been treated with lithium and noted a decline in relapse rate similar to that observed by Baastrup and Schou (1967) and by Angst et al. (1969). It appears that if, as in these investigations, only patients with very frequent recent episodes are studied there will tend to be a decline in relapse rate whatever the treatment, and hence perhaps only double-blind controlled prospective studies can determine whether or not lithium has any prophylactic effect. Certainly not all studies have shown that lithium prevents relapse; Spring, Schweid, Steinberg and Bond (1969) have reported a series of nine patients given long-term lithium therapy, of whom five relapsed while taking the drug in apparently adequate doses.

Adverse Effects of Lithium

Lithium Intoxication

The untoward effects of lithium have been reviewed by Christodoulou (1968) and by Schou (1968) and are listed in Table 1.5. During the initial stages of treatment, as has already been mentioned, patients may complain of gastro-intestinal disturbances, fine tremor of the hands and tiredness. These are probably due to the steep rise in serum lithium concentration coincident with the absorption of each dose; they are intermittent and do not occur when the drug is given in the form of slow release tablets (Amdisen, 1969; Coppen et al., 1969). They usually disappear within one or two weeks of starting treatment, but they may indicate toxic accumulation of lithium within the body, especially if they become continuous or more severe. Pruritic maculo-papular rashes and cutaneous ulceration in the lower anterior tibial region have also been reported to develop sometimes during the first three weeks of treatment (Callaway, Hendrie and Luby, 1968).

Table 1.5

ADVERSE EFFECTS OF LITHIUM
(Christodoulou, 1968)

Gastro-intestinal	*Mental*
Anorexia	Retardation
Nausea	Somnolence
Vomiting	Confusion
Diarrhoea	Restlessness
Dry mouth	Stupor
Weight loss	Coma

	Cardiovascular
Neuromuscular	Irregular pulse
Muscular weakness	Low blood pressure
Tremor	ECG changes
Ataxia	Peripheral circulatory failure
Muscular hyperirritability	Circulatory collapse
with fasciculation	
Choreo-athetotic movements	*Endocrine*
Hyperactive tendon reflexes	Non-toxic goitre

	Other
Central nervous system	Polyuria
Skin anaesthesia	Polydypsia
Incontinence	Dehydration
Dysarthria	Glycosuria
Blurred vision	Fatigue
Dizziness	Lethargy and sleepiness
Vertigo	Morphogenetic effects
Epileptiform seizures	(not seen in humans)
EEG changes	Rashes

Intoxication occurs when the dose of lithium is greater than that which can be excreted by the kidneys and is most likely with large doses, or when the renal clearance is impaired as in patients with renal disease or in the elderly, or when the patient is taking a low-salt diet. Premonitory symptoms are feelings of sluggishness and drowsiness, coarse tremor or muscle twitching, dysarthria, loss of appetite, vomiting and diarrhoea (Schou, Amdisen and Trap-Jensen, 1968). More severe intoxication leads to an encephalopathy with impairment of consciousness, confusion, ataxia, widespread muscular tremor, brisk tendon reflexes and characteristic sudden jerking movements of the arms and legs; less commonly there are epileptic fits (Schou, Amdisen and Trap-Jensen, 1968; Allgén, 1969). There do not seem to be any serious effects on the heart and kidneys although ECG changes (flattening or inversion of the T waves) have been reported in human subjects, and animal studies have shown evidence of renal damage. Severe toxic effects are almost always associated with serum lithium levels of 3-6 mEq/l and values above 4 mEq/l usually indicate a fatal outcome (Schou, 1959).

Treatment of lithium poisoning is unsatisfactory since there is no specific antidote, but forced diuresis induced by intravenously administered urea combined with alkalinization of the urine with sodium lactate increases the lithium excretion and has been used with good effect in two cases of intoxication by Thomsen (1969). Horowitz and Fisher (1969) have noted a good response in a patient with lithium intoxication treated by acetazolamide, sodium bicarbonate, potassium chloride and mannitol while Gaind and Saran (1970) have reported another patient presenting as status epilepticus who improved remarkably after intravenous administration of M/6 lactate. In severe cases haemodialysis may be used (Amdisen and Skjoldborg, 1969).

Thyroid Disturbances

Schou, Amdisen, Jensen and Olsen (1968) have reported the development of diffuse non-toxic goitres in 12 patients receiving lithium and they have estimated that about 4 per cent of patients taking the drug continuously for one year will have this complication. In nine cases the enlarged thyroid was noted after several months' treatment (range, 5 months to 2 years) with doses of 900-2100 mg lithium carbonate daily. In the other three cases the goitre may have been present before treatment but became more prominent when the drug was administered. The enlargement led to dysphagia in four patients, and in two of these partial thyroidectomy was undertaken to relieve the pressure. Discontinuing the lithium led to a diminution in the size of the goitre over a period of two or three months, and in two of three patients who were given thyroid hormone while the lithium was continued, the gland became smaller. One of the patients who was pregnant while receiving lithium gave birth to a child with a very large goitre which disappeared within two months. Shopsin, Blum and Gershon (1969) have reported a patient with unsuspected Hashimoto's thyroiditis who developed a goitre and signs of hypothyroidism after two years' treatment with lithium and who reverted to her previous state when lithium was discontinued. In the cases so far described the thyroid enlarged only after several months' treatment, but Fries (1969) has reported a case where a goitre appeared after three weeks' therapy and the gland became normal one week after withdrawing the drug.

Lithium has been shown to affect thyroid function. Its administration causes a fall in serum protein bound iodine concentration and a well-marked increase in radio-iodine uptake by the gland, and these effects are reversed on discontinuing the drug (Schou, Amdisen, Jensen et al., 1968; Sedvall, Jönsson and Petterson, 1969; Cooper and Simpson, 1969). Schou, Amdisen, Jensen et al. (1968) suggest that these findings indicate that lithium may act on the thyroid primarily by inhibiting hormone production and that this leads to a compensatory increase in TSH secretion with consequent hyperplasia of the gland.

B

Lithium in Pregnancy

Developmental abnormalities have been observed in certain lowly organisms cultured in lithium-containing media (Schou, 1968) and this raises the possibility of a teratogenic effect in humans. Johansen and Ulrich (1969), however, have administered lithium to albino rats throughout pregnancy and have noted no abnormality in the offspring. Schou and Amdisen (1969) have reported 20 children (all normal) born to mothers who had been treated with lithium during pregnancy; in 16 cases the drug had been administered throughout the pregnancy and in four cases during the first trimester only. Further instances of normal children born to women receiving lithium have been reported by Nassr (1969) and by Weinstein and Goldfield (1969), and there is now little reason to suppose that there is a serious risk to the foetus by administering lithium during pregnancy.

Mode of Action of Lithium

Although the mechanism by which lithium exerts its therapeutic action is unknown, lithium has been shown to have some effects which fit in with existing biochemical theories of affective disorder.

First, Schildkraut, Schanberg, Breese and Kopin (1967) have made a number of observations in animal experiments which suggest that lithium may decrease the amount of noradrenaline available to brain adrenergic receptors, by promoting its intraneuronal inactivation. A study by Colburn, Goodwin, Bunney and Davis (1967) also suggests that the therapeutic effect of lithium is due to a decrease in available noradrenaline, but their findings indicate a different mechanism, namely that lithium increases the re-uptake of noradrenaline at nerve endings. A second kind of effect of lithium is on sodium and water metabolism (Coppen, Malleson and Shaw, 1965; Coppen and Shaw, 1967; Hullin *et al.*, 1968). This may be relevant to the therapeutic action of lithium, since the distribution of sodium appears to be severely disturbed in mania (Coppen, Shaw, Malleson and Costain, 1966).

REFERENCES

ALLGÉN, L-G. (1969). Laboratory experience of lithium toxicity in man. *Acta psychiat. scand.* Supplement 207, pp. 98-104.

AMDISEN, A. (1967). Serum lithium determination for clinical use. *Scand. J. clin. Lab. Invest.* 20, 104-108.

AMDISEN, A. (1969). Variation of serum lithium concentration during the day in relation to treatment control, absorptive side-effects and the use of slow-release tablets. *Acta psychiat. scand.* Supplement 207, pp. 55-57.

AMDISEN, A. and SKJOLDBORG, H. (1969). Haemodialysis for lithium poisoning. *Lancet*, 2, 213.

ANGST, J., DITTRICH, A. and GROF, P. (1969). Course of endogenous affective psychoses and its modification by prophylactic administration of imipramine and lithium. *Int. Pharmacopsychiat.* 2, 1-11.

BAASTRUP, P. C. and SCHOU, M. (1967). Lithium as a prophylactic agent. *Arch. gen. Psychiat.* **16**, 162-172.

BAASTRUP, P. C. and SCHOU, M. (1968). Prophylactic lithium. *Lancet*, **1**, 1419-1422.

BAER, L., DURELL, J., BUNNEY, W. E., LEVY, B. S., MURPHY, D. L., GREENSPAN, K. and CARDON, P. V. (1970). Sodium balance and distribution in lithium carbonate therapy. *Arch. gen. Psychiat.* **22**, 40-44.

BAKER, M. A. and WINOKUR, G. (1966). Cerebrospinal fluid lithium in manic illness. *Brit. J. Psychiat.* **112**, 163-165.

BLACKWELL, B. and SHEPHERD, M. (1968). Prophylactic lithium. Another therapeutic myth? An examination of the evidence to date. *Lancet*, **1**, 968-971.

BLIJENBERG, B. G. and LEIJNSE, B. (1968). The determination of lithium in serum by atomic absorption spectroscopy and flame emission spectroscopy. *Clin. chim. Acta*, **19**, 97-99.

CADE, J. F. J. (1949). Lithium salts in the treatment of psychotic excitement. *Med. J. Aust.* **2**, 349-352.

CALLAWAY, C. L., HENDRIE, H. C. and LUBY, E. D. (1968). Cutaneous conditions observed in patients during treatment with lithium. *Amer. J. Psychiat.* **124**, 1124-1125.

CHRISTODOULOU, G. N. (1968). The use of lithium in psychiatry. *Hosp. Med.* **2**, 1181-1184.

COLBURN, R. W., GOODWIN, F. K., BUNNEY, W. E. and DAVIS, J. M. (1967). Effect of lithium on the uptake of noradrenaline by synaptosomes. *Nature (Lond.)*, **215**, 1395-1397.

COOPER, T. B. and SIMPSON, G. M. (1969). Preliminary report of a longitudinal study on the effects of lithium on iodine metabolism. *Curr. ther. Res.* **11**, 603-608.

COPPEN, A., BAILEY, J. E. and WHITE, S. G. (1969). Slow-release lithium carbonate. *J. clin. Pharmacol.* **9**, 160-162.

COPPEN, A., MALLESON, A. and SHAW, D. M. (1965). Effects of lithium carbonate on electrolyte distribution in man. *Lancet*, **1**, 682-683.

COPPEN, A. and SHAW, D. M. (1967). The distribution of electrolytes and water in patients after taking lithium carbonate. *Lancet*, **2**, 805-806.

COPPEN, A., SHAW, D. M., MALLESON, A. and COSTAIN, R. (1966). Mineral metabolism in mania. *Brit. med. J.* **1**, 71-75.

DYSON, W. L. and MENDELS, J. (1968). Lithium and depression. *Curr. ther. Res.* **10**, 601-608.

FANN, W. E., ASHER, H. and LUTON, F. H. (1969). Use of lithium in mania. *Dis. nerv. Syst.* **30**, 605-610.

FIEVE, R. R., PLATMAN, S. R. and PLUTCHIK, R. R. (1968). The use of lithium in affective disorders. I. Acute endogenous depression. *Amer. J. Psychiat.* **125**, 487-491.

FRIES, H. (1969). Experience with lithium carbonate treatment at a psychiatric department in the period 1964-1967. *Acta psychiat. scand.* Supplement 207, pp. 41-43.

GAIND, R. and SARAN, B. M. (1970). Acute lithium poisoning. *Postgrad. med. J.* **46**, 629-631.

GERSHON, S. (1970). Lithium in mania. *Clin. Pharmacol. Ther.* **11**, 168-187.

GOODWIN, F. K., MURPHY, D. L. and BUNNEY, W. E. (1969). Lithium carbonate treatment in depression and mania. *Arch. gen. Psychiat.* **21**, 486-496.

HOROWITZ, L. C. and FISHER, G. U. (1969). Acute lithium toxicity. *New Engl. J. Med.* **281**, 1369.

HULLIN, R. P., SWINSCOE, J. C., McDONALD, R. and DRANSFIELD, G. A. (1968). Metabolic balance studies on the effect of lithium salts in manic-depressive psychosis. *Brit. J. Psychiat.* **114**, 1561-1573.

JOHANSEN, K. T. and ULRICH, K. (1969). Preliminary studies of the possible teratogenic effect of lithium. *Acta psychiat. scand.* Supplement 207, pp. 91-95.

JOHNSON, G., GERSHON, S. and HEKIMIAN, L. J. (1968). Controlled evaluation of lithium and chlorpromazine in the treatment of manic states: an interim report. *Comprehens. Psychiat.* 9, 563-573.

MAGGS, R. (1963). Treatment of manic illness with lithium carbonate. *Brit. J. Psychiat.* 109, 56-65.

MELIA, P. I. (1967). A pilot trial of lithium carbonate in recurrent affective disorders. *J. Irish med. Ass.* 60, 160-170.

NASSR, D. G. (1969). Use of lithium in pregnancy. *Brit. J. Psychiat.* 115, 1102.

NOYES, R. (1969). Lithium carbonate. (A review.) *Dis. nerv. Syst.* 30, 318-321.

PLATMAN, S. R. and FIEVE, R. R. (1969a). Lithium retention and excretion. The effect of sodium and fluid intake. *Arch. gen. Psychiat.* 20, 285-289.

PLATMAN, S. R. and FIEVE, R. R. (1969b). The effect of lithium carbonate on the electroencephalogram of patients with affective disorders. *Brit. J. Psychiat.* 115, 1185-1188.

PLATMAN, S. R., ROHRLICH, J. and FIEVE, R. R. (1968). Absorption and excretion of lithium in manic-depressive disease. *Dis. nerv. Syst.* 29, 733-738.

RIMÓN, R. and RÄKKÖLÄINEN, V. (1968). Lithium iodide in the treatment of confusional states. *Brit. J. Psychiat.* 114, 109-110.

SARAN, B. M. (1969). Lithium. *Lancet*, 1, 1208-1209.

SCHILDKRAUT, J. J., SCHANBERG, S. M., BREESE, G. R. and KOPIN, I. J. (1967). Norepinephrine metabolism and drugs used in the affective disorders: A possible mechanism of action. *Amer. J. Psychiat.* 124, 600-608.

SCHOU, M. (1959). Lithium in psychiatric therapy. Stock-taking after ten years. *Psychopharmacologia (Berl.)*, 1, 65-78.

SCHOU, M. (1968). Lithium in psychiatric therapy and prophylaxis. *J. psychiat. Res.* 6, 67-95.

SCHOU, M. (1969). Lithium: elimination rate, dosage, control, poisoning, goitre, mode of action. *Acta psychiat. scand.* Supplement 207, pp. 49-54.

SCHOU, M. and AMDISEN, A. (1969). Lithium and foetal abnormalities. *Brit. med. J.* 1, 316.

SCHOU, M., AMDISEN, A., JENSEN, S. E. and OLSEN, T. (1968). Occurrence of goitre during lithium treatment. *Brit. med. J.* 3, 710-713.

SCHOU, M., AMDISEN, A. and TRAP-JENSEN, J. (1968). Lithium poisoning. *Amer. J. Psychiat.* 125, 520-527.

SCHOU, M. and BAASTRUP, P. C. (1967). Lithium treatment of manic-depressive disorder. Dosage and control. *J. Amer. med. Ass.* 201, 696-698.

SCHOU, M., JUEL-NIELSEN, N., STRÖMGREN, E. and VOLDBY, H. (1954). The treatment of manic psychoses by the administration of lithium salts. *J. Neurol. Neurosurg. Psychiat.* 17, 250-260.

SEDVALL, G., JÖNSSON, B. and PETTERSON, U. (1969). Evidence of an altered thyroid function in man during treatment with lithium carbonate. *Acta psychiat. scand.* Supplement 207, pp. 59-66.

SERRY, M. (1969). Lithium retention and response. *Lancet*, 1, 1267-1268.

SHOPSIN, B., BLUM, M. and GERSHON, S. (1969). Lithium-induced thyroid disturbance: case report and review. *Comprehens. Psychiat.* 10, 215-223.

SPRING, G. K., SCHWEID, D., STEINBERG, J. and BOND, D. (1969). Prophylactic use of lithium carbonate? More data concerning its use in manic-depressive illness. *J. Amer. med. Ass.* 208, 1901-1903.

THOMSEN, K. (1969). Renal lithium elimination in man and active treatment of lithium poisoning. *Acta psychiat. scand.* Supplement 207, pp. 83-84.

WEINSTEIN, M. R. and GOLDFIELD, M. (1969). Lithium carbonate treatment during pregnancy. *Dis. nerv. Syst.* 30, 828-832.

WOLPERT, E. A. and MUELLER, P. (1969). Lithium carbonate in the treatment of manic-depressive disorders. *Arch. gen. Psychiat.* **21**, 155-159.

MONOAMINES AND AFFECTIVE DISORDERS

Monoamine Theory of Affective Disturbances

There are now a large number of observations indicative of quantitative abnormalities in the metabolism of brain monoamines (i.e. catecholamines such as noradrenaline and dopamine, and indolalkylamines such as 5-hydroxytryptamine) in depression and mania. These observations which have been reviewed recently by Schildkraut and Kety (1967), Coppen (1967), Gibbons (1968) and Schildkraut (1969) have given rise to the theory that monoamines have a central role in the aetiology of the affective disorders. In particular, the catecholamine theory postulates that depression arises when there is a relative deficiency of noradrenaline at functionally important adrenergic receptors in the brain and that states of elation are associated with an excess of noradrenaline (Rosenblatt, Chanley, Sobotka and Kaufman, 1960; Schildkraut, 1965; Schildkraut and Kety, 1967). Alternatively, it has been proposed that 5-hydroxytryptamine (serotonin, 5-HT) deficiency and excess are of greater relevance (Lapin and Oxenkrug, 1969; Curzon, 1969).

These hypotheses are based on the as yet largely unproven assumption that cerebral monoamines are involved in neurohumoral transmission at synapses. There is no doubt that monoamines are present in high concentrations in certain parts of the brain—noradrenaline and 5-HT in the hypothalamus and brain-stem, and dopamine in the extrapyramidal system—where they are stored as intraneuronal granules at the nerve endings, a situation ideally suited for release into the synaptic cleft. Nevertheless there is little direct evidence that they are liberated with nerve stimulation, although Jouvet (1969) has shown that 5-HT is intimately involved in neural pathways mediating sleep.

The interpretation of abnormalities in monoamine metabolism depends on a knowledge of the normal biochemical pathways. Metabolism relevant to the study of affective disorders is summarized in Figures 1.2, 1.3, 1.4 and 1.5, but knowledge is undoubtedly incomplete and further investigation may show other pathways to be important.

Noradrenaline is synthesized from phenylalanine, with tyrosine, dopa and dopamine as intermediaries (Figure 1.2). Noradrenaline is metabolized by catechol-O-methyl transferase (COMT) and monoamine oxidase (MAO) to form normetanephrine and vanillylmandelic acid, while dopamine is degraded by the same enzymes to homovanillic acid (Figure 1.3).

Noradrenaline is concentrated in two stores within the neurone (Pletscher, 1965). One (NA_1, Figure 1.4) is localized close to the nerve ending and is liberated into the synapse in response to a nerve stimulus (pathway 1, Figure 1.4); after release 95 per cent or more of this noradrenaline is taken up again by the nerve ending for re-use (pathway 2, Figure 1.4), while the remainder is inactivated by COMT (pathway 3, Figure 1.4). Another store (NA_2, Figure

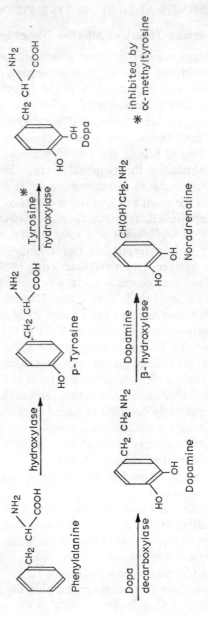

Figure 1.2 Synthesis of noradrenaline

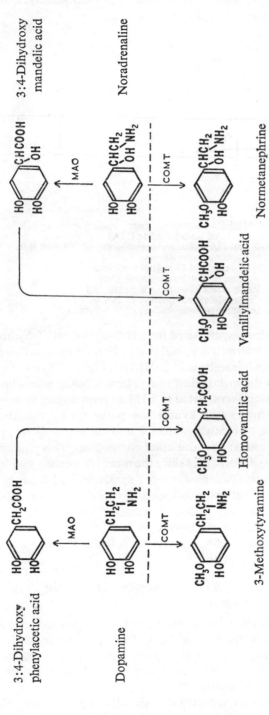

Figure 1.3 Metabolism of catecholamines in the brain. Reactions above the broken line take place within the neurone. *Note:* 3-methoxytyramine and normetanephrine are metabolized by MAO, to homovanillic acid and vanillylmandelic acid respectively. (Shepherd, Lader and Rodnight, 1968)

1.4), in equilibrium with the first, is localized near mitochondria and its size is regulated by MAO (pathway 4, Figure 1.4).

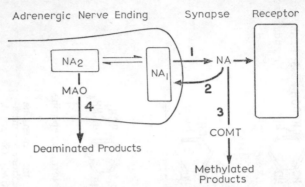

Figure 1.4 Model of adrenergic nerve ending showing fate
of noradrenaline (NA)
NA$_1$ and NA$_2$—intraneuronal stores of NA (see text)
MAO—monoamine oxidase
COMT—catechol-O-methyl transferase
1. Release of NA into synaptic cleft
2. Re-uptake of NA from synaptic cleft
3. Extracellular methylation of NA by COMT
4. Intracellular deamination of NA by MAO

5-hydroxytryptamine is synthesized from tryptophan with 5-hydroxytryptophan (5-HTP) as an intermediary, and is metabolized by enzymes (including MAO) to 5-hydroxyindoleacetic acid (5-HIAA). Figure 1.5 sets out this pathway and also shows the metabolism of tryptamine. Only a small proportion of tryptophan, however, is converted to 5-HT or tryptamine; most is metabolized along another route (the kynurenine pathway) by the liver enzyme tryptophan pyrrolase to formylkynurenine and subsequently to kynurenine, xanthenuric acid, nicotinic acid and other compounds. This pathway may be important in affective disturbances since the more tryptophan that is metabolized along it, the less is available for 5-HT synthesis, and it has been shown that the administration of hydrocortisone to experimental animals increases tryptophan pyrrolase activity with consequent inhibition of the formation of brain 5-HT (Curzon and Green, 1968; Green and Curzon, 1968).

The most important findings in favour of the monoamine theory of affective disorders are as follows:

1. *Chemical substances which cause depression decrease the amount of monoamines available at synapses*

(*a*) Treatment with reserpine or tetrabenazine is associated with depression in a proportion of cases (Bunney and Davis, 1965; Lingjaerde, 1963). In animal studies their administration has been shown to liberate noradrenaline and 5-HT from the intracellular stores and hence (via pathway 4, Figure 1.4) to the depletion of these stores (Shore, 1962).

(*b*) Depression has been reported occasionally as a side-effect of α-methyldopa when used in the treatment of hypertension (see Chapter 7). Alpha-methyl-dopa displaces dopa so that α-methyl-noradrenaline is synthesized instead of noradrenaline and the normal catecholamine stores are reduced (Day and Rand, 1963).

Alpha-methyl-tyrosine also interferes with catecholamine synthesis, but by a different mechanism; it inhibits the conversion of tyrosine to dopa. Although there have been no reports that its administration induces depression, anxiety and tremulousness have been noted as side-effects and insomnia and increased alertness may occur when it is withdrawn (Sjoerdsma, Engelman, Spector and Undenfriend, 1965; Engelman, Horwitz, Jéquier and Sjoerdsma, 1968).

The synthesis of 5-HT is inhibited by para-chlorophenylalanine which interferes with the conversion of tryptophan to 5-HTP. Of five patients with the carcinoid syndrome treated with para-chlorophenylalanine by Engelman, Lovenberg and Sjoerdsma (1967), one became depressed and mentally confused, one deluded and hallucinated and a third became confused and anxious.

(c) Progestogen-oestrogen formulations, used as oral contraceptives, sometimes cause depression (see Chapter 9). The tendency to depression varies with the preparation, but is greatest with those compounds which show the greatest MAO-inducing activity (Grant and Pryse-Davies, 1968). Interference with tryptophan metabolism has however also been implicated and Baumblatt and Winston (1970), in an uncontrolled study, have found that the administration of pyridoxine 50 mg/day by mouth relieves the mental side-effects.

2. *Physical treatments that are effective in depression tend to increase the amount of monoamines available to central receptors*

(a) MAO inhibitors prevent the intraneuronal deamination of monoamines (i.e. inhibit pathway 4, Figure 1.4) and increase their concentration in the brain; this has been demonstrated both in animals (Spector, Prockop, Shore and Brodie, 1958) and in man (Maclean, Nicholson, Pare and Stacey, 1965). The clinical response of depressed patients to this class of compounds appears to be related, at least in part, to their ability to inhibit MAO, since the more anti-MAO activity a drug has, the greater is its antidepressant effect (Feldstein, Hoagland, Oktem and Freeman, 1965; Dunlop, DeFelice, Bergen and Resnick, 1965). Furthermore Maclean et al. (1965) found that there is a delay between the beginning of MAO treatment and the rise in brain 5-HT concentration of approximately the same duration as the delay in therapeutic response.

MAO inhibitors, however, have other actions which may determine their antidepressant effect. In particular they inhibit the re-uptake of noradrenaline (pathway 2, Figure 1.4) and Hendley and Snyder (1968) have found that their clinical efficacy correlates better with this action than with MAO inhibition. A third possible mode of action has been proposed by Schildkraut (1970) who has found evidence that tranylcypromine liberates noradrenaline at adrenergic nerve endings.

(b) Tricyclic antidepressants, such as imipramine, potentiate the response to sympathetic nerve stimulation and to administered catecholamines and

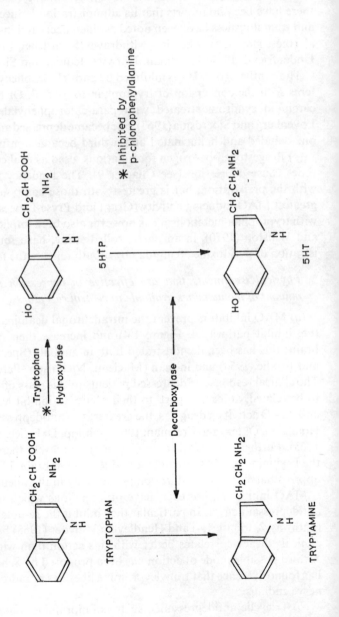

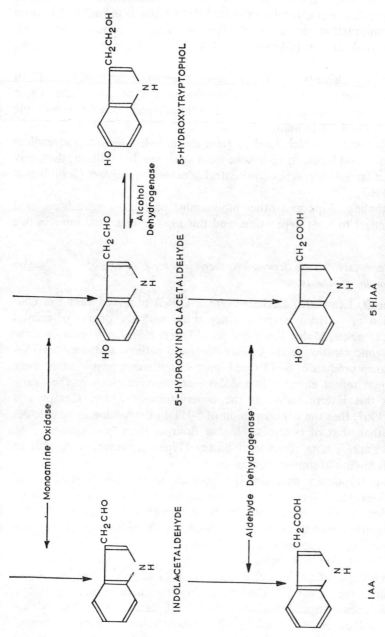

Figure 1.5 Metabolism of tryptophan along the indolalkylamine pathways (after Ashcroft, 1969)

5-HT (Sigg, Soffer and Gyermek, 1963; Kitazawa and Langham, 1968). The most probable mechanism, which could also account for the antidepressant effect, is inhibition of the re-uptake of liberated noradrenaline (pathway 2, Figure 1.4) so that noradrenaline released from brain neurones in response to nervous stimulation remains in the synapse in higher concentrations and for longer periods of time (Glowinski and Axelrod, 1964; Klerman and Cole, 1965).

(c) Electroconvulsive stimulation in animals increases the level of 5-HT in the brain-stem and facilitates the neuronal discharge of noradrenaline. These effects, which have been discussed earlier in this chapter, may be responsible for the efficacy of ECT in man.

(d) Amphetamines, which tend to raise the mood, release noradrenaline from neurones and block its re-uptake from synapses. In addition, they may have a direct stimulating action on central adrenergic receptors (Schildkraut and Kety, 1967).

(e) Tryptophan, dopa and other monoamine precursors have been used with good effect to treat depression, and this topic is discussed later in this chapter.

3. *In spontaneously arising depression, there is some evidence of a diminution in monoamine synthesis*

(a) Ashcroft, Crawford, Eccleston *et al.* (1966) observed that the CSF concentration of 5-HIAA correlated negatively with the degree of mental depression. Dencker, Malm, Roos and Werdinius (1966) also noted a decrease in 5-HIAA concentration in the CSF of depressed patients and since 5-HIAA is a breakdown product of 5-HT (see Figure 1.5), it seems possible that these findings might reflect changes in indoleamine concentrations in the brain. Supporting this interpretation is the observation of Shaw, Camps and Eccleston (1967) that the concentration of 5-HT in the hindbrain of suicides was lower than that of controls. Neither Bourne, Bunney, Colburn *et al.* (1968) nor Pare, Yeung, Price and Stacey (1969), however, were able to confirm this finding in similar studies.

(b) Urinary tryptamine excretion is abnormally low during depression, and rises by an average of 70 per cent to approximately normal values on recovery (Coppen, Shaw, Malleson *et al.*, 1965). Although this finding probably reflects a disturbance of tryptophan metabolism in the kidney, there may be a similar disturbance in the brain during depression.

(c) Schildkraut, Green, Gordon and Durell (1966) have noted an increase in the urinary excretion of normetanephrine (a degradation product of noradrenaline—see Figure 1.3) during recovery from depression suggesting a relative deficiency of noradrenaline during the illness. There is some doubt about the significance of this and similar observations however since most urinary normetanephrine is derived from the peripheral sympathetic nervous system and urinary levels may therefore be a reflection of general bodily activity rather than changes within the brain.

4. *Physical treatments that are effective in mania tend to reduce stimulation by monoamines of central receptors*

(*a*) Lithium, the efficacy of which in mania has been discussed earlier in this chapter, possibly acts by decreasing the amount of noradrenaline available at brain adrenergic synapses.

(*b*) Methysergide is a 5-HT antagonist, and there have been some reports that its administration to manic patients leads to immediate and striking improvement in the mental state (see below).

REFERENCES

ASHCROFT, G. W. (1969). Amine metabolism in brain. *Proc. roy. Soc. Med.* **62**, 1099-1101.

ASHCROFT, G. W., CRAWFORD, T. B. B., ECCLESTON, D., SHARMAN, D. F., MACDOUGALL, E., STANTON, J. B. and BINNS, J. K. (1966). 5-hydroxyindole compounds in the cerebrospinal fluid of patients with psychiatric or neurological diseases. *Lancet*, **2**, 1049-1052.

BAUMBLATT, M. J. and WINSTON, F. (1970). Pyridoxine and the pill. *Lancet*, **1**, 832-833.

BOURNE, H. R., BUNNEY, W. E., COLBURN, R. W., DAVIS, J. M., DAVIS, J. N., SHAW, D. M. and COPPEN, A. J. (1968). Noradrenaline, 5-hydroxytryptamine and 5-hydroxyindoleacetic acid in hindbrains of suicidal patients. *Lancet*, **2**, 805-808.

BUNNEY, W. E. and DAVIS, J. M. (1965). Norepinephrine in depressive reactions. *Arch. gen. Psychiat.* **13**, 483-494.

COPPEN, A. (1967). The biochemistry of affective disorders. *Brit. J. Psychiat.* **113**, 1237-1264.

COPPEN, A., SHAW, D. M., MALLESON, A., ECCLESTON, E. and GUNDY, G. (1965). Tryptamine metabolism in depression. *Brit. J. Psychiat.* **111**, 993-998.

CURZON, G. (1969). Tryptophan-pyrrolase—a biochemical factor in depressive illness? *Brit. J. Psychiat.* **115**, 1367-1374.

CURZON, G. and GREEN, A. R. (1968). Effect of hydrocortisone on rat brain 5-hydroxytryptamine. *Life Sci.* **7** (part 1), 657-663.

DAY, M. D. and RAND, M. J. (1963). A hypothesis for the mode of action of α-methyldopa in relieving hypertension. *J. Pharm. Pharmacol.* **15**, 221-224.

DENCKER, S. J., MALM, U., ROOS, B-E. and WERDINIUS, B. (1966). Acid monoamine metabolites of cerebrospinal fluid in mental depression and mania. *J. Neurochem.* **13**, 1545-1548.

DUNLOP, E., DEFELICE, E. A., BERGEN, J. R. and RESNICK, O. (1965). The relationship between MAO inhibition and improvement of depression. *Psychosomatics*, **6**, 1-7.

ENGELMAN, K., HORWITZ, D., JÉQUIER, E. and SJOERDSMA, A. (1968). Biochemical and pharmacologic effects of α-methyltyrosine in man. *J. clin. Invest.* **47**, 577-594.

ENGELMAN, K., LOVENBERG, W. and SJOERDSMA, A. (1967). Inhibition of serotonin synthesis by parachlorophenylalanine in patients with carcinoid syndrome. *New Engl. J. Med.* **277**, 1103-1108.

FELDSTEIN, A., HOAGLAND, H., OKTEM, M. R. and FREEMAN, H. (1965). MAO inhibition and antidepressant activity. *Int. J. Neuropsychiat.* **1**, 384-387.

GIBBONS, J. L. (1968). Biochemistry of depressive illness. In *Recent Developments in Affective Disorders* (Editors Coppen, A. and Walk, A.), pp. 55-64. British Journal of Psychiatry Special Publication No. 2. Ashford.

GLOWINSKI, J. and AXELROD, J. (1964). Inhibition of uptake of tritiated-noradrenaline in the intact rat brain by imipramine and structurally related compounds. *Nature (Lond.)*, **204**, 1318-1319.

GRANT, E. C. G. and PRYSE-DAVIES, J. (1968). Effect of oral contraceptives on depressive mood changes and on endometrial monoamine oxidase and phosphatases. *Brit. med. J.* **3**, 777-780.

GREEN, A. R. and CURZON, G. (1968). Decrease of 5-hydroxytryptamine in the brain provoked by hydrocortisone and its prevention by allopurinol. *Nature (Lond.)*, **220**, 1095-1097.

HENDLEY, E. D. and SNYDER, S. H. (1968). Relationship between the action of monoamine oxidase inhibitors on the noradrenaline uptake system and their antidepressant activity. *Nature (Lond.)*, **220**, 1330-1331.

JOUVET, M. (1969). Biogenic amines and the states of sleep. *Science*, **163**, 32-41.

KITAZAWA, Y. and LANGHAM, M. E. (1968). Influence of an adrenergic potentiator on the ocular response to catecholamines in primates and man. *Nature (Lond.)*, **219**, 1376-1378.

KLERMAN, G. L. and COLE, J. O. (1965). Clinical pharmacology of imipramine and related antidepressant compounds. *Pharmacol. Rev.* **17**, 101-141.

LAPIN, I. P. and OXENKRUG, G. F. (1969). Intensification of the central serotoninergic processes as a possible determinant of the thymoleptic effect. *Lancet*, **1**, 132-136.

LINGJAERDE, O. (1963). Tetrabenazine (Nitoman) in the treatment of psychoses. *Acta psychiat. scand.* Supplement 170.

MACLEAN, R., NICHOLSON, W. J., PARE, C. M. B. and STACEY, R. S. (1965). Effect of monoamine oxidase inhibitors on the concentrations of 5-hydroxytryptamine in the human brain. *Lancet*, **2**, 205-208.

PARE, C. M. B., YEUNG, D. P. H., PRICE, K. and STACEY, R. S. (1969). 5-hydroxytryptamine, noradrenaline and dopamine in brainstem, hypothalamus, and caudate nucleus of controls and of patients committing suicide by coal-gas poisoning. *Lancet*, **2**, 133-135.

PLETSCHER, A. (1965). Pharmacology of monoamine oxidase inhibitors. In *The Scientific Basis of Drug Therapy in Psychiatry* (Editors Marks, J. and Pare, C. M. B.), pp. 115-126. Oxford.

ROSENBLATT, S., CHANLEY, J. D., SOBOTKA, H. and KAUFMAN, M. R. (1960). Interrelationships between electroshock, the blood-brain barrier, and catecholamines. *J. Neurochem.* **5**, 172-176.

SCHILDKRAUT, J. J. (1965). The catecholamine hypothesis of affective disorders: a review of supporting evidence. *Amer. J. Psychiat.* **122**, 509-522.

SCHILDKRAUT, J. J. (1969). Neuropsychopharmacology and the affective disorders. *New Engl. J. Med.* **281**, 197-201; 248-255; 302-308.

SCHILDKRAUT, J. J. (1970). Tranylcypromine: effects on norepinephrine metabolism in rat brain. *Amer. J. Psychiat.* **126**, 925-931.

SCHILDKRAUT, J. J., GREEN, R., GORDON, E. K. and DURELL, J. (1966). Normetanephrine excretion and affective state in depressed patients treated with imipramine. *Amer. J. Psychiat.* **123**, 690-700.

SCHILDKRAUT, J. J. and KETY, S. S. (1967). Biogenic amines and emotion. *Science*, **156**, 21-28.

SHAW, D. M., CAMPS, F. E. and ECCLESTON, E. G. (1967). 5-hydroxytryptamine in the hind-brain of depressive suicides. *Brit. J. Psychiat.* **113**, 1407-1411.

SHEPHERD, M., LADER, M. and RODNIGHT, R. (1968). *Clinical Psychopharmacology*, p. 221. London.

SHORE, P. A. (1962). Release of serotonin and catecholamines by drugs. *Pharmacol. Rev.* **14**, 531-550.

SIGG, E. B., SOFFER, L. and GYERMEK, L. (1963). Influence of imipramine and related psychoactive agents on the effect of 5-hydroxytryptamine and catecholamines on the cat nictitating membrane. *J. Pharmacol. exp. Ther.* **142**, 13-20.

SJOERDSMA, A., ENGELMAN, K., SPECTOR, S. and UNDENFRIEND, S. (1965). Inhibition of catecholamine synthesis in man with alpha-methyl-tyrosine, an inhibitor of tyrosine hydroxylase. *Lancet*, **2**, 1092-1094.

SPECTOR, S., PROCKOP, D., SHORE, P. A. and BRODIE, B. B. (1958). Effect of iproniazid on brain levels of norepinephrine and serotonin. *Science*, **127**, 704.

Effects of Tryptophan, 5-HTP and Dopa on Depression

The administration of noradrenaline and 5-HT or of their precursors might be expected, on the monoamine theory of affective disorders, to relieve depression or produce elation. Noradrenaline and 5-HT do not pass the blood-brain barrier and they are not effective; this perhaps explains why 5-HT-producing carcinoid tumours are not usually associated with mental disturbances and why the mental abnormalities noted with noradrenaline-producing phaeochromocytomata are more probably due to peripheral than central effects. However the precursors of the catecholamines, i.e. dihydroxyphenylalanine (dopa), and of 5-HT (i.e. tryptophan and 5-HTP) do pass the blood-brain barrier and their effect on depression has been investigated.

Tryptophan and 5-HTP

Pollin, Cardon and Kety (1961) studied the effects of tryptophan on the mental state of chronic schizophrenic patients. They gave iproniazid at the same time in order to inhibit MAO and hence to prevent the breakdown of any 5-HT formed from the tryptophan and they noted that this drug combination produced a quite definite elevation of mood. Coppen, Shaw and Farrell (1963) treated 12 randomly chosen depressed patients with DL-tryptophan (214 mg/kg body weight per day) and 13 similar patients with a placebo mixture indistinguishable in taste and appearance from the active preparation. All patients received an MAO inhibitor (tranylcypromine) throughout the period of administration of tryptophan or placebo and for one week before; in addition all patients received pyridoxine hydrochloride 20 mg daily and other B vitamins, since these are required in tryptophan metabolism. Patients receiving tryptophan showed much greater improvement of their depression than those receiving placebo, but tryptophan administration was associated with side-effects, particularly hypotension, drowsiness and ataxia. Pare (1963) added L-tryptophan (7·5-15 g/day) to the treatment of 14 depressed patients receiving an MAO inhibitor and noted a striking improvement within two or three days in six cases, and relapse within two to seven days of substituting placebo for the tryptophan. Side-effects, particularly drowsiness, nausea, muscular jactitation and hyper-reflexia, and perceptual changes, were however common and their severity necessitated withdrawal of the tryptophan in five patients. Pare also treated 10 similar patients with a tricyclic antidepressant (imipramine or amitriptyline) but only one showed significant improvement when L-tryptophan was added; moreover the side-effects of L-tryptophan were very much less notable in these patients compared with those observed in subjects receiving an MAO inhibitor. Coppen, Shaw, Herzberg and Maggs (1967) have described a further clinical trial of DL-tryptophan in depression and they found that it was as effective a treatment as ECT. Patients receiving tranylcypromine (30 mg daily) in addition to tryptophan showed slightly greater improvement than those receiving tryptophan alone. Supplementing the diet with potassium and glucose in an attempt to increase tryptophan transport and metabolism enhanced slightly the efficacy of tryptophan and tranylcypromine. In yet another study, Glassman and Platman (1969) also showed that tryptophan potentiates the effects of MAO inhibition in depression. Of 10 patients receiving DL-tryptophan, 12-18 g daily, and phenelzine, 60 mg/day, six improved markedly within three weeks, while of 10 similar severely depressed patients taking phenelzine and placebo, only two were improved.

In contrast to these consistent reports that tryptophan benefits depression, it seems doubtful whether 5-HTP has any antidepressant action. Although Persson and Roos (1967) have reported a case where its administration appeared to lead to a notable improvement within a few days, other workers (e.g. Pare and Sandler, 1959) have found no such effect. Both tryptophan and 5-HTP cross the blood-brain barrier, but only tryptophan administration is followed by a rise in brain 5-HT concentration, and this may explain the difference in therapeutic effect between these two precursors of 5-HT (Ashcroft, 1969).

Dihydroxyphenylalanine (Dopa)

Dopa, a precursor of noradrenaline, crosses the blood-brain barrier and in theory might be expected to relieve depression; in practice, however, it seems to be of uncertain value. Using relatively small doses of DL-dopa, Pare and Sandler (1959) noted no improvement in depressed patients, whereas Klerman, Schildkraut, Hasenbush et al. (1963) found that doses of 400-1200 mg per day were effective. Bunney and his colleagues administered L-dopa to 10 depressed patients and observed a favourable response in only two; in four patients the drug was without effect and in two delusions and behavioural disturbances became more obvious (Bunney, Janowsky, Goodwin et al., 1969; Bunney, Murphy, Brodie and Goodwin, 1970). Furthermore, there have been a number of reports of L-dopa, used in the treatment of Parkinsonism, giving rise to mental side-effects. While hypomania has been observed (consistent with the monoamine theory), confusional states and aggressive behaviour have also been reported and severe depression has sometimes been precipitated (Cotzias, Papavasiliou and Gellene, 1969; Calne, Stern, Laurence et al., 1969; Godwin-Austen, Tomlinson, Frears and Kok, 1969; Wagshul and Daroff, 1969; Yahr, Duvoisin, Schear et al., 1969; McDowell, Lee, Swift et al., 1970). Bunney et al. (1970) have pointed out that L-dopa seems to be converted in the brain to dopamine rather than to noradrenaline, and this may explain its failure to have a consistent antidepressant action.

REFERENCES

ASHCROFT, G. W. (1969). Amine metabolism in brain. *Proc. roy. Soc. Med.* **62**, 1099-1101.

BUNNEY, W. E., JANOWSKY, D. S., GOODWIN, F. K., DAVIS, J. M., BRODIE, H. K. H., MURPHY, D. L. and CHASE, T. N. (1969). Effect of L-dopa on depression. *Lancet*, **1**, 885-886.

BUNNEY, W. E., MURPHY, D. L., BRODIE, H. K. H. and GOODWIN, F. K. (1970). L-dopa in depressed patients. *Lancet*, **1**, 352.

CALNE, D. B., STERN, G. M., LAURENCE, D. R., SHARKEY, J. and ARMITAGE, P. (1969). L-dopa in postencephalitic Parkinsonism. *Lancet*, **1**, 744-746.

COPPEN, A., SHAW, D. M. and FARRELL, J. P. (1963). Potentiation of the anti-depressive effect of a monoamine-oxidase inhibitor by tryptophan. *Lancet*, **1**, 79-81.

COPPEN, A., SHAW, D. M., HERZBERG, B. and MAGGS, R. (1967). Tryptophan in the treatment of depression. *Lancet*, **2**, 1178-1180.

COTZIAS, G. C., PAPAVASILIOU, P. S. and GELLENE, R. (1969). Modification of Parkinsonism—chronic treatment with L-dopa. *New Engl. J. Med.* **280**, 337-345.

GLASSMAN, A. H. and PLATMAN, S. R. (1969). Potentiation of a monoamine oxidase inhibitor by tryptophan. *J. psychiat. Res.* **7**, 83-88.

GODWIN-AUSTEN, R. B., TOMLINSON, E. B., FREARS, C. C. and KOK, H. W. L. (1969). Effects of L-dopa in Parkinson's disease. *Lancet*, **2**, 165-168.

KLERMAN, G. L., SCHILDKRAUT, J. J., HASENBUSH, L. L., GREENBLATT, M. and FRIEND, D. G. (1963). Clinical experience with dihydroxyphenylalanine (dopa) in depression. *J. psychiat. Res.* **1**, 289-297.

McDOWELL, F., LEE, J. E., SWIFT, T., SWEET, R. D., OGSBURY, J. S. and KESSLER, J. T. (1970). Treatment of Parkinson's syndrome with L-dihydroxyphenylala-nine (levodopa) *Ann. intern. Med.* **72**, 29-35.

PARE, C. M. B. (1963). Potentiation of mono-amine oxidase inhibitors by tryptophan. *Lancet*, **2**, 527-528.

PARE, C. M. B. and SANDLER, M. (1959). A clinical and biochemical study of a trial of iproniazid in the treatment of depression. *J. Neurol. Neurosurg. Psychiat.* **22**, 247-251.

PERSSON, T. and ROOS, B-E. (1967). 5-hydroxytryptophan for depression. *Lancet*, **2**, 987-988.

POLLIN, W., CARDON, P. V. and KETY, S. S. (1961). Effects of aminoacid feedings in schizophrenic patients treated with iproniazid. *Science*, **133**, 104-105.

WAGSHUL, A. M. and DAROFF, R. B. (1969). Depression during L-dopa treatment. *Lancet*, **2**, 592.

YAHR, M. D., DUVOISIN, R. C., SCHEAR, M. J., BARRETT, R. E. and HOEHN, M. M. (1969). Treatment of Parkinsonism with levodopa. *Arch. Neurol. (Chic.)* **21**, 343-354.

Other Theories of Affective Disorder involving Monoamines

Dewhurst's Theory and the Use of Methysergide in Mania

While the findings summarized in the previous sections are consistent with the hypothesis that mood is related to the amount of noradrenaline and 5-HT available to central receptors, they are also consistent with a more recent theory, proposed by Dewhurst (1968a, b, 1969a). In animal studies, Dewhurst and his colleagues noted the cerebral effects of a large number of synthetic and naturally occurring amines and concluded that there were two types of amines (type A and type C) with opposing actions. Type A amines tend to excite the brain, and in man to elevate the mood. They are lipophilic compounds, soluble in fat as well as in water and their action (on specific type A receptors in the brain) is antagonized by methysergide. Naturally occurring type A amines include tryptamine and β-phenylethylamine. In contrast, type C amines tend to depress the brain; they dissolve poorly in fat and act on specific (type C) cerebral receptors which resemble peripheral α-adrenergic receptors and which are antagonized (though only in large doses) by α-adrenergic blocking agents such as phenoxybenzamine. Naturally occurring type C amines include adrenaline and noradrenaline. Dewhurst proposes that some forms of depressive illness may be caused by deficiency of type A amines or by a diminished sensitivity of type A receptors, and that mania may be caused by an excess of these amines or by an increased sensitivity of the receptors to their action.

On Dewhurst's theory, the observation that MAO inhibitors relieve depression is explained because they inhibit the degradation of tryptamine and other type A amines while the efficacy of tricyclic antidepressants is due to their potentiation of type A amines. Dewhurst argues that amphetamines elevate the mood because they directly stimulate type A receptors, that reserpine causes depression because it leads to depletion of type A amines, and that tryptophan is effective in depression because it is a precursor of tryptamine. Thus most experimental findings to date are consistent with both the classical monoamine theory and Dewhurst's hypothesis, but one recent finding, if substantiated, strongly supports the latter, namely that methysergide has a beneficial effect in mania. Methysergide is a 5-HT antagonist which blocks type A receptors and Dewhurst predicted that its administration should relieve mania.

Several trials of methysergide ("Deseril", "Sansert") in mania have now been reported. Verster (1963) gave it intrathecally in a single dose of 2·5 mg to four manic patients and noted some relief of symptoms within 60 to 90 minutes of the injection and complete recovery within a few days. Dewhurst (1968c) observed a rapid response (within 48 hours) in all the five manic patients he treated with methysergide 3-6 mg/day, and noted that relapse occurred in two patients when the drug was withdrawn, while Haškovek and Souček (1968, 1969), who gave the drug intramuscularly at first, noted a similar dramatic improvement in eight of the ten patients they treated. Kane (1970) has reported an uncontrolled trial of cinanserin, an antiserotonin agent which has now been withdrawn from use in humans because of its tendency to produce liver tumours in animals. Of seven manic patients receiving the drug in a dose of 200 mg three times daily, five improved within 24 to 48 hr and treatment was stopped after three to four days in two patients because no response was apparent.

Two controlled studies have reported that methysergide is without effect in mania. Coppen, Prange, Whybrow *et al.* (1969) treated 10 manic subjects in a double-blind balanced cross-over study with oral methysergide 6 mg/day and placebo, each for eight days, and noted no difference between the efficacy of the treatments, while Fieve, Platman and Fleiss (1969) observed no benefit in six manic patients when treated by oral methysergide 8 mg/day for 7 days, although subsequently each improved markedly on lithium therapy. In both these studies methysergide was given by mouth, and Haškovek (1969) has suggested that it may be more effective when given parenterally. Dewhurst (1969*b*) has also pointed out that there may be variation in absorption of the drug when given orally and suggests that if there is no quick response to the drug when taken by mouth, the dose can be increased up to 12 mg per day or more, or it can be given by injection. Dewhurst (1969*b*) also suggests that methysergide may be potentiated by other drugs, particularly by pheno-thiazines, and that this might account for some of the variation in response.

The principal side-effects of methysergide are, first, that it may precipitate severe depression (Serry, 1969; Dewhurst, 1969*b*) which may necessitate treatment with ECT, and secondly, that its long-continued use is associated with fibrosis in the retroperitoneal, pleural or pulmonary tissues. Graham, Suby, LeCompte and Sadowsky (1966) have reported 27 cases of retroperitoneal fibrosis in patients receiving methysergide as prophylaxis against migraine. This complication was never noted less than nine months after starting treatment, but quite small doses (2 mg/day) were sometimes responsible. Stopping the drug led to complete or partial regression of symptoms. It seems unlikely that patients receiving short courses of methysergide for acute mania run any risk of developing fibrotic changes.

Tryptophan Pyrrolase and Depression

It has already been pointed out that hydrocortisone appears to divert tryptophan from 5-HT synthesis to the kynurenine pathway. Altman and Greengard (1966) obtained liver biopsies before and five hours after the administration of 250 mg hydrocortisone hemisuccinate to human subjects and noted a two- to four-fold increase in tryptophan pyrrolase activity and a three- to five-fold increase in kynurenine excretion after giving the drug. In rats, adrenalectomy reduces liver tryptophan pyrrolase activity (Knox and Auerbach, 1955) while the administration of hydrocortisone induces the enzyme and is followed by a fall in brain concentration of both 5-HT and 5-HIAA indicating decreased brain synthesis of 5-HT (Curzon and Green, 1968; Green and Curzon, 1968). Inhibiting tryptophan pyrrolase by yohimbine or allopurinol prevents the fall in brain 5-HT, suggesting that the latter is secondary to the effect on the liver (Green and Curzon, 1968). These actions of hydrocortisone have been linked with the now well-attested observation that adreno-cortical activity is increased in severe depression (Gibbons and McHugh, 1962; Butler and Besser, 1968; Carroll, Martin and Davies, 1968) and have given rise to a theory which postulates that the primary change in depressive illness is an increased production of corticosteroids with subsequent induction of tryptophan pyrrolase and increased metabolism of tryptophan along the kynurenine pathway, and hence to a reduction in brain 5-HT (Lapin and Oxenkrug, 1969; Curzon, 1969). Consistent with this are observations that the conversion of tryptophan to kynurenine is much greater than normal in depression (Rubin, 1967; Curzon, 1969).

Cyclic Adenosine Monophosphate

The urinary excretion of 3',5'cyclic adenosine monophosphate (cyclic A.M.P.) is lower than normal in severely depressed patients, and is higher than normal in patients with mania (Paul, Ditzion, Pauk and Janowsky, 1970; Abdulla and Hamadah, 1970). The significance of these findings is as yet uncertain and they may reflect merely differences in general body activity. But cyclic A.M.P. does mediate the actions of various hormones including the catecholamines and 5-HT and hence these observations might be consistent with monoamine theories of affective disorder.

REFERENCES

ABDULLA, Y. H. and HAMADAH, K. (1970). 3',5'cyclic adenosine monophosphate in depression and mania. *Lancet*, 1, 378-381.

ALTMAN, K. and GREENGARD, O. (1966). Tryptophan pyrrolase induced in human liver by hydrocortisone: effect on excretion of kynurenine. *Science*, 151, 332-333.

BUTLER, P. W. P. and BESSER, G. M. (1968). Pituitary-adrenal function in severe depressive illness. *Lancet*, 1, 1234-1236.

CARROLL, B. J., MARTIN, F. I. R. and DAVIES, B. (1968). Resistance to suppression by dexamethasone of plasma 11-O.H.C.S. levels in depressive illness. *Brit. med. J.* 3, 285-287.

COPPEN, A., PRANGE, A. J., WHYBROW, P. C., NOGUERA, R. and PAEZ, J. M. (1969). Methysergide in mania. *Lancet*, 2, 338-340.

CURZON, G. (1969). Tryptophan-pyrrolase—a biochemical factor in depressive illness? *Brit. J. Psychiat.* 115, 1367-1374.

CURZON, G. and GREEN, A. R. (1968). Effect of hydrocortisone on rat brain 5-hydroxytryptamine. *Life Sci.* 7 (Part 1), 657-663.

DEWHURST, W. G. (1968a). Cerebral amine functions in health and disease. In *Studies in Psychiatry* (Editors Shepherd, M. and Davies, D. L.), pp. 289-317. London.

DEWHURST, W. G. (1968b). New theory of cerebral amine function and its clinical application. *Nature (Lond.)*, 218, 1130-1133.

DEWHURST, W. G. (1968c). Methysergide in mania. *Nature (Lond.)*, 219, 506-507.

DEWHURST, W. G. (1969a). Amines and abnormal mood. *Proc. roy. Soc. Med.* 62, 1102-1107.

DEWHURST, W. G. (1969b). Methysergide in mania. *Lancet*, 1, 624-625.

FIEVE, R. R., PLATMAN, S. R. and FLEISS, J. L. (1969). A clinical trial of methysergide and lithium in mania. *Psychopharmacologia (Berl.)*, 15, 425-429.

GIBBONS, J. L. and McHUGH, P. R. (1962). Plasma cortisol in depressive illness. *J. psychiat. Res.* 1, 162-171.

GRAHAM, J. R., SUBY, H. I., LeCOMPTE, P. R. and SADOWSKY, N. L. (1966). Fibrotic disorders associated with methysergide therapy for headache. *New Engl. J. Med.* **274**, 359-368.

GREEN, A. R. and CURZON, G. (1968). Decrease of 5-hydroxytryptamine in the brain provoked by hydrocortisone, and its prevention by allopurinol. *Nature (Lond.)*, **220**, 1095-1097.

HAŠKOVEK, L. (1969). Methysergide in mania. *Lancet*, **2**, 902.

HAŠKOVEK, L. and SOUČEK, K. (1968). Trial of methysergide in mania. *Nature (Lond.)*, **219**, 507-508.

HAŠKOVEK, L. and SOUČEK, K. (1969). The action of methysergide in manic states. *Psychopharmacologia (Berl.)*, **15**, 415-424.

KANE, F. J. (1970). Treatment of mania with cinanserin, an antiserotonin agent. *Amer. J. Psychiat.* **126**, 1020-1023.

KNOX, W. E. and AUERBACH, V. H. (1955). The hormonal control of tryptophan peroxidase in the rat. *J. biol. Chem.* **214**, 307-313.

LAPIN, I. P. and OXENKRUG, G. F. (1969). Intensification of the central serotoninergic processes as a possible determinant of the thymoleptic effect. *Lancet*, **1**, 132-136.

PAUL, M. I., DITZION, B. R., PAUK, G. L. and JANOWSKY, D. S. (1970). Urinary adenosine 3'-5'-monophosphate excretion in affective disorders. *Amer. J. Psychiat.* **126**, 1493-1497.

RUBIN, R. T. (1967). Adrenal cortical activity changes in manic-depressive illness. Influence on intermediary metabolism of tryptophan. *Arch. gen. Psychiat.* **17**, 671-679.

SERRY, D. (1969). Methysergide in mania. *Lancet*, **1**, 417.

VERSTER, J. P. (1963). Preliminary report on the treatment of mentally disordered patients by intrathecally administered phenothiazine drugs and an antiserotonin substance. *S. Afr. med. J.* **37**, 1086-1089.

HYPERTENSIVE REACTIONS WITH
MONOAMINE OXIDASE INHIBITORS

A major complication of treatment with monoamine oxidase (MAO) inhibiting drugs is a sudden rise in blood pressure, sometimes severe enough to cause intracranial haemorrhage or heart failure. Most commonly these hypertensive crises are precipitated by the ingestion of certain foodstuffs, especially cheese, less often by the administration of sympathomimetic drugs.

Blackwell, Marley, Price and Taylor (1967) have described 25 patients undergoing treatment with MAO inhibitors who developed acute hypertension after eating certain foods. The symptoms, beginning 10 to 135 minutes after a meal, were of precordial palpitations and throbbing of the neck vessels, followed after some minutes by severe pulsating headache, at first occipital or temporal, later becoming generalized. Nine of the 25 patients felt flushed or perspired profusely, seven had neck stiffness or photophobia (but no evidence of subarachnoid haemorrhage) and eight vomited or complained of nausea. Systolic blood pressure, where measured during the attack, was always raised, usually to more than 200 mm Hg, and the headache remitted as the pressure fell. The duration of the crisis varied from 10 minutes to 6 hours, but in four patients there was evidence on lumbar puncture of subarachnoid haemorrhage, and these patients continued to have symptoms.

One of these died and one developed a left hemiplegia which lasted for six weeks. Further mild headache occurred for several days after the acute episode in one-third of the series and in two subjects there was a period of hypotension, lasting 12 and 36 hours respectively, with systolic blood pressures of less than 90 mm Hg.

The main hazard of the reaction is that it may precipitate intracranial haemorrhage, but acute pulmonary oedema due to left ventricular failure has also been reported (Sherman, Hauser and Glover, 1964). De Villiers (1966) has reviewed 29 cases of intracranial haemorrhage in patients treated with MAO inhibitors, including 16 previously unreported, and of these five died. Only one patient showed any evidence of a pre-existing vascular abnormality but of those who survived eight had permanent neurological disabilities.

A wide variety of foodstuffs has been implicated as precipitants of the hypertensive reaction, and Blackwell *et al.* (1967) have summarized previous reports from the literature (Table 1.6). Cheese is the most common precipitant—it accounted for 17 of the 25 reactions reported by Blackwell *et al.* (1967)—but alcohol (particularly beer and red wines such as Chianti), yeast

Table 1.6

FOOD PRECIPITANTS OF HYPERTENSIVE REACTIONS
IN PATIENTS TREATED WITH MONOAMINE OXIDASE
INHIBITORS
(Blackwell *et al.*, 1967)

Precipitant	No. of cases reported
Cheese	67
Alcohol	5
Yeast products	3
Cream	3
Broad beans	2
Pickled herring	2
Chocolate	1

extracts (particularly "Marmite" when taken as a beverage, and "Bovril", a meat product containing added "Marmite") and broad beans have also been implicated and are best avoided by patients on MAO inhibitors. Less commonly, cream, pickled herring, chocolate and "Complan" (a dehydrated high protein preparation) may precipitate a crisis (Blackwell *et al.*, 1967) while Hedberg, Gordon and Glueck (1966) have reported six cases where chicken liver seemed to be responsible. Some of these foods so rarely cause trouble that it is not necessary to warn patients to avoid all of them and most psychiatrists are content to give each patient a card, to be kept on his person, which lists those foods which are most likely to precipitate a crisis (Figure 1.6).

The experimental production of hypertension in animals and humans taking MAO inhibitors following the ingestion of cheese, yeast extracts and broad beans (Blackwell, 1963; Hodge, Nye and Emerson, 1964; Blackwell, Marley and Mabbitt, 1965; Blackwell and Marley, 1966a, b; Blackwell *et al.*, 1967) leaves no doubt that these foods have a pressor action. The responsible substance in the majority of foodstuffs which precipitate hypertension has been identified as tyramine (Asatoor, Levi and Milne, 1963; Horwitz, Lovenberg, Engelman and Sjoerdsma, 1964; Blackwell and Mabbitt, 1965; Blackwell, Marley *et al.*, 1965), a sympathomimetic amine which has a pressor

You are taking a

MONO-AMINE

OXIDASE INHIBITOR

You should not eat

CHEESE, MARMITE,

BOVRIL OR BROAD BEANS

and you should drink

ALCOHOL in moderation only.

Do not take any drugs except those prescribed for you.

ST. MARY'S HOSPITAL
PADDINGTON

NAME

CASE No.

YOU MUST CARRY THIS CARD WITH YOU AND SHOW IT TO ANY DOCTOR OR DENTIST WHOM YOU CONSULT.

DRUG	Date Started	Date Stopped

Figure 1.6 Front (*above*) and back (*below*) of card carried by patients taking monoamine oxidase inhibitors

effect markedly potentiated by MAO inhibitors. In broad beans, however, dihydroxyphenylalanine (dopa) appears to be the responsible constituent (Hodge *et al.*, 1964).

Tyramine acts indirectly by liberating noradrenaline from adrenergic nerve endings. The hypertension is due to stimulation, by the released noradrenaline, of α-adrenergic receptors, and hence can be controlled by α-receptor blocking drugs such as phentolamine which is usually effective when given intravenously in a dose of 5 mg, repeated if necessary. Pethidine and other opiate analgesics are absolutely contraindicated for the treatment of the headache, because of the undue sensitivity of some patients on MAO inhibitors to these drugs (Taylor, 1962; Vigran, 1964).

There are a number of mechanisms by which MAO inhibitors could enhance the pressor effect of tyramine. First, MAO inhibitors increase the peripheral stores of noradrenaline, making more available for release by tyramine (Sjöqvist, 1965; Pettinger and Oates, 1968). Certainly, the pressor response to tyramine may depend on the size of the catecholamine stores, and in patients with phaeochromocytoma the response is large enough to be of diagnostic use (Engelman and Sjoerdsma, 1964). However, this explanation is not wholly satisfactory since the urinary excretion of catecholamine metabolites is not increased after a hypertensive crisis (Blackwell *et al.*, 1967). Secondly, MAO inhibitors might augment the effect of tyramine by decreasing the rate of breakdown of released noradrenaline, but noradrenaline is metabolized mainly by catechol-O-methyl transferase and inhibition of MAO should not affect its rate of degradation (Sjöqvist, 1965). Thirdly, Blackwell *et al.* (1967) have suggested that inhibition of MAO in the gut, and possibly in the liver as well, allows tyramine to be absorbed unchanged into the systemic circulation, where it exerts its pressor action, but MAO inhibitors augment the effect of tyramine even when the latter is given intravenously (Horwitz *et al.*, 1964), so that this mechanism cannot account wholly for the development of acute hypertension following oral ingestion. Lastly, it has been suggested by Rand and Trinker (1968) that MAO inhibitors may affect hepatic enzymes other than MAO which are responsible for the breakdown of tyramine.

Only a minority of patients treated with MAO inhibitors develop acute hypertension. Blackwell *et al.* (1967) estimate the proportion to be about 4 per cent, and many patients give a history of eating potentially dangerous foodstuffs with impunity. Age, sex, premorbid personality, liability to headache and type of depressive illness do not appear to affect the likelihood of hypertensive reactions, but duration of treatment, type of MAO taken and the amount of pressor amine in the food eaten do seem to be important (Blackwell *et al.*, 1967). With tranylcypromine hypertensive crises usually occur early in treatment, often within the first two weeks, but in patients taking phenelzine, they tend to appear later, usually after a minimum period of four weeks. The risk of hypertensive reactions is greatest among patients receiving tranylcypromine where it is 8 per cent, five times greater than among patients on phenelzine. Tranylcypromine also produces more severe reactions than other MAO inhibitors. Of the 29 cases of intracranial haemorrhage reviewed by de Villiers (1966), all but two had taken tranylcypromine and all the five deaths occurred in patients on this drug. That tranylcypromine may be associated with such serious reactions may be related to its particularly powerful inhibition of gut MAO and to its intrinsic pressor actions related to its amphetamine-like structure.

The amount of tyramine required to produce a hypertensive crisis in patients taking MAO inhibitors is of the order of 10 to 25 mg. The content of different foods varies (Table 1.7) but is highest in cheese, particularly Cheddar, though even here there is variation since the tyramine content varies in different samples. It should be pointed out, however, that even when a patient receiving an MAO inhibitor has ingested an apparently critical dose of tyramine, hypertensive symptoms may not develop if absorption from the gut has been delayed by the presence of other food eaten at the same time or if the last dose of MAO inhibitor has not been taken sufficiently recently to prevent the breakdown of tyramine in the intestine (Blackwell *et al.*, 1967).

Table 1.7

TYRAMINE CONTENT OF VARIOUS FOODS
(Horwitz *et al.*, 1964; Blackwell and Mabbitt, 1965; Blackwell, Marley and Mabbitt, 1965)

Product	Tyramine content (*microgrammes/g*)
Cheeses	
Camembert	86
Stilton	466
Brie	180
Emmentaler	225
N.Y. State Cheddar	1416
English Cheddar	0-1620
Canadian Cheddar	231-535
New Zealand Cheddar	417-580
Australian Cheddar	226
Gruyère	516
Processed American	50
Cream	Not detected
Cottage	Not detected
Wensleydale	0-132
Cheshire	84-216
Caerphilly	0-138
Yeast	Not detected
"Marmite"	1500
Yoghurt	Not detected
Beer	1·8-4·4
Wines	
Sherry	3·6
Sauternes	0·4
Riesling	0·6
Chianti	25·4
Port	Not detected

Hypertensive crises in patients undergoing treatment with MAO inhibitors may also occur after the administration of sympathomimetic amines. Examples, sometimes fatal, have been reported after intravenous injection of methylamphetamine (Dally, 1962; Mason, 1962; Cooper, Magnus and Rose, 1964) or of mephentermine (Stark, 1962) and after the oral ingestion of amphetamine (Tonks and Livingston, 1963). Elis, Laurence, Mattie and Prichard (1967) found that phenelzine and tranylcypromine strongly potentiated the pressor effect of oral or intravenous ephedrine and phenylephrine in human volunteers, but that intravenously administered noradrenaline was not potentiated. The pressor effect of phenylpropanolamine is also strongly augmented by inhibition of MAO (Cuthbert, Greenberg and Morley, 1969) and hypertensive crises have been reported (Tonks and Lloyd, 1965; Mason and Buckle, 1969; Humberstone, 1969). Phenylephrine and phenylpropanolamine are common constituents of cough and cold remedies, some of which are available without prescription, and patients undergoing treatment with MAO inhibitors should be warned not to take drugs which have not been medically prescribed. When hypertension does occur it may be relieved by the injection of phentolamine (Elis *et al.*, 1967; Cuthbert *et al.*, 1969).

REFERENCES

ASATOOR, A. M., LEVI, A. J. and MILNE, M. D. (1963). Tranylcypromine and cheese. *Lancet*, 2, 733-734.

BLACKWELL, B. (1963). Hypertensive crisis due to mono-amine oxidase inhibitors. *Lancet*, 2, 849-851.

BLACKWELL, B. and MABBITT, L. A. (1965). Tyramine in cheese related to hypertensive crisis after monoamine-oxidase inhibition. *Lancet*, 1, 938-940.

BLACKWELL, B. and MARLEY, E. (1966a). Interactions of cheese and of its constituents with monoamine oxidase inhibitors. *Brit. J. Pharmacol.* 26, 120-141.

BLACKWELL, B. and MARLEY, E. (1966b). Interactions of yeast extracts and their constituents with monoamine oxidase inhibitors. *Brit. J. Pharmacol.* 26, 142-161.

BLACKWELL, B., MARLEY, E. and MABBITT, L. A. (1965). Effects of yeast extract after monoamine-oxidase inhibition. *Lancet*, 1, 940-943.

BLACKWELL, B., MARLEY, E., PRICE, J. and TAYLOR, D. (1967). Hypertensive interactions between monoamine oxidase inhibitors and foodstuffs. *Brit. J. Psychiat.* 113, 349-365.

COOPER, A. J., MAGNUS, R. V. and ROSE, M. J. (1964). A hypertensive syndrome with tranylcypromine medication. *Lancet*, 1, 527-529.

CUTHBERT, M. F., GREENBERG, M. P. and MORLEY, S. W. (1969). Cough and cold remedies: a potential danger to patients on monoamine oxidase inhibitors. *Brit. med. J.* 1, 404-406.

DALLY, P. J. (1962). Fatal reaction associated with tranylcypromine and methylamphetamine. *Lancet*, 1, 1235-1236.

DE VILLIERS, J. C. (1966). Intracranial haemorrhage in patients treated with monoamine oxidase inhibitors. *Brit. J. Psychiat.* 112, 109-118.

ELIS, J., LAURENCE, D. R., MATTIE, H. and PRICHARD, B. N. C. (1967). Modification by monoamine oxidase inhibitors of the effect of some sympathomimetics on blood pressure. *Brit. med. J.* 2, 75-78.

ENGELMAN, K. and SJOERDSMA, A. (1964). A new test for phaeochromocytoma. Pressor responsiveness to tyramine. *J. Amer. med. Ass.* 189, 81-86.

HEDBERG, D. L., GORDON, M. W. and GLUECK, B. C. (1966). Six cases of hypertensive crisis in patients on tranylcypromine after eating chicken livers. *Amer. J. Psychiat.* 122, 933-937.

HODGE, J. V., NYE, E. R. and EMERSON, G. W. (1964). Monoamine-oxidase inhibitors, broad beans, and hypertension. *Lancet*, 1, 1108.

HORWITZ, D., LOVENBERG, W., ENGELMAN, K. and SJOERDSMA, A. (1964). Mono-amine oxidase inhibitors, tyramine and cheese. *J. Amer. med. Ass.* **188**, 1108-1110.

HUMBERSTONE, P. M. (1969). Hypertension from "cold" remedies. *Brit. med. J.* **1**, 846.

MASON, A. (1962). Fatal reaction associated with tranylcypromine and methyl-amphetamine. *Lancet*, **1**, 1073.

MASON, A. M. S. and BUCKLE, R. M. (1969). "Cold" cures and monoamine-oxidase inhibitors. *Brit. med. J.* **1**, 845-846.

PETTINGER, W. A. and OATES, J. A. (1968). Supersensitivity to tyramine during monoamine oxidase inhibition in man. Mechanism at the level of the adrenergic neuron. *Clin. Pharmacol. Ther.* **9**, 341-344.

RAND, M. J. and TRINKER, F. R. (1968). The mechanism of the augmentation of responses to indirectly acting sympathomimetic amines by monoamine oxidase inhibitors. *Brit. J. Pharmacol.* **33**, 287-303.

SHERMAN, M., HAUSER, G. C. and GLOVER, B. H. (1964). Toxic reactions to tranylcypromine. *Amer. J. Psychiat.* **120**, 1019-1021.

SJÖQVIST, F. (1965). Interaction between monoamine oxidase (MAO) inhibitors and other substances. *Proc. roy. Soc. Med.* **58**, 967-978.

STARK, D. C. C. (1962). Effects of giving vasopressors to patients on monoamine-oxidase inhibitors. *Lancet*, **1**, 1405-1406.

TAYLOR, D. C. (1962). Alarming reaction to pethidine in patients on phenelzine. *Lancet*, **2**, 401-402.

TONKS, C. M. and LIVINGSTON, D. (1963). Monoamineoxidase inhibitors. *Lancet*, **1**, 1323-1324.

TONKS, C. M. and LLOYD, A. T. (1965). Hazards with monoamine-oxidase in-hibitors. *Brit. med. J.* **1**, 589.

VIGRAN, I. M. (1964). Dangerous potentiation of meperidine hydrochloride by pargyline hydrochloride. *J. Amer. med. Ass.* **187**, 953-954.

CHAPTER 2

THE DIAGNOSIS OF SCHIZOPHRENIA

The Phenomenology of Schizophrenia. Schizophrenic Thought Disorder. Clinical Diagnosis of Schizophrenia

THE PHENOMENOLOGY OF SCHIZOPHRENIA

SCHIZOPHRENICS, like other patients with serious mental disorder, may have abnormal psychic experiences such as hallucinations. Since these are subjective they are not amenable to the same type of study as are physical (objective) phenomena, but nevertheless careful description of these abnormalities allows them to be classified and distinguished and their interrelationships to be determined in a clinically useful way. This study of abnormal psychic phenomena (phenomenology or descriptive psychopathology) is concerned with observations on the *form* that the phenomena take and contrasts with dynamic psychopathology which deals with the significance of the *content* of the experiences. Thus delusions of the same form but with different content have the same phenomenological significance but possibly differ from one another in their psychodynamic interpretation, while phenomenologically different experiences may be equivalent psychodynamically, as, for example, an obsession, an hallucination and a delusion with similar content.

Until recently phenomenology was of interest mainly to Continental psychiatrists, but the translation into English of Schneider's *Clinical Psychopathology* (1959) and of Jaspers' *General Psychopathology* (1963) has brought this subject to the attention of the English-speaking world and has evoked interest there. Taylor (1966) and Fish (1967a) have produced textbooks, Anderson and Trethowan (1967) have prepared a useful summary, while Taylor (1967) and Jaspers (1968) have written on the role of phenomenology in psychiatry.

Hallucinatory Experiences

Phenomenology

The phenomenology of hallucinatory experiences has been described by Sedman (1966a, c.) He defines true hallucinations (hallucinations proper) as experiences which are perceived through the sense organs and which are accepted by the subject as real perceptions but which occur in the absence of any sensory stimuli. Hallucinated objects look, sound, smell, feel or taste like real objects, they appear in the same dimensions of space (external objective space) as normal perceptions and they are independent of the will in that they cannot voluntarily be brought to consciousness nor dismissed from it (Jaspers, 1963). Most commonly, true hallucinations are auditory, sometimes olfactory, gustatory or tactile and less commonly, visual. When occurring in clear consciousness they are strongly suggestive, though not diagnostic, of schizophrenia. Thus, of 24 patients with true hallucinations arising in clear consciousness studied by Sedman (1966a), 12 were diagnosed as schizophrenic and four as suffering from schizo-affective psychosis. There were three patients with organic psychoses, two with affective psychoses and two whose hallucinations were associated with epilepsy; the diagnosis of one patient was uncertain. True hallucinations occurring during a half-awake state (i.e. hypnagogic or hypnopompic hallucinations) or when consciousness is clouded do not have the same diagnostic significance (Sedman, 1966a).

True hallucinations must be distinguished from pseudohallucinations and imagery. Pseudohallucinations (Sedman, 1966a, c) are like true hallucinations in that they are perceived through the senses, arise in external objective space and cannot be evoked at will. But, unlike true hallucinations, they are recognized by the patient as not being true perceptions. Sedman (1966a) reported 25 patients with pseudohallucinations (mainly visual or auditory) in clear consciousness and of these only four were suffering from schizophrenia or schizo-affective psychosis. He noted that they were significantly more common in women and that they were associated with self-insecurity and attention-seeking traits in the premorbid personality and with sexual frigidity. Because of these traits many of these patients are diagnosed as "hysteric".

Imagery refers to those experiences (usually auditory or visual) which occur in inner subjective space (i.e. in the "mind's eye", the "mind's ear", etc.) and which are easily recognized by the patient to be the product of his own mind and to have no basis in external reality; they are usually under the control of the will. Sedman (1966a) reported 15 patients who had this type of experience in clear consciousness and only one was schizophrenic. He found that they were more common among patients with obsessive-compulsive symptoms and where the premorbid personality showed attention-seeking and obsessional traits, and he regards these experiences, particularly those auditory in type, as being obsessive-compulsive in nature.

Hallucinations in Schizophrenia

Small, Small and Andersen (1966) studied 50 newly hospitalized schizophrenics and noted that 38 (76 per cent) were hallucinated. Most of their patients had hallucinations involving more than one sensory modality, but the most common was of auditory type. Table 2.1 shows the type of hallucination experienced by their patients and also by 50 hallucinated schizophrenics reported in a comparable series by Higashi and Koshika (1967).

Auditory Hallucinations

Thirty-three of the schizophrenic patients studied by Small et al. (1966)

Table 2.1

TYPES OF HALLUCINATION AMONG SCHIZOPHRENICS

	Small et al. (1966) (n=38)	*Higashi and Koshika* (1967) (n=50)
	%	%
Auditory	87	98
Visual	40	20
Tactile	26	8
Bodily	30	20
Olfactory	50	12

reported hearing hallucinatory voices in clear consciousness. The voices were identified by the patients as follows:

Family	14
Friends	10
God	2
President of U.S.	1
Unknown	6

The major themes discussed by the voices were:

Family affairs	16
Accusations and/or threats	8
Religion	5
Instructions	3
Predictions of future	1

About one-third of the patients were afraid of the voices while most of the others had no definite emotional reaction to them, but a few did derive comfort.

As has been pointed out, true auditory hallucinations arising in clear consciousness are strongly suggestive of schizophrenia, but they can occur in almost any type of severe mental disorder. Schneider (1959) has asserted that certain types of auditory hallucination are diagnostic of schizophrenia, if organic brain disease can be excluded. These are: (*a*) hearing one's own thoughts (there is no generally accepted English term for this phenomenon which is often known as *gedankenlautwerden* or *echo de la pensée*); (*b*) hearing hallucinatory voices conversing with one another, particularly when they argue and refer to the patient in the third person; and (*c*) hearing hallucinatory voices that keep up a running commentary, usually critical, on the patient's behaviour. Sedman (1966*b*) has however indicated that Schneider's view of the significance of *gedankenlautwerden* needs to be modified, and that it is only diagnostic of schizophrenia when the experience is a true hallucination, that is, when the patient feels that the voices are alien and that some external agency is responsible for them. Sedman describes a number of non-schizophrenic patients who recognized that the voices were those of their own consciences or who felt responsible for them in the same way as ordinary thoughts. He regards these experiences as imagery or pseudohallucinations allied to obsessions, and not diagnostic of schizophrenia even when located in bizarre places such as in the patient's chest or abdomen.

Visual Hallucinations

The phenomenology of visual hallucinatory experiences has been investigated by Frieske and Wilson (1966) who compared their characteristics in 50 schizophrenics with those experienced by 30 patients with organic psychoses and by 15 patients with affective disorders (4 manic and 11 depressive). The visual hallucinations were very similar in the three groups, but some statistically significant differences were noted:

(a) Most schizophrenics tended to hallucinate continuously except when asleep, and patients experiencing visual hallucinations only at night were most likely to have an organic illness.

(b) All the schizophrenics experienced abnormal sensations in other modalities; in descending order of frequency these were auditory, tactile, olfactory and gustatory. Visual hallucinations occurring alone almost always indicated a diagnosis of organic psychosis. (Thirty-three per cent of patients with organic reactions had no hallucinations other than visual compared with 7 per cent of patients with affective disorders; among schizophrenics visual hallucinations were always accompanied by other sensory disturbances.)

(c) The majority of hallucinations were accepted by the patients as being completely real, and they were experienced passively and were not under the control of the will or imagination; these characteristics did not vary with the diagnosis. Most of the hallucinations were frightening, but those of organic cause were very much less likely to have a special personal significance for the patient than those due to functional mental disorder.

(d) Other characteristics of the hallucinations were similar in the three diagnostic groups. The majority tended to be three-dimensional, in bright colour and normal in size, and appeared to be moving. These qualities were independent of the diagnosis except that movement in the hallucination was significantly more common in organic states.

In a similar study, Higashi and Koshika (1967) compared the visual hallucinations of 10 patients with typical schizophrenia with those of 31 patients with organic psychoses and noted that they were more often coloured, complex and moving when organic in aetiology.

The content of schizophrenic visual hallucinations has been studied by Small et al. (1966) whose 15 patients identified their visions as follows:

Family members	7
Religious, Saints or Virgin	3
Animals	2
Other	3

Higashi and Koshika (1967) also noted that relatives and other familiar persons figured prominently in the hallucinations of their schizophrenic patients and that unknown persons and animals were less common.

Somatic Hallucinations

In schizophrenia various types of abnormal bodily sensations may be reported. First, there may be simple hallucinations of the bodily senses, for example of touch (Small *et al.*, 1966; Higashi and Koshika, 1967) or of heat. Secondly, there may be passivity experiences in the form of bodily sensations, where the patient has hallucinatory feelings such as of pain, electricity or sexual excitement which are attributed to an external agency (these are discussed further later). Thirdly, there are coenaesthetic hallucinations in which part or the whole of the body feels distorted or changed in some bizarre way (Lunn, 1965). Of 50 patients with this type of complex disturbance of body image studied by Lukianowicz (1967) 23 were schizophrenic, but bizarre somatic hallucinations forming the basis of delusions are not uncommon in other functional psychoses and in organic mental states and Lukianowicz cites a number of such cases.

Delusions

Phenomenology

Delusions may be defined as false unshakeable beliefs of morbid origin (Fish, 1967*a*). Their characteristics include:

(*a*) non-acceptance by people of the same social, religious, educational and cultural background;

(*b*) the absolute conviction with which they are held and their incorrigibility by experience or argument;

(*c*) their content is often, though not always, absurd or impossible.

Delusions may be classified as primary (also known as autochthonous delusions, delusions proper or true delusions) and secondary (delusion-like ideas or delusional ideas). The distinction between these two types of delusion is that secondary delusions can be understood as arising from some other morbid experience; for example, schizophrenics may have delusions of persecution secondary to auditory hallucinations while in depressive psychosis secondary delusions of guilt or bodily illness consistent with the mood may occur. In contrast, primary delusions cannot be understood in terms of preceding morbid experiences. Fish (1967*b*) has likened them to the "brain waves" of normal individuals where an idea presents itself suddenly in consciousness. A primary delusion differs from a normal "brain wave", however, in that the presenting idea has the characteristics of a delusion. They are sometimes preceded by a delusional mood (*wahnstimmung*) in which the patient vaguely feels that something unusual is happening in his environment, yet has no idea what it is until the delusion itself appears.

Secondary delusions occur in all forms of serious mental disorder but primary delusions are almost always diagnostic of schizophrenia, although rarely they may be seen in other functional disorders and in organic mental reactions. One type of primary delusion, namely delusional perception, is however probably pathognomonic of schizophrenia if organic brain disease can be excluded (Schneider, 1959). Delusional perception denotes a primary delusion arising in response to a normal perception. Jaspers (1963) gives as an example the experience of a woman who on seeing a man in the street knew immediately that he was an ex-lover who had disguised himself. Another example is given by Fish (1967*b*) of a man standing at a bar who was offered a biscuit by his brother-in-law; immediately the man realized that his brother-in-law believed him to be homosexual and that he was conspiring against him. Secondary delusions, like primary delusions, may arise in response to normal perceptions, but these, of course, are not delusional perceptions and are better called delusional misinterpretations. For example, a paranoid patient, hearing an actual knock at the door may believe that his persecutors have come; this type of experience is not diagnostic of schizophrenia.

Delusions in Schizophrenia

Lucas, Sainsbury and Collins (1962) studied an unselected series of 405 hospitalized schizophrenics and noted that 71 per cent were deluded; delusions were significantly more common among females (77 per cent of 209) than among males (65 per cent of 196). Fourteen per cent of their patients showed no evidence of delusions and the remaining 15 per cent were either mute or their speech incomprehensible because of gross thought disorder, so that the presence or absence of delusions could not be determined. Lucas and his colleagues categorized the delusions by their content (Table 2.2) and found that paranoid delusions (delusions of persecution) were the most common by far. Delusions of a sexual nature were almost twice as frequent among women

Table 2.2

CONTENT OF DELUSIONS AMONG 288 SCHIZOPHRENICS
(Lucas *et al.*, 1962)

	Males (n=127)		Females (n=161)	
	No.	%	*No.*	%
Religious	23	18	38	24
Grandiose	52	41	75	47
Paranoid	93	73	112	70
Sexual	38	30	88	55
Hypochondriacal	25	20	34	21
Inferiority	20	16	14	9
Other	3	2	20	12

as among men but there were no other significant differences between the sexes. Many patients expressed more than one type of delusion. Grandiose delusions were noted in 127 patients and most commonly these consisted of false beliefs in their superior social status or in their having some special skill or ability (Table 2.3). Delusions of authority and power were significantly

C

Table 2.3

CONTENT OF GRANDIOSE DELUSIONS OF 127 SCHIZOPHRENICS
(Lucas *et al.*, 1962)

	No.	%
Authority and power	17	13
Wealth	20	16
Social status	59	46
Skill	46	36
Other	21	17

more common among males than females but no other sex differences were observed. The most common types of sexual delusion reported were false beliefs of imposed heterosexual activity and, in women, of being married or pregnant (Table 2.4). Men, but not women sometimes expressed delusions involving masturbation. Of the 205 patients with paranoid delusions the

Table 2.4

CONTENT OF SEXUAL DELUSIONS OF 126 SCHIZOPHRENICS
(Lucas *et al.*, 1962)

	Males (n=38)		Females (n=88)	
	No.	%	No.	%
Heterosexual activity imposed on patient	11	29	31	35
Homosexual activity imposed on patient	2	5	5	6
Infidelity of spouse	6	16	6	7
Marriage or betrothal	8	21	23	26
Pregnancy or having children	3	8	27	31
Masturbation	7	18	0	0
Other	4	11	14	16

majority could identify their alleged persecutors as relatives, neighbours, work-mates etc or as members of a defined group such as the Jews, Freemasons, Communists or police, but 34 per cent cited unspecified people (Table 2.5).

Table 2.5

IDENTITY OF ALLEGED PERSECUTORS OF 205 SCHIZOPHRENICS
WITH PARANOID DELUSIONS
(Lucas *et al.*, 1962)

	No.	%
Family	43	21
Close associates, workmates, neighbours	66	32
Defined group	52	25
People not further specified	69	34

Passivity Experiences

Normal individuals are aware that the psychic events which they experience are their own and they take responsibility for them. Schizophrenics however may experience thoughts, emotions or actions as not being their own, and it is this type of phenomenon that is denoted by the term passivity experience.

Thus a schizophrenic may have a thought, yet at the same time feel that it is not his own thought, that it has been forced on him, that he has been made to think it and that it has interrupted his own stream of thought ("thought insertion", "made" thoughts). It is important to distinguish this type of passivity thinking from obsessional phenomena where the patient cannot rid himself of ideas that intrude into his consciousness. The distinguishing features are first, that the patient accepts that obsessional ideas are his own thoughts, even though he may regard them as ludicrous or at complete variance with his own personality; secondly, obsessions are not attributed to some outside influence; and thirdly, obsessions, unlike "made" thoughts, are associated with the feeling that they must be resisted.

Thought withdrawal (or interruption of thought) is another example of passivity thinking, where the patient experiences the withdrawal of his thoughts—the thought suddenly vanishes and he feels that this is due to outside action.

Just as thoughts may be experienced by a patient as being foreign or as manufactured against his will, so also may bodily sensations, moods and volitional behaviour such as walking or talking. Thus schizophrenics may experience, as alien, pains and other symptoms due to physical illness, sexual feelings, somatic hallucinations, depression, ecstasy, or motor acts. Since the patient is certain that these phenomena do not arise from his own mind, he may account for their occurrence by delusional ideas, that he is being hypnotized or bewitched or that he is being controlled by electrical apparatus, earth satellites etc.

Clear evidence that a patient is having passivity experiences is strongly suggestive of schizophrenia, although they may arise sometimes in organic mental reactions. Schneider (1959) asserts that if relevant physical disease can be excluded, their occurrence is pathognomonic of schizophrenia. Fish (1967a) however points out that anxious and bewildered patients sometimes feel "as if" they are being controlled by alien influences, and unless these patients are questioned very carefully, they may be diagnosed erroneously as schizophrenic.

REFERENCES

ANDERSON, E. W. and TRETHOWAN, W. H. (1967). *Psychiatry*, 2nd edition. London.
FISH, F. (1967a). *Clinical Psychopathology*. Bristol.
FISH, F. (1967b). Clinical presentation and classification of schizophrenia. *Hosp. Med.* 1, 566-571.
FRIESKE, D. A. and WILSON, W. P. (1966). Formal qualities of hallucinations: a comparative study of the visual hallucinations in patients with schizophrenic, organic and affective psychoses. In *Psychopathology of Schizophrenia*. (Editors Hoch, P. H. and Zubin, J.), pp. 49-62. New York.
HIGASHI, H. and KOSHIKA, K. (1967). On the comparative study of hallucinations in the schizophrenias and organic psychoses. *Bull. Osaka med. Sch.* Supplement 12, pp. 155-161.
JASPERS, K. (1963). *General Psychopathology* (7th edition, translated by Hoenig, J. and Hamilton, M. W.). Manchester.

JASPERS, K. (1968). The phenomenological approach in psychopathology. *Brit. J. Psychiat.* **114**, 1313-1323.

LUCAS, C. J., SAINSBURY, P. and COLLINS, J. G. (1962). A social and clinical study of delusions in schizophrenia. *J. ment. Sci.* **108**, 747-758.

LUKIANOWICZ, N. (1967). "Body image" disturbances in psychiatric disorders. *Brit. J. Psychiat.* **113**, 31-47.

LUNN, V. (1965). On body hallucinations. *Acta psychiat. scand.* **41**, 387-399.

SCHNEIDER, K. (1959). *Clinical Psychopathology* (5th revised edition, translated by Hamilton, M. W.). New York.

SEDMAN, G. (1966a). A comparative study of pseudohallucinations, imagery and true hallucinations. *Brit. J. Psychiat.* **112**, 9-17.

SEDMAN, G. (1966b). "Inner voices". Phenomenological and clinical aspects. *Brit. J. Psychiat.* **112**, 485-490.

SEDMAN, G. (1966c). A phenomenological study of pseudohallucinations and related experiences. *Acta psychiat. scand.* **42**, 35-70.

SMALL, I. F., SMALL, J. G. and ANDERSEN, J. M. (1966). Clinical characteristics of hallucinations of schizophrenics. *Dis. nerv. Syst.* **27**, 349-353.

TAYLOR, F. K. (1966). *Psychopathology, its Causes and Symptoms*. London.

TAYLOR, F. K. (1967). The role of phenomenology in psychiatry. *Brit. J. Psychiat.* **113**, 765-770.

SCHIZOPHRENIC THOUGHT DISORDER

A proportion of schizophrenics show disturbances in the thinking process and in the use of concepts which are unlike those seen in other mental illness. The main characteristic of this schizophrenic thought disorder (formal thought disorder) is a disconnection of thought such that the patient puts together ideas which are not obviously related; his speech seems incoherent and he appears unable to focus on the main point of an argument. Cameron (1944) investigated schizophrenic thought disorder and noted a number of specific abnormalities:

(a) a lack of causal links between successive thoughts or statements ("*asyndetic thinking*");

(b) the use of imprecise approximations ("*metonyms*") where some substitute term or phrase is used instead of a more usual or correct one;

(c) an inability to differentiate between personal preoccupations and what is going on in the outside world, so that statements about both tend to occur in the course of a single sentence ("*interpenetration of themes*");

(d) "*overinclusive thinking*", an inability to preserve the boundaries of a concept, so that distantly related or wholly irrelevant ideas are incorporated into it.

A further abnormality of schizophrenic thinking has been noted by Goldstein (1944), namely an impairment of ability to think in an abstract way. This impairment has two consequences, both of which have been utilized for diagnostic purposes; first, there is a difficulty in grouping and categorizing objects (as in object-sorting tests) and secondly there is a tendency to interpret proverbs concretely rather than by making acceptable generalizations. Payne and Hewlett (1960) have, however, produced evidence which suggests that concrete thinking is not a fundamental characteristic of schizophrenia and that it is more closely related to lack of intelligence than to any particular diagnostic category.

Tests of Overinclusion

Payne and his colleagues have investigated the significance of overinclusive thinking in schizophrenia and have devised a clinically useful battery of tests to measure this disturbance (Payne and Hewlett, 1960; Payne and Friedlander, 1962; Payne, 1966). The battery consists of three tests:

Object Classification Test

The material comprises twelve objects varying in weight, thickness, size, material, and in the hue and brightness of the colours in which they are painted. They are designed to be grouped logically in ten different ways, for example by shape (there are four triangles, four squares and four circles), by size (six objects are large and six are small), by material (some are made of wood, some of metal and some of light plastic material) or by colour; each of these ten logical ways of grouping is known, for the purposes of the test, as an "A" response. The objects can however be grouped in unusual and unintended ways, for example by the shadows cast by the objects on the table, by the slight scratches that have appeared by chance on the objects, or by some personal associations of the sorter, and this type of grouping is known as a "non-A" response.

The test is administered by asking the subject to group the objects in as many ways as he can and to explain his reason for each sorting. Schizophrenics do not differ significantly from normal subjects or from patients suffering from other psychiatric disorders in the number of "A" responses, but they do produce significantly more "non-A" responses; this is to be expected if schizophrenics are more overinclusive since overinclusion implies seeing relationships which normal subjects would regard as unusual or irrelevant.

Proverbs Test

The tester reads 14 proverbs and the subject is asked for the meaning of each. The overinclusion score is the average number of words the subject uses to explain the proverbs; (if the subject says that he does not know the meaning of a particular proverb, it is excluded from the test). Schizophrenic subjects use significantly more words in their explanations than do normal persons or other patients, presumably because overinclusive subjects include, in their answers, associations to a proverb which a normal person would think unnecessary for its explanation.

Goldstein Object-Sorting Test

This is a modification of a test devised by Goldstein and Scheerer. The test material consists of about 30 different objects (e.g. table-knife, apple, sugar cubes, screwdriver, pair of pincers, matchbox, etc). On four separate occasions one of the objects is selected and each time the subject is asked to hand to the examiner all those other objects which the subject thinks could be grouped, for any reason at all, with the original one. The score of overinclusion is the number of objects handed to the examiner. Schizophrenics give significantly higher overinclusion scores than do other subjects, because their over-inclusive thinking allows them to see unusual relationships between the objects.

Payne and Friedlander (1962) have suggested that by combining the scores of the three tests in their battery a clinically useful measure of overinclusion is obtained, and that this might be helpful in diagnosis. The possible usefulness of these tests is however limited for a number of reasons. First, only a proportion of schizophrenics (about one-half) score highly on them. Hence while a high score probably indicates a diagnosis of schizophrenia, a low score does not rule it out. Secondly, only schizophrenics who are acutely ill score highly; with recovery or if the disease becomes chronic the test results may fall into the normal range (Payne, 1966). Thirdly, there is some doubt about the validity of the tests since a patient's score on one test does not necessarily correlate with his scores on the others, suggesting that the tests are not measuring the same variable (Hawks, 1964; Foulds, Hope, McPherson and Mayo, 1967). Lastly, McGhie, Chapman and Lawson (1964) have reported two hypomanic and obsessional patients who gave even higher scores of overinclusion than schizophrenics, suggesting that the tests may not be diagnosis-specific.

Payne, Caird and Laverty (1964) have found an association in schizo-phrenics between overinclusive thinking and the presence of delusions and they put forward the hypothesis that the association is that of cause and effect. Their hypothesis suggests that overinclusive thinking leads the patient to perceive relationships where none exist and hence to have beliefs based on evidence that is unacceptable to normal people. Foulds, Hope, McPherson and Mayo (1968) have also found an association between the presence of delusions in schizophrenics and high scores on tests for overinclusion but Lloyd (1967) has thrown doubt on the theoretical basis for the association.

The Repertory Grid

A completely different type of test of schizophrenic thought disorder makes use of the Repertory Grid technique (Bannister, 1965b; Slater, 1969), a sorting test which measures the relationships between concepts. It is based on Kelly's Personal Construct Theory which states that each individual, as a result of his experience, develops a personal repertoire of concepts (or constructs) and of relationships between these concepts, by means of which he construes his environment in general and new situations in particular. The technique consists of getting the subject to apply a set of *constructs* (concepts such as, for example, *kind* or *honest*) to a set of *elements* (e.g. people he knows or photographs of people). In one commonly used method, the subject ranks the elements in order, according to each of several constructs in turn, and scores are derived from the statistical correlations between the various rankings.

Bannister (1960, 1962) has developed this technique into a test which attempts to discriminate between thought-disordered schizophrenics and other psychiatric patients. The most recent version of the test is that published by Bannister and Fransella (1966). The subject is shown eight photographs (the elements) of persons unknown to him and he is asked, in the first place, to rank them according to how *kind* each person seems. When this has been done, the elements are then ranked using the following constructs in turn: *stupid, selfish, sincere, mean* and *honest*. The whole procedure is then repeated using the same elements and the same constructs.

Normal subjects tend to show high correlations (either positive or negative) between the rank orders. Thus one person who ranks the elements in a particular way as regards *kind* may give similar rank orders as regards *sincere* and *honest* and may tend to give the reverse rank orders in respect of *stupid, selfish* and *mean*. Different subjects have different personal construct systems so that another normal, though perhaps cynical, subject who regards *kind* persons as not *honest* may give negatively correlated rank orders for these two constructs. Thus the pattern of correlations will vary from one normal subject to another and no particular pattern is more correct than any other. But what is characteristic of the normal is a tendency to show strong inter-relationships between the constructs, and hence to generate, on the Bannister and Fransella test, high statistical correlations (positive or negative) between the various rank orders. The higher these correlations the greater the intensity of the interrelationships between the constructs and Bannister and Fransella have shown how the correlations can be combined to form a single score of Intensity. During the second presentation of the elements, normal subjects tend to maintain the same pattern of relationships that were shown during the first presentation, and by comparing the rank order correlations on the two occasions a second score (of Consistency) can be derived.

Bannister and Fransella (1966) tested a group of 30 thought-disordered schizophrenics and compared their scores of Intensity and Consistency with those of five other groups of patients (non-thought-disordered schizophrenics, depressives, neurotics, patients with organic mental reactions and patients with subnormal intelligence) and with a group of normal subjects without any history of psychiatric disorder. They found highly significant differences between the scores of thought-disordered schizophrenics and those of the other groups. Thought disorder was associated with low scores of Intensity and Consistency suggesting that it is due to a pathological loosening of the construct system; indeed, Bannister (1960) has shown how the clinical features of thought disorder might arise from such loosening. Bannister and Fransella indicate that their test might be used as a diagnostic test of thought disorder, but they point out that it is not a valid test of schizophrenia itself, since only a proportion of schizophrenics are thought-disordered. If the test indicates the presence of thought disorder, the diagnosis is probably schizophrenia, but if there is no evidence of thought disorder the possibility of schizophrenia cannot be ruled out.

Corroboration of the findings of Bannister and Fransella (1966) has been reported by Foulds *et al.* (1967) who tested 48 schizophrenics and obtained somewhat higher scores of Intensity and Consistency than did Bannister and Fransella, but Foulds' patients were probably less thought-disordered and there is no reason to doubt the validity of the test. McPherson (1969) has adduced some evidence that thought disorder, as detected by the Repertory Grid, correlates better with delusions of "non-integration" (characterized by solipsistic preoccupation, disturbances of body-image and by visual and auditory hallucinations) than with delusions of persecution.

Bannister (1963, 1965a) has sought to explain thought disorder as the outcome of serial invalidation. He argues that if a person is repeatedly invalidated in his construing of an element, an eventual response may be to loosen and weaken the relationships of the construct. Bannister's theory of the genesis of thought disorder is therefore a psychogenic one since it implies that it is experience that determines the loosening of the construct system.

REFERENCES

BANNISTER, D. (1960). Conceptual structure in thought disordered schizophrenics. *J. ment. Sci.* **106**, 1230-1249.

BANNISTER, D. (1962). The nature and measurement of schizophrenic thought disorder. *J. ment. Sci.* **108**, 825-842.

BANNISTER, D. (1963). The genesis of schizophrenic thought disorder. A serial invalidation hypothesis. *Brit. J. Psychiat.* **109**, 680-686.

BANNISTER, D. (1965a). The genesis of schizophrenic thought disorder: retest of the serial invalidation hypothesis. *Brit. J. Psychiat.* **111**, 377-382.

BANNISTER, D. (1965b). The rationale and clinical relevance of Repertory Grid technique. *Brit. J. Psychiat.* **111**, 977-982.

BANNISTER, D. and FRANSELLA, F. (1966). A grid test of schizophrenic thought disorder. *Brit. J. soc. clin. Psychol.* **5**, 95-102.

CAMERON, N. (1944). Experimental analysis of schizophrenic thinking. In *Language and Thought in Schizophrenia*. (Editor Kasanin, J. S.), pp. 50-63. Berkeley.

FOULDS, G. A., HOPE, K., McPHERSON, F. M. and MAYO, P. R. (1967). Cognitive disorder among the schizophrenias. I. The validity of some tests of thought process disorder. *Brit. J. Psychiat.* **113**, 1361-1368.

FOULDS, G. A., HOPE, K., McPHERSON, F. M. and MAYO, P. R. (1968). Paranoid delusions, retardation and overinclusive thinking. *J. clin. Psychol.* **24**, 177-178.

GOLDSTEIN, K. (1944). Methodological approach to the study of schizophrenic thought disorder. In *Language and Thought in Schizophrenia* (Editor Kasanin, J. S.), pp. 17-39. Berkeley.

HAWKS, D. V. (1964). The clinical usefulness of some tests of overinclusive thinking in psychiatric patients. *Brit. J. soc. clin. Psychol.* **3**, 186-195.

LLOYD, D. N. (1967). Overinclusive thinking and delusions in schizophrenic patients. *J. abnorm. Psychol.* **72**, 451-453.

McGHIE, A., CHAPMAN, J. and LAWSON, J. S. (1964). Disturbances in selective attention in schizophrenia. *Proc. roy. Soc. Med.* **57**, 419-422.

McPHERSON, F. M. (1969). Thought process disorder, delusions of persecution and "non-integration" in schizophrenia. *Brit. J. med. Psychol.* **42**, 55-57.

PAYNE, R. W. (1966). The measurement and significance of overinclusive thinking and retardation in schizophrenic patients. In *Psychopathology of Schizophrenia* (Editors Hoch, P. H. and Zubin, J.), pp. 77-97. New York.

PAYNE, R. W., CAIRD, W. K. and LAVERTY, S. G. (1964). Overinclusive thinking and delusions in schizophrenic patients. *J. abnorm. soc. Psychol.* **68**, 562-566.

PAYNE, R. W. and FRIEDLANDER, D. (1962). A short battery of simple tests for measuring overinclusive thinking. *J. ment. Sci.* **108**, 362-367.

PAYNE, R. W. and HEWLETT, J. H. G. (1960). Thought disorder in psychotic patients. In *Experiments in Personality*, Volume II (Editor Eysenck, H. J.). London.

SLATER, P. (1969). Theory and technique of the Repertory Grid. *Brit. J. Psychiat.* **115**, 1287-1296.

CLINICAL DIAGNOSIS OF SCHIZOPHRENIA

Problems of Diagnosis

In essence, diagnosis means allotting a patient (or his illness) to one category in a classificatory system. Hempel (1961) has pointed out that a classification divides a given set of objects, the *universe of discourse*, into subclasses. In an ideal classification, every object in the universe of discourse can be allotted to one and only one subclass, that is the subclasses are mutually exclusive and jointly exhaustive. In addition, in an ideal system the classificatory terms are defined, preferably by using operational definitions which lay down strict criteria for allocating any given object to its appropriate subclass. In applying such an ideal system, there will be no inter-observer or intra-observer variation, so that different observers will allocate objects in exactly the same way, and the same observer will, on different occasions, always allocate the same object to the same category.

In psychiatric diagnosis, the universe of discourse comprises all mentally disturbed persons and the subclasses are the diagnostic categories, but it is clear that no system of psychiatric classification is ideal. Indeed, the fact that Stengel (1959) was able to collect together 17 different psychiatric classifications in use in different countries, indicates this. It is therefore not surprising that there is considerable inter-observer variation in psychiatric diagnosis (Kreitman, Sainsbury, Morrissey *et al.*, 1961; Zubin, 1967; Shepherd, Brooke, Cooper and Lin, 1968) or that the diagnosis of a mental illness may vary with time even when there does not seem to have been any notable change in the patient's condition (Cooper, 1967). Part of this variation is due to differences between clinicians in the use of the diagnostic terms and to remedy this both the American Psychiatric Association and the General Register Office in Great Britain have produced glossaries defining the psychiatric terms used in the World Health Organization International Classification of Disease (I.C.D.) (World Health Organization, 1967). Even so, the glossaries sometimes differ in their definitions. For example, the term *latent schizophrenia* (I.C.D. code number 295.5) is used in Great Britain "to designate those abnormal states in which, in the absence of obvious schizophrenic symptoms, the suspicion is strong that the condition is in fact a schizophrenia" (General Register Office, 1968). In the United States, however, the same term in the same system of classification is defined as "a category for patients having clear symptoms of schizophrenia but no history of a psychotic schizophrenic episode" (American Psychiatric Association, 1968). These two definitions are operationally incompatible and a patient satisfying one would always be excluded by the other. But even where different psychiatrists appear to agree on the definition of the categories, there is still considerable inter-observer variation, both as regards diagnosis (Kreitman *et al.*, 1961) and as regards observations on the history and mental state of patients (Grosz and Granville-Grossman, 1964, 1968) and this seems to be due, at least in part, to variation between individual clinicians in their judgmental biases and in their response styles.

Diagnostic Criteria of Schizophrenia

In Great Britain the clinical diagnosis of schizophrenia is usually based on an assessment of the mental state, and if at any time during the course of the illness there is good evidence that certain specific abnormalities have been present, the diagnosis can be made with some confidence. These abnormalities include schizophrenic thought disorder, passivity phenomena, catatonic symptoms, flattening of affect and certain types of delusions and hallucinations; they are listed in textbooks of psychiatry and a useful summary appears in the British glossary (General Register Office, 1968). Since these symptoms sometimes occur in organic mental reactions, schizophrenia is not usually diagnosed if there is evidence of an organic basis for the illness. Willis and Bannister (1965) asked a number of senior psychiatrists in England and Wales to indicate which mental abnormalities they thought were important in diagnosing schizophrenia and found that there was considerable agreement. The most important abnormality was thought disorder followed in order of decreasing significance by incongruity of affect, the use of neologisms, thought block, passivity feelings, paranoid delusions, stereotypy and delusions in general. Many other symptoms were ranked as of less importance.

A different approach is that of Fish (1967) who defines a schizophrenic symptom as "a symptom other than an abnormal mood state or delusions of persecution which cannot be understood as arising rationally or emotionally from the patient's mood state or the interaction of his personality with the environment". If such a symptom is present then the diagnosis is schizophrenia unless there is evidence of physical disease of the brain. But since different observers differ in their "understanding" (in Fish's sense of the term), his criterion is not widely used.

Schneider (1959) has listed those symptoms which he regards as being of first-rank importance in distinguishing schizophrenia from other functional psychoses and he asserts that if a person with no relevant somatic disease experiences any of them, the diagnosis is schizophrenia. Schneider's first-rank symptoms are:

(a) certain types of auditory hallucinations, i.e audible thoughts, voices heard arguing and voices giving a running commentary on the patient's actions;

(b) somatic passivity phenomena—the experience of influences playing on the body;

(c) thought withdrawal and other interferences with thought;

(d) diffusion of thought (or thought broadcasting) where the patient experiences his thoughts as being also thought by others;

(e) delusional perceptions;

(f) all feelings, impulses (drives) and volitional acts that are experienced by the patient as the work or influence of others.

All other abnormal subjective experiences in schizophrenia are, according to Schneider, of much less diagnostic importance, and he calls them second-rank symptoms.

Mellor (1970) has elaborated on Schneider's assertions. He classifies the abnormal experiences listed in (f) above as:

(i) "made" affect, i.e. emotion expressed by the patient yet felt to be imposed from without and not experienced by him as his own;

(ii) "made" impulses (drives), where a patient experiences an impulse as coming from outside himself which he is forced to carry out;

(iii) "made" voluntary acts, where the patient experiences his actions as being completely under outside control.

Schneider's list of first-rank symptoms has limitations since failure to obtain evidence that they are present does not necessarily preclude the possibility of schizophrenia. Mellor (1970) studied 166 newly-admitted patients diagnosed as schizophrenic and noted the presence of one or more first-rank symptoms in 119 (71·7 per cent). There were 12 further patients (7·2 per cent) who had no first rank symptoms when seen but who gave a history of experiencing them at some time in the past. They appeared to be more common in patients with a short duration of mental disturbance, suggesting that as the illness progresses they become less evident. In a further study Mellor (1970) investigated 173 schizophrenic patients with one or more first-rank symptoms. The observed frequencies of the different phenomena are set out in Table 2.6. The incidence of each symptom is low, ranging from 21·4 per cent for *thought broadcasting* to 2·9 per cent for *"made" impulses*; among schizophrenics in general the incidences are lower, since Mellor's patients were all experiencing at least one of them. He further showed that certain symptoms were significantly related to one another and to other characteristics. Thus the experience of hearing hallucinatory *voices heard arguing* was associated with *voices commenting* and with auditory hallucinations of second rank importance; *thought insertion* was associated with *thought withdrawal* and with schizophrenic thought disorder in general. *Somatic passivity* tended to be associated with haptic and olfactory hallucinations and *"made" affect* with disturbances of mood.

Table 2.6

FREQUENCY OF FIRST RANK SYMPTOMS IN 173 SCHIZOPHRENICS
(Mellor, 1970)

Symptom	No.	%
Audible thoughts	20	11·6
Voices arguing	23	13·3
Voices commenting	23	13·3
Somatic passivity	20	11·6
Thought broadcasting	37	21·4
Thought insertion	34	19·7
Thought withdrawal	17	9·8
"Made" affect	11	6·4
"Made" impulse	5	2·9
"Made" volition	16	9·2
Delusional perception	11	6·4

Another useful catalogue of symptoms is that prepared by Parkes (1963). He lists (A) symptoms strongly supporting a diagnosis of schizophrenia and (B) symptoms detracting from the diagnosis, as follows:

A.1. *Ideas of change of self* attributed to external influence.
   2. *Feelings of passivity*, control from without or under external influence, *Abulia*.
   3. *Feelings of telepathy*, of thoughts being read or of reading the thoughts of others.
   4. *Disorder of speech and thinking*, characterized by lack of connection between one thought and the next, dysymbole, blocking, stereotypy, ellipsis, metonymy, asyndesis, interpenetration, bizarre content, neologisms, inappropriateness, lack of consensual validation, overinclusion.
   5. *Catatonic disturbance* of motor functions and behaviour.
   6. *Incongruity, inappropriateness or flattening of affect.*
   7. *Delusions of persecution* (plus hallucinations of persecutory voices or ideas of reference) provided they are not believed to be deserved or to be a punishment for some real or imagined crime.
   8. *Bizarre delusions, impossible or extracampine hallucinations.*
B.1. *Prominent affective symptoms*, not describable as labile (lasting less than 12 hours), incongruous or flat.
   2. *Clouding of consciousness or disorientation.*
   3. *Neurotic manifestations.*

Parkes (1963) suggests that a diagnosis of *probable schizophrenia* can be made if there is clear evidence of symptoms in list A and none in list B, and a diagnosis of *doubtful schizophrenia* if there are symptoms in both lists A and B. The reliability of the diagnoses derived from these criteria is discussed later.

While most clinicians have very little difficulty in diagnosing typical cases of schizophrenia there are many patients whose mental disorder is not typical but seems to merge with other mental illnesses. Thus there may be difficulty in distinguishing paranoid schizophrenia (I.C.D. code 295.3) from involutional paraphrenia (297.1), paranoia (297.0) and from acute paranoid reactions (298.3). Schizo-affective psychosis (295.7) and affective psychosis (296) are sometimes hard to differentiate as are latent schizophrenia (295.5) and schizoid personality (301.2). Occasionally the mental abnormalities seen in other conditions such as hysteria or obsessive compulsive neurosis may be unusual and raise the possibility that the illness is schizophrenic, and in organic conditions such as chronic alcoholism and temporal lobe epilepsy, the schizophrenia-like mental symptoms may hinder the correct diagnosis. These difficulties are reflected in the inter-observer variation shown when clinicians attempt to diagnose the disorder.

The Reliability of the Diagnosis of Schizophrenia

Both inter-observer and intra-observer correlation of diagnosis are commonly used as measures of its reliability (Hempel, 1961) while Zubin (1967) has suggested a third method, namely a comparison of the frequencies with which the diagnosis is made in two random samples of the same population.

There are now a number of published reports on the inter-observer variation in the diagnosis of schizophrenia. Parkes (1963) and a colleague examined the case records of 211 patients who had been diagnosed as schizophrenic by other psychiatrists. They had agreed on the criteria for allocating these patients to the three diagnostic categories: "probable schizophrenia", "doubtful schizophrenia", and "schizophrenia not confirmed" (these criteria are as detailed above in the section on Diagnostic Criteria of Schizophrenia. The two observers showed complete diagnostic agreement in 68 per cent of the patients (Table 2.7). Disagreement was most

Table 2.7

RELIABILITY OF CERTAINTY OF DIAGNOSIS OF SCHIZOPHRENIA BY TWO OBSERVERS
(Parkes, 1963)

		Ratings by first observer			Total
		Probable schiz.	Doubtful schiz.	Schiz. not confirmed	
Ratings by second observer	Probable schiz.	64	6	8	78
	Doubtful schiz.	13	5	7	25
	Schiz. not confirmed	17	16	75	108
	Total	94	27	90	211

notable in the "doubtful schizophrenia" category and Parkes suggested that this was due to difficulty in deciding in these patients whether symptoms strongly supporting the diagnosis of schizophrenia were present or not. He further suggested that the reliability could be increased if each symptom were explicitly defined and if the raters were trained in the use of the definitions. Wing, Birley, Cooper *et al.* (1967) introduced a structured interview technique using prepared definitions in an attempt to improve the reliability. They studied 172 patients, each of whom was interviewed by two psychiatrists experienced in the technique and found that of 75 patients diagnosed as schizophrenic by one psychiatrist, 69 (92 per cent) were similarly diagnosed by the other.

Sandifer, Hordern, Timbury and Green (1968) prepared cinematic records of interviews with 30 patients and showed them to a number of psychiatrists in North Carolina (U.S.A.), London and Glasgow. Very high inter-observer correlation might be expected with this technique but it was not found. Indeed if an American psychiatrist made a diagnosis of schizophrenia only 62 per cent of his American colleagues and 56 per cent of the British psychiatrists agreed with him. Similar levels of concordance were obtained when British diagnoses were considered, suggesting international disagreement in the concept of schizophrenia as well as disagreement between individual psychiatrists. A number of other studies on the inter-observer reliability of the diagnosis of schizophrenia have been reviewed by Zubin (1967) who noted on average a concordance of 70-80 per cent.

The inter-observer variation demonstrated in these studies seems to indicate that schizophrenia is not a clear-cut diagnostic entity, and that this state of affairs is likely to persist until some objective method of diagnosis, for example the demonstration of a specific biochemical or psychological disturbance, is discovered. But although a diagnosis of schizophrenia at present carries with it a degree of uncertainty it may yet have some value. Indeed, Hare (1967) has pointed out that prior to the introduction of the Wassermann reaction, the diagnosis of dementia paralytica, like that of schizophrenia nowadays, was based on clinical phenomena; yet its syphilitic basis was strongly suspected. Hence our knowledge of schizophrenia may continue to increase even though diagnosis is uncertain.

REFERENCES

AMERICAN PSYCHIATRIC ASSOCIATION (1968). *Diagnostic and Statistical Manual of Mental Disorders* (2nd Edition). Washington.

COOPER, J. E. (1967). Diagnostic change in a longitudinal study of psychiatric patients. *Brit. J. Psychiat.* **113**, 129-142.

FISH, F. (1967). Clinical presentation and classification of schizophrenia. *Hosp. Med.* **1**, 566-571.

GENERAL REGISTER OFFICE (1968). A glossary of mental disorders. *Studies on Medical and Population Subjects No. 22.* H.M.S.O. London.

GROSZ, H. J. and GRANVILLE-GROSSMAN, K. L. (1964). The sources of observer variation and bias in clinical judgments. I. The item of psychiatric history. *J. nerv. ment. Dis.* **138**, 105-113.

GROSZ, H. J. and GRANVILLE-GROSSMAN, K. L. (1968). Clinician's response style: a source of variation and bias in clinical judgments. *J. abnorm. Psychol.* **73**, 207-214.

HARE, E. H. (1967). The epidemiology of schizophrenia. In *Recent Developments in Schizophrenia* (Editors Coppen, A. and Walk, A.) British Journal of Psychiatry Special Publication No. 1. Ashford.

HEMPEL, C. G. (1961). Introduction to problems of taxonomy. In *Field Studies in the Mental Disorders* (Editor Zubin, J.). New York.

KREITMAN, N., SAINSBURY, P., MORRISSEY, J., TOWERS, J. and SCRIVENER, J. (1961). The reliability of psychiatric assessment: an analysis. *J. ment. Sci.* **107**, 887-908.

MELLOR, C. S. (1970). First rank symptoms of schizophrenia. I. The frequency in schizophrenics on admission to hospital. II. Differences between individual first rank symptoms. *Brit. J. Psychiat.* **117**, 15-23.

PARKES, C. M. (1963). Interhospital and intrahospital variations in the diagnosis and severity of schizophrenia. *Brit. J. prev. soc. Med.* **17**, 85-89.

SANDIFER, M. G., HORDERN, A., TIMBURY, G. C. and GREEN, L. M. (1968). Psychiatric diagnosis: a comparative study in North Carolina, London and Glasgow. *Brit. J. Psychiat.* **114**, 1-9.

SCHNEIDER, K. (1959). *Clinical Psychopathology* (Translated by Hamilton, M. W.). New York.

SHEPHERD, M., BROOKE, E. M., COOPER, J. E. and LIN, T. (1968). An experimental approach to psychiatric diagnosis. *Acta psychiat. scand.* Supplement 201.

STENGEL, E. (1959). Classification of mental disorders. *Bull. Wld. Hlth. Org.* **21**, 601-663.

WILLIS, J. H. and BANNISTER, D. (1965). The diagnosis and treatment of schizophrenia. A questionnaire study of psychiatric opinion. *Brit. J. Psychiat.* **111**, 1165-1171.

WING, J. K., BIRLEY, J. L. T., COOPER, J. E., GRAHAM, P. and ISAACS, A. D. (1967). Reliability of a procedure for measuring and classifying "present psychiatric state". *Brit. J. Psychiat.* **113**, 499-515.

WORLD HEALTH ORGANIZATION (1967). *Manual of the International Statistical Classification of Diseases, Injuries and Causes of Death.* Eighth revision. Geneva.

ZUBIN, J. (1967). Classification of the behaviour disorders. *Ann. Rev. Psychol.* **18**, 373-406.

CHAPTER 3

DRUG DEPENDENCE

The Characteristics of Drug Dependence. Tolerance and Physical Dependence. The Epidemiology of Heroin Dependence in Great Britain. Morbidity and Mortality of Heroin Addiction. New Drug Treatments of Morphine-type Dependence

THE CHARACTERISTICS OF DRUG DEPENDENCE

VARIOUS terms, particularly "drug addiction" and "drug dependence", have been used to denote some of the conditions which may result from the consumption of drugs for non-medical purposes. The World Health Organization Expert Committee on Addiction-producing Drugs (1957) defined "drug addiction" and "drug habituation" but later (World Health Organization, 1964) recommended their replacement by the term "drug dependence". The 1957 definitions were as follows:

"*Drug addiction* is a state of periodic or chronic intoxication produced by the repeated consumption of a drug (natural or synthetic). Its characteristics include (1) an overwhelming desire or need (compulsion) to continue taking the drug and to obtain it by any means; (2) a tendency to increase the dose; (3) a psychic (psychological) and generally a physical dependence on the effects of the drug; (4) detrimental effect on the individual and on society.

"*Drug habituation* (*habit*) is a condition resulting from the repeated consumption of a drug. Its characteristics include: (1) a desire (but not a compulsion) to continue taking the drug for the sense of improved well-being which it engenders; (2) little or no tendency to increase the dose; (3) some degree of psychic dependence on the effect of the drug, but absence of physical dependence and hence of an abstinence syndrome; (4) detrimental effects, if any, primarily on the individual."

The recommended change in terminology in 1964 followed the observation that there had been confusion in the application of the older terms, and that they had been misused. The component common to the various types of drug abuse appeared to be dependence (psychic or physical, or both) and the new term "drug dependence" was defined (World Health Organization, 1964, as slightly modified by Eddy, Halbach, Isbell and Seevers, 1965), as follows: "*Drug dependence* is a state of psychic or physical dependence, or both, on a drug, arising in a person following administration of that drug on a periodic or continuous basis." The characteristics of drug dependence often vary considerably with the agent involved. Thus morphine dependence differs markedly from dependence on cannabis, but resembles closely dependence on pethidine. The type of drug dependence (e.g. morphine type, cannabis type, etc.) should therefore always be specified. These recommendations have been

70

widely accepted, but nevertheless terms such as "addiction" and "addict" are still commonly used, both in clinical practice, and by official bodies such as the United Nations Commission on Narcotic Drugs and the Advisory Committee on Drug Dependence in the United Kingdom (Home Office, 1968).

Eight types of drug dependence have been described by the World Health Organization (Eddy *et al.*, 1965), namely:

1. *Morphine type*—dependence on opium and its preparations, morphine, heroin and other morphine derivatives; or on synthetic substances with morphine-like effects, such as pethidine, methadone, dextromoramide, etc.

2. *Barbiturate type*—dependence on pentobarbitone, amylobarbitone, quinalbarbitone and other barbiturates; paraldehyde; chloral hydrate; meprobamate; glutethimide; methaqualone; chlordiazepoxide; diazepam, etc.

3. *Alcohol type*—dependence on ethyl alcohol, beer, wine, spirits, etc. (*Note:* there is a substantial affinity with the barbiturate type of dependence.)

4. *Amphetamine type*—dependence on amphetamine, dexamphetamine, phenmetrazine, diethylpropion, methylamphetamine, etc.

5. *Cocaine type*—dependence on coca leaf and preparations of cocaine.

6. *Cannabis type*—dependence on cannabis leaf and resin, and its preparations (marihuana, hashish, etc.)

7. *Khat type*—dependence on Khat leaf (*Catha edulis*).

8. *Hallucinogen type*—dependence on lysergic acid diethylamide (LSD); mescaline and mescal cactus; morning glory; psylocybin; dimethyltryptamine; diethyltryptamine, atropine-like drugs, etc.

This list is not an exhaustive one and dependence on many other types of drugs and chemical substances has been reported, e.g. petrol, glue, nutmeg, salicylates, bromides, etc. Tobacco smoking also involves dependence.

Certain characteristics of drug dependence are shared by a number of different types.

1. In all types of drug dependence there is *psychic dependence* characterized by a psychological need to continue to take the drug either to produce a feeling of pleasure or well-being, or to avoid discomfort.

2. *Physical dependence*, occurring particularly in morphine, alcohol and barbiturate types, is characterized by an altered physiological state which shows itself by the development of physical disturbances on withdrawal of the drug or when a specific antagonist is administered, and by the relief of these withdrawal symptoms by the drug itself or by other drugs of the same type.

3. Drug dependence is often associated with the development of *tolerance* which is characterized by a diminution in the effect of the drug after repeated administration of the same dose, and by a need to increase the dose to produce the same initial pharmacological effect.

4. Drugs producing dependence tend to have a detrimental effect on the individual taking them, and on the society in which he lives. The hallucinogens

in particular tend to alter the mental state and lead to a derangement of normal mental function with consequent disturbance in behaviour. Legislation restricting the use of drugs is usually based on these adverse effects on society.

Drug dependence of morphine type is characterized by (*a*) strong psychic dependence, an overpowering drive or compulsion to continue to take the drug; (*b*) the development of tolerance and a notable tendency to increase the dose; (*c*) the early development of physical dependence which increases in intensity as the dose increases, with a specific abstinence syndrome on withdrawal or on administration of a morphine antagonist such as nalorphine; (*d*) detriment to the individual (personal neglect, physical complications, etc.) and to society (disruption of interpersonal relationships, economic loss, crime, etc.).

Drug dependence of barbiturate type is characterized by (*a*) strong psychic dependence; (*b*) the development of tolerance, and of some cross-tolerance with alcohol; (*c*) very slowly developing physical dependence with a specific abstinence syndrome similar to that associated with alcohol dependence; (*d*) an adverse effect on the individual (impairment of mental ability, confusion, emotional instability, etc.) and a slightly detrimental effect on society.

Drug dependence of alcohol type is characterized by (*a*) psychic dependence which tends to be periodic and to vary markedly in intensity; (*b*) the development of a slight degree of tolerance, and of cross-tolerance with barbiturate type drugs; (*c*) the very slow development of physical dependence with an abstinence syndrome similar to that seen with barbiturates; (*d*) a strongly adverse effect on the individual (mentally and physically) and on society (neglect of family, decline in productivity, etc.).

Drug dependence of cocaine type is characterized by (*a*) strong psychic dependence with (*b*) no physical dependence and (*c*) no tolerance. It is usually associated with dependence on other drugs, particularly on opiates.

Drug dependence of cannabis type is characterized by (*a*) moderate to strong psychic dependence; (*b*) absence of physical dependence and (*c*) absence of tolerance. There is no definite evidence of a detrimental effect on the individual or on society, but it possibly predisposes to the morphine type of dependence.

Drug dependence of amphetamine type is characterized by (*a*) psychic dependence of variable degree; (*b*) no definite physical dependence although some mental and physical symptoms may develop on withdrawal; (*c*) the slow development of tolerance to certain of its pharmacological actions, and (*d*) an adverse effect on the individual (mental and physical complications) and on society.

Drug dependence of Khat type is characterized by (*a*) moderate but often persistent psychic dependence; (*b*) lack of physical dependence; (*c*) absence of tolerance and (*d*) damage to the individual's health and to society.

Drug dependence of hallucinogenic type is characterized by (*a*) a slight to moderate degree of psychic dependence; (*b*) no physical dependence; (*c*) rapid development and decline of tolerance; (*d*) adverse psychological effects on the individual (impairment of judgment, delusions, hallucinations, etc.) and detriment to society.

REFERENCES

EDDY, N. B., HALBACH, H., ISBELL, H. and SEEVERS, M. H. (1965). Drug dependence: its significance and characteristics. *Bull. Wld. Hlth. Org.* **32**, 721-733.
HOME OFFICE (1968). *The Rehabilitation of Drug Addicts. Report of the Advisory Committee on Drug Dependence.* H.M.S.O. London.
WORLD HEALTH ORGANIZATION (1957). Expert Committee on Addiction-producing Drugs. Seventh Report. *Wld. Hlth. Org. techn. Rep. Ser.* No. 116.
WORLD HEALTH ORGANIZATION (1964). Expert Committee on Addiction-producing Drugs. Thirteenth Report. *Wld. Hlth. Org. techn. Rep. Ser.* No. 273.

TOLERANCE AND PHYSICAL DEPENDENCE

Tolerance

With the repeated administration of certain drugs (particularly those leading to dependence of morphine or barbiturate type) the effect of the drug gradually diminishes and increasingly large doses are required to produce the same effect (Seevers and Deneau, 1963). With the development of such tolerance, a given dose of a morphine-type drug has less analgesic, sedative and other central depressant effects and these last for shorter periods of time. In addition, the lethal dose increases. In clinical practice, addicts who take 500 mg or more daily of heroin are not uncommon, while Isbell (1967) has encountered patients who have taken 5 grammes of morphine in the course of twenty-four hours. Tolerance to barbiturates (particularly those with short durations of action) is also frequently observed and 2 grammes daily or more of drugs such as quinalbarbitone sodium may be taken by addicts without undue sedation. Tolerance to the hypnotic effect of barbiturates does not however confer any protection against lethal doses.

Tolerance to a particular drug is associated with tolerance to other drugs of the same type. Thus heroin addicts show increased tolerance to morphine, pethidine, etc., as well as to heroin, and tolerance to one sedative drug is generally accompanied by tolerance to others; there is also some cross-tolerance between alcohol and drugs producing dependence of barbiturate type.

Development of Tolerance to Opiates

The continued therapeutic use of morphine-type analgesics is usually associated with the development of obvious tolerance. Eddy, Lee and Harris (1959) observed that the daily dose of morphine required to relieve the pain of cancer patients gradually increased by about 30 per cent over the course of several weeks. Ferguson and Mitchell (1969) have reported a more rapid development of tolerance—within a few days—in human volunteers subjected to experimentally-induced ischaemic pain, and their results suggest that this tolerance occurs more readily in the presence of pain. Animal studies indicate that tolerance to morphine may develop even more quickly—over the course of a few hours—if the drug is administered continuously (Cox, Ginsburg and Osman, 1968; Way, Loh and Shen, 1969) or even as the result of a single injection (Kornetsky and Bain, 1968), but the relevance of these findings to the clinical situation is at present uncertain.

REFERENCES

Cox, B. M., Ginsburg, M. and Osman, O. H. (1968). Acute tolerance to narcotic analgesic drugs in rats. *Brit. J. Pharmacol.* 33, 245-256.

Eddy, N. B., Lee, L. E. and Harris, C. A. (1959). The rate of development of physical dependence and tolerance to analgesic drugs in patients with chronic pain. Comparison of morphine, oxymorphone and anilerdine. *Bull. Narcot.* 11, No. 1, 3-17.

Ferguson, R. K. and Mitchell, C. L. (1969). Pain as a factor in the development of tolerance to morphine analgesia in man. *Clin. Pharmacol. Ther.* 10, 372-382.

Isbell, H. (1967). Drug dependence (addiction). In *Cecil-Loeb Textbook of Medicine*, 12th Edition (Editors, Beeson, P. B. and McDermott, W.), pp. 1494-1500. Philadelphia.

Kornetsky, C. and Bain, G. (1968). Morphine: single-dose tolerance. *Science*, 162, 1011-1012.

Seevers, M. H. and Deneau, G. A. (1963). Physiological aspects of tolerance and physical dependence. In *Physiological Pharmacology* (Editors Root, W. S. and Hoffman, F. G.), Volume I, pp. 565-640. New York.

Way, E. L., Loh, H. H. and Shen, F-H. (1969). Simultaneous quantitative assessment of morphine tolerance and physical dependence. *J. Pharmacol. exp. Ther.* 167, 1-8.

Physical Dependence

Physical dependence is characterized by the development of specific physical disturbances when the drug is withdrawn such that continued administration is necessary for the subject's well-being. It is commonly observed with abuse both of alcohol and sedative drugs (Chapter 4) and of opiates (discussed below), but it has also been found in dependence of amphetamine type. Oswald and Thacore (1963) studied six patients, four of whom were dependent on amphetamine and two on phenmetrazine and they noted that when the drugs were withdrawn the proportion of REM sleep increased markedly at first and only slowly returned to normal over the course of several weeks; re-introduction of the drugs abolished the abnormality. (These changes are similar to those observed on withdrawal of barbiturate-alcohol type drugs from dependent subjects—see Chapter 4.) Symptoms after amphetamine withdrawal are however relatively mild and are limited to listlessness, depression, sleepiness and intense craving for the drug.

Effects of Opiate Withdrawal

When morphine-like drugs are abruptly withdrawn from subjects physically dependent on them, a variety of disturbances occur, many of which are mediated through the autonomic nervous system. Table 3.1 lists these symptoms and signs in the order they occur. The time course varies with the drug

Table 3.1

SYMPTOMS AND SIGNS OF WITHDRAWAL IN MORPHINE-TYPE DEPENDENCE
(Blachly, 1966)

Grade	Symptoms and signs	Hours after last dose		
		Morphine	Heroin	Methadone
0	Craving for drug Anxiety	6	4	12
1	Yawning Perspiration Lacrimation Rhinorrhoea "Yen" sleep*	14	8	34-48
2	Mydriasis Piloerection Muscle twitches Aching bones and muscles Anorexia	16	12	48-72
3	Insomnia Hypertension Fever Tachypnoea Tachycardia Restlessness Nausea	24-36	18-24	—
4	Vomiting Diarrhoea Spontaneous ejaculation Haemoconcentration	36-48	24-36	—

* Restless, tossing sleep.

and is most rapid (and most severe) after withdrawal of heroin, and slowest (and least severe) on withdrawal of methadone. In addition to the phenomena listed in Table 3.1, the following have also been noted: quarrelsomeness and irritability, the adoption of peculiar postures, strabismus, hiccough, convulsions, hyperglycaemia, cough and salivation (Seevers and Deneau, 1963). The incidences of the more common signs are given in Table 3.2 (from Quock, Cheng, Chan and Way, 1968). Maximum distress occurs after about 36 hours of heroin abstinence and after some 48 hours of morphine abstinence, and thereafter the symptoms gradually subside so that one week after withdrawal there is relatively little in the way of clinical abnormality and tolerance to the drug is lost. A subsequent chronic phase of abstinence characterized by gradually decreasing insomnia, irritability and muscular aches and pains lasting two to four months has been described by Isbell (1967).

The abstinence syndrome may be modified by the administration of drugs of the same type, and this phenomenon of cross-dependence is the basis of the current practice of using methadone to alleviate the symptoms of heroin or morphine withdrawal. Blachly (1966) suggests giving methadone when

Table 3.2

INCIDENCE OF WITHDRAWAL PHENOMENA IN 26 NARCOTIC ADDICTS
(Quock *et al.*, 1968)

Phenomenon	Per cent incidence
Yawning	88·5
Lacrimation	88·5
Mydriasis	84·5
Anorexia	65·3
Piloerection	65·3
Rhinorrhoea	61·5
Perspiration	57·6
Vomiting	38·5
Restlessness	26·9
Tremor	15·4

Grade 2 signs (Table 3.1) appear, and he points out that of these signs, piloerection of the hair of the chest is the most valuable since it is more objective than the others. He advocates a dose of 10 mg in syrup form, but if this is vomited it may be given parenterally. If after 1-2 hours Grade 2 signs persist a further 10 mg of the drug may be given. A daily dose of 30-40 mg normally controls the symptoms and this may then be reduced by about 10 mg daily. It should be pointed out that the majority of narcotic addicts who are admitted to hospital for withdrawal do not develop such severe symptoms that methadone substitution is necessary. Cross-dependence is also the rationale of using barbiturate-type drugs in the treatment of delirium tremens and related conditions (see Chapter 4).

Effect of Narcotic Antagonists in Dependent Subjects

There are now a large number of synthetic compounds which antagonize the effects of morphine-type drugs. These include nalorphine, naloxone, levallorphan, cyclazocine and pentazocine (Martin, 1967) and their administration to morphine-dependent subjects will precipitate typical withdrawal symptoms. Wikler, Fraser and Isbell (1953) gave nalorphine 15 mg subcutaneously to ex-addict volunteers who had been made dependent on morphine, methadone or heroin and noted the development of a severe abstinence syndrome over the course of 30-45 minutes, gradually subsiding over the next one to two hours. In general, smaller doses of nalorphine are sufficient to produce some disturbance in dependent subjects and Eddy, Lee and Harris (1959) found that 1·0 mg was sufficient to cause increases in blood pressure, temperature and respiration rate. In non-dependent subjects, nalorphine causes constriction of the pupils, but in addicts it produces dilatation and Terry and Baumoeller (1956) have introduced a test based on this observation in which change in pupil size is noted 30 minutes after the subcutaneous injection of 3 mg nalorphine; this test is now widely used in California for the detection of opiate abuse (Elliot, Nomof, Parker and Turgeon, 1968).

The Development of Opiate Dependence

The intensity of the withdrawal symptoms depends on the drug taken, on the duration of the abuse and on the daily dose. Heroin and morphine produce much greater physical dependence than do less addicting drugs such as pethidine, methadone or codeine. Isbell (1967) states that only the mildest of symptoms arise during withdrawal after one month of taking 40-80 mg morphine daily and that as the daily dose increases so does the intensity of the abstinence syndrome; maximum intensity is reached when withdrawal occurs after taking about 360 mg daily for at least one month. It is however possible to detect physical dependence much earlier and on much lower doses by administering a narcotic antagonist. Thus, by giving nalorphine Wikler et al. (1953) found evidence of some dependence after the administration of 60 mg daily morphine or heroin or of 40 mg daily methadone for as short a period as two or three days, while Eddy et al. (1959) precipitated signs of withdrawal in cancer patients after 2-4 weeks' treatment with morphine.

REFERENCES

BLACHLY, P. H. (1966). Management of the opiate abstinence syndrome. Amer. J. Psychiat. 122, 742-744.

EDDY, N. B., LEE, L. E. and HARRIS, C. A. (1959). The rate of development of physical dependence and tolerance to analgesic drugs in patients with chronic pain. Comparison of morphine, oxymorphone and anilerdine. Bull. Narcot. 11, No. 1, 3-17.

ELLIOT, H. W., NOMOF, N., PARKER, K. D. and TURGEON, G. R. (1968). Detection of narcotic use—comparison of the Nalorphine (pupil) test with chemical tests. Calif. Med. 109, 121-125.

ISBELL, H. (1967). Drug dependence (addiction). In Cecil-Loeb Textbook of Medicine, 12th Edition (Editors, Beeson, P. B. and McDermott, W.), pp. 1494-1500. Philadelphia.

MARTIN, W. R. (1967). Opioid antagonists. Pharmacol. Rev. 19, 463-521.

OSWALD, I. and THACORE, V. R. (1963). Amphetamine and phenmetrazine addiction. Physiological abnormalities in the abstinence syndrome. Brit. med. J. 2, 427-431.

QUOCK, C. P., CHENG, J., CHAN, S. C. and WAY, E. L. (1968). The abstinence syndrome in long term high dosage narcotic addiction. Brit. J. Addict. 63, 261-270.

SEEVERS, M. H. and DENEAU, G. A. (1963). Physiological aspects of tolerance and physical dependence. In Physiological Pharmacology (Editors Root, W. S. and Hoffman, F. G.), Volume I, pp. 565-640. New York.

TERRY, J. G. and BAUMOELLER, F. L. (1956). Nalline: an aid in detecting narcotic users. Calif. Med. 85, 299-301.

WIKLER, A., FRASER, H. F. and ISBELL, H. (1953). N-allylnormorphine: effects of single doses and precipitation of acute "abstinence syndromes" during addiction to morphine, methadone or heroin in man (post-addicts). *J. Pharmacol. exp. Ther.* **109**, 8-20.

Theories of Tolerance and Dependence

There is now good evidence that there are two quite distinct mechanisms responsible for the development of tolerance to barbiturates and other sedative drugs (Remmer, 1969). First, short-acting barbiturates such as quinalbarbitone appear to stimulate those hydroxylating enzymes in the liver which are responsible for their degradation, so that with repeated administration the rate at which the blood barbiturate level falls is increased; alcohol also induces these enzymes, although this does not seem to be responsible for the development of tolerance to alcohol itself. Secondly, tolerance to drugs of the alcohol-barbiturate type is due, at least in part, to a reduction in sensitivity of the nerve cells; tolerance to long-acting barbiturates such as phenobarbitone, which are not metabolized by the liver to any great extent, is almost entirely of this type. Opiate tolerance is wholly at a cellular level and there is no consistent evidence of any differences in drug metabolism, excretion or distribution within the body between tolerant and non-tolerant subjects (Way and Adler, 1960; Mulé, 1969).

The mechanisms by which cellular tolerance and physical dependence are produced are unknown, but current theories take into account four observations. First, both tolerance and physical dependence develop in step, suggesting that they have modes of production in common. Secondly, drug withdrawal in a physically dependent subject leads to excitation of those functions which are depressed by the ordinary pharmacological action of the drug. (The administration of morphine causes, for example, drowsiness, constipation and miosis, while withdrawal leads to insomnia, diarrhoea and mydriasis; barbiturates have sedative and anticonvulsant actions, while withdrawal may cause sleeplessness and epileptic seizures.) Thirdly, both the direct pharmacological effects of addictive drugs and their abstinence syndromes appear to be mediated through the nervous system, and fourthly, withdrawal symptoms are relieved by the administration of the drug.

Most current theories postulate an adaptive mechanism, that, under the influence of an addictive drug, neurones develop responses which oppose the direct actions of the drug. Such a homoeostatic mechanism would explain the development of tolerance because the adaptive responses would lessen the effect of the drug, while their persistence after withdrawal of the drug would account for both the occurrence and the character of the abstinence syndrome.

Various suggestions have been made concerning the exact nature of the homoeostatic mechanism. Paton (1969) has pointed out that opiates interfere with neurotransmitter release and he proposes a "surfeit" theory which postulates that with continued drug administration neurotransmitter accumulates in the terminal axones. As the concentration rises more becomes available for release in response to a nerve stimulus and the drug will therefore have less effect, while withdrawal symptoms arise as a result of an abnormally great output of neurotransmitter.

A second theory has been formulated by Jaffe and Sharpless (1965, 1968; Sharpless and Jaffe, 1969) and by Collier (1968, 1969), based on observations made by Emmelin (1961, 1965) that the continued administration of drugs which block neurotransmission leads to the development of heightened sensitivity of the neuroreceptors—the so-called supersensitivity of pharmacological denervation—similar to that seen after surgical denervation. Since opiates and barbiturates interfere with neurotransmitter release, the hypothesis predicts that their administration will cause the relevant receptors to become supersensitive so that the reduced amount of neurotransmitter that is available will be more potent than normal and tolerance will be observed. Furthermore when the drug is withdrawn and release no longer inhibited, the normal amounts of neurotransmitter then available will cause excessive stimulation of the supersensitive receptors and hence the appearance of abstinence phenomena, which persist for the few days that it takes for sensitivity to decline to normal. Paton (1969) has criticized this theory on the grounds that supersensitivity develops over the course of some days, whereas tolerance has been observed within a few hours, and he suggests that his "surfeit" hypothesis more readily explains early tolerance and physical dependence; he acknowledges, however, that at a later stage supersensitivity may be the more important mechanism.

A further suggestion, alternative to both the above theories, has been proposed by Martin (1968). It postulates that where there is more than one neural pathway mediating a particular physiological function, one of them may be depressed by the drug, and the others will then hypertrophy and take over the function of the first. Tolerance will be observed and on withdrawal of the drug the first pathway will no longer be depressed and the function in question will be enhanced with the production of symptoms.

Recent animal studies have demonstrated the possibility of modifying the development of morphine tolerance and physical dependence. First, it has been shown that the administration of actinomycin D, cycloheximide or other similar drugs which inhibit protein synthesis, prevents the development of acute tolerance to morphine (Cox, Ginsburg and Osman, 1968; Cox and Osman, 1969), and that cycloheximide prevents physical dependence also (Way, Loh and Shen, 1968). Secondly, it has been claimed that it is possible to induce tolerance in animals who have not received morphine by the injection of brain extracts from tolerant animals (Ungar and Cohen, 1966; Ungar and Galvan, 1969), but other workers have been unable to confirm this (Tirri, 1967; Smits and Takemori, 1968). Lastly, there is some evidence that monoamines may be involved. Way et al. (1968) found that p-chlorophenylalanine, an inhibitor of 5-hydroxytryptamine synthesis, interferes with the development of tolerance and physical dependence, while Takagi and

Kuriki (1969) have reported that tetrabenazine—which, like reserpine, depletes neurones of monoamines—has similar suppressive actions, and that these effects are antagonized by the administration of dopa.

REFERENCES

COLLIER, H. O. J. (1968). Supersensitivity and dependence. *Nature (Lond.)*, **220**, 228-231.

COLLIER, H. O. J. (1969). Humoral transmitters, supersensitivity, receptors and dependence. In *Scientific Basis of Drug Dependence* (Editor Steinberg, H.), pp. 49-66. London.

COX, B. M., GINSBURG, M. and OSMAN, O. H. (1968). Acute tolerance to narcotic analgesic drugs in rats. *Brit. J. Pharmacol.* **33**, 245-256.

COX, B. M. and OSMAN, O. H. (1969). The role of protein synthesis inhibition in the prevention of morphine tolerance. *Brit. J. Pharmacol.* **35**, 373P-374P.

EMMELIN, N. (1961). Supersensitivity following "pharmacological denervation". *Pharmacol. Rev.* **13**, 17-37.

EMMELIN, N. (1965). Action of transmitters on the responsiveness of effector cells. *Experientia (Basel)*, **21**, 57-65.

JAFFE, J. H. and SHARPLESS, S. K. (1965). The rapid development of physical dependence on barbiturates. *J. Pharmacol. exp. Ther.* **150**, 140-145.

JAFFE, J. H. and SHARPLESS, S. K. (1968). Pharmacological denervation supersensitivity in the central nervous system: a theory of physical dependence. *Res. Publ. Ass. Res. nerv. ment. Dis.* **46**, 226-243.

MARTIN, W. R. (1968). A homeostatic and redundancy theory of tolerance to and dependence on narcotic analgesics. *Res. Publ. Ass. Res. nerv. ment. Dis.* **46**, 206-223.

MULÉ, S. J. (1969). The relationship of the disposition and metabolism of morphine in the CNS to tolerance. In *Scientific Basis of Drug Dependence* (Editor Steinberg, H.), pp. 97-109. London.

PATON, W. D. M. (1969). A pharmacological approach to drug dependence and drug tolerance. In *Scientific Basis of Drug Dependence* (Editor Steinberg, H.), pp. 31-47. London.

REMMER, H. (1969). Tolerance to barbiturates by increased breakdown. In *Scientific Basis of Drug Dependence* (Editor Steinberg, H.), pp. 111-128. London.

SHARPLESS, S. and JAFFE, J. (1969). Withdrawal phenomena as manifestations of disuse supersensitivity. In *Scientific Basis of Drug Dependence* (Editor Steinberg, H.), pp. 67-76. London.

SMITS, S. E. and TAKEMORI, A. E. (1968). Lack of transfer of morphine tolerance by administration of rat cerebral homogenates. *Proc. Soc. exp. Biol. (N.Y.)*, **127**, 1167-1171.

TAKAGI, H. and KURIKI, H. (1969). Suppressive effect of tetrabenazine on the development of tolerance to morphine and its reversal by dopa. *Int. J. Neuropharmacol.* **8**, 195-196.

TIRRI, R. (1967). Transfer of induced tolerance to morphine and promazine by brain homogenate. *Experientia (Basel)*, **23**, 278.

UNGAR, G. and COHEN, M. (1966). Induction of morphine tolerance by material extracted from brain of tolerant animals. *Int. J. Neuropharmacol.* **5**, 183-192.

UNGAR, G. and GALVAN, L. (1969). Conditions of transfer of morphine tolerance by brain extracts. *Proc. Soc. exp. Biol. (N.Y.)*, **130**, 287-291.

WAY, E. L. and ADLER, T. K. (1960). The pharmacological implications of the fate of morphine and its surrogates. *Pharmacol. Rev.* **12**, 383-446.

WAY, E. L., LOH, H. H. and SHEN, F-H. (1968). Morphine tolerance, physical dependence and synthesis of 5-hydroxytryptamine. *Science*, **162**, 1290-1292.

THE EPIDEMIOLOGY OF HEROIN DEPENDENCE IN GREAT BRITAIN

The Growth of Heroin Addiction

Until about 10 years ago dependence on opiates in the United Kingdom created relatively few problems. Home Office statistics (Spear, 1969) show that in 1958 there were 442 known opiate addicts of whom 349 (79 per cent) had become dependent as the result of prolonged treatment of physical illness with morphine-type drugs. In general, these patients were middle-aged or elderly and did not abuse the drugs prescribed for them, and the so-called British System, which allowed established addicts to have the drugs they needed, worked very well. Relatively few addicts became dependent while physically fit (in 1958 there were 68 known to the Home Office) but the existence of these "non-therapeutic" addicts did not cause undue concern in official circles (Ministry of Health and Department of Health for Scotland, 1961). A high proportion of known addicts were in professions which allowed access to Dangerous Drugs (i.e. medical, dental, nursing, pharmaceutical and veterinary personnel) but here again there was no social problem since these addicts usually obtained drugs solely for their own use; in 1958, 16 per cent of addicts were in medical and allied professions.

Since 1961, the total number of known persons dependent on Dangerous Drugs in Great Britain has risen steadily (Spear, 1969). Figure 3.1 demonstrates that this growth is entirely attributable to an enormous increase in the numbers of "non-therapeutic" addicts using heroin. In 1958, there were 62 heroin addicts known to the Home Office of whom 43 were "non-therapeutic", whereas in 1968, of the 2240 known heroin addicts, all except eight were "non-therapeutic". The number of morphine and pethidine users has remained fairly constant over the years, and while there has been a recent increase in numbers of methadone-dependent subjects, this is due, at least in part, to the prescription of this drug by doctors for heroin addicts as a substitute for heroin. Addiction to Dangerous Drugs in medical personnel has not increased in recent years; indeed, there has been a significant decrease (Figure 3.2).

Two further recent notable changes have been in relation to the sex and age of opiate addicts. In 1958 less than half (45 per cent) were male, compared with more than three-quarters (78 per cent) in 1968. Figure 3.3 demonstrates the steady increase in the proportion of men since 1960. The change in the age distribution of the addicts is shown in Figure 3.4. In 1959, 66 per cent of all persons dependent on Dangerous Drugs and 38 per cent of heroin addicts were aged 50 years or over, and no case under the age of 20 years was known to the Home Office, whereas nine years later the vast majority were below the age of 35.

These data show that the recent opiate problem in Great Britain has been due to the spread of heroin addiction in physically fit young persons. There is good evidence that this has been caused by users of heroin obtaining more of the drug than is required for their own use and giving or selling the surplus to non-addicted friends or acquaintances. De Alarcón and Rathod (1968)

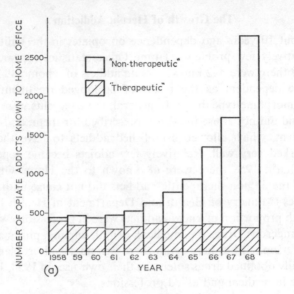

(a)

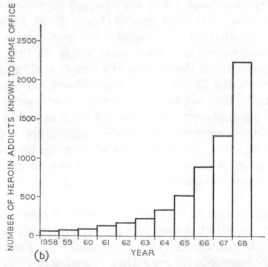

(b)

Figure 3.1 Number of persons known to be addicted to Dangerous
Drugs in the United Kingdom, 1958-68 (Spear, 1969)
(a) "Therapeutic" and "non-therapeutic" addicts
(b) Heroin addicts

carried out a survey of heroin abuse among young people in Crawley, a new town south of London with a population of 62,000, and they calculated that the 1967 prevalence of confirmed users was 8·50 per 1000 of the population

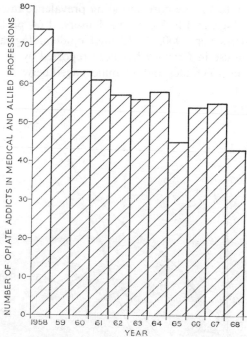

Figure 3.2 Addicts in the medical and allied professions known to Home Office, United Kingdom, 1958-68 (Spear, 1969)

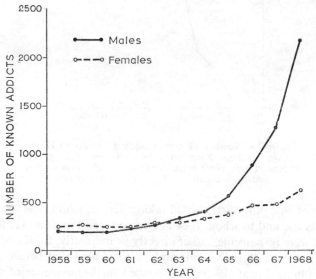

Figure 3.3 Male and female addicts known to Home Office, United Kingdom, 1958-68 (Spear, 1969)

aged 15 to 20 years, with a further 0·85 probable users per 1000 and 6·29 suspected users per 1000. The corresponding prevalence rates among young males were much higher: 14·75 confirmed users, 1·64 probable users and 10·82 suspected users per 1000. A detailed epidemiological study on the spread of heroin abuse in Crawley has been reported by de Alarcón (1969). Fifty-eight drug users (53 males and 5 females) aged between 15 and 20 years

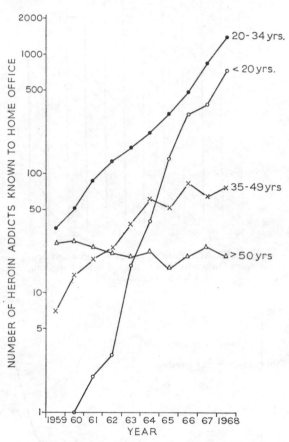

Figure 3.4 Number of heroin addicts known to Home Office, United Kingdom, 1959-68, by age group (Spear, 1969). Note logarithmic scale. The exponential growth is greatest in the younger age groups

gave details of when they first started taking heroin, who it was who initiated them into its use and to whom they had introduced the drug. He found that two addicts were responsible, either directly or indirectly, for the initiation of the habit in at least 48 individuals and he concluded that heroin abuse is a contagious illness. Spear (1969) has adduced further evidence of contagion. In 1951, a large quantity of heroin and cocaine was stolen from a hospital pharmacy near London and he was able to show that there had been contact (either directly or through intermediaries) between the thief and about 40 heroin addicts who came to official notice for the first time after the theft. Indeed, Spear argues that it was the appearance of this stolen heroin and cocaine that may have started the present epidemic of addiction among young people in Great Britain.

A further factor which encouraged the spread of heroin use has been described by the Interdepartmental Committee on Drug Addiction (Ministry of Health and Scottish Home and Health Department, 1965), which found that a few doctors were prescribing excessively for addicts. As an example, it reported that one doctor had prescribed 600,000 tablets of heroin (i.e. 6 kilogrammes) for addicts in the course of one year and that the same doctor had written prescriptions for one individual for several grammes of the drug within a few days of one another. The Committee argued that supplies on this scale would easily provide a surplus and lead to an increase in the number of addicts. Quite clearly, greater control over the prescription of Dangerous Drugs was needed, but the Committee pointed out that the degree of control was crucial, since if the restrictions were too severe, addicts might be seriously discouraged from obtaining legitimate supplies and resort to, and thereby encourage, illicit sources, while if the controls were too lax addicts would continue to obtain more than they required and the abuse would spread further. During the early part of 1968, the Dangerous Drugs (Notification of Addicts) Regulations and the Dangerous Drugs (Supply to Addicts) Regulations came into operation in an attempt to solve this dilemma. These require all medical practitioners to notify particulars (name, address, sex, date of birth and drugs used) to the Chief Medical Officer of the Home Office of persons addicted to drugs specified in Part I of the Schedule to the Dangerous Drugs Act of 1965 (including cocaine and natural and synthetic drugs of morphine type). They also restrict the authority of doctors to prescribe or supply heroin or cocaine to addicts, to those holding Home Office licences. Later in 1968, legislation was introduced permitting methyl-amphetamine for intravenous use to be supplied by hospitals only, with the purpose of preventing its reckless prescription. A further development has been the establishment of drug dependency centres staffed by licensed doctors, to enable established addicts to obtain legitimate supplies of heroin.

It is still too early to know whether these measures will stem the spread of heroin abuse, but already there are indications that they may not be having the desired effect and illicit ("Chinese") heroin is now being introduced into the United Kingdom, a development which the new regulations were specifically designed to prevent (Glatt, 1969). Both Connell (1969) and Edwards (1969) have argued that the rationale of the new approach rests on a number of assumptions which may be unwarranted. It is assumed that licensed doctors will only supply drugs to established addicts and in just the right quantity so that each patient has no surplus to give or sell to others and yet has sufficient to make it unlikely that he will try to obtain illicit supplies. But, as these authors point out, the experts at the special centres are not infallible;

they have no accurate way of estimating the critical dose and they may on occasions even be led unwittingly to prescribe heroin for non-addicted persons. Furthermore, the new clinics have been established as treatment centres, on the assumption that addiction is an expression of mental disorder and that withdrawal of the drugs is possible. But few patients are so co-operative that their drugs can be withdrawn and Edwards (1969) foresees the possibility of further legislation allowing compulsory treatment.

REFERENCES

CONNELL, P. H. (1969). Drug dependence in Great Britain: a challenge to the practice of Medicine. In *Scientific Basis of Drug Dependence* (Editor, Steinberg, H.), pp. 291-299. London.

DE ALARCÓN, R. (1969). The spread of heroin abuse in a community. *Bull. Narcot.* **21**, No. 3, 17-22.

DE ALARCÓN, R. and RATHOD, N. H. (1968). Prevalence and early detection of heroin abuse. *Brit. med. J.* **2**, 549-553.

EDWARDS, G. (1969). The British approach to the treatment of heroin addiction. *Lancet*, **1**, 768-772.

GLATT, M. M. (1969). The changing British drug scene. *Lancet*, **2**, 429-430.

MINISTRY OF HEALTH AND DEPARTMENT OF HEALTH FOR SCOTLAND (1961). *Drug Addiction. Report of the Interdepartmental Committee.* H.M.S.O. London.

MINISTRY OF HEALTH AND SCOTTISH HOME AND HEALTH DEPARTMENT (1965). *Drug Addiction. The Second Report of the Interdepartmental Committee.* H.M.S.O. London.

SPEAR, H. B. (1969). The growth of heroin addiction in the United Kingdom. *Brit. J. Addict.* **64**, 245-255.

The Characteristics of British Heroin Addicts

Various recent reports have described the characteristics of the new type of drug addict in the United Kingdom (Glatt, Pittman, Gillespie and Hills, 1967; Bewley and Ben-Arie, 1968; Kosviner, Mitcheson, Myers *et al.*, 1968; Willis, 1969*a, b*; Hawks, Mitcheson, Ogborne and Edwards, 1969).

Family Background

The distribution by social class of the parents of addicts does not appear to differ significantly from that found in the general population, although in the study by Kosviner *et al.* (1968) there was a highly significant tendency for the subjects to have parents in the professions. Profound disturbance in the home during childhood appears to be much more common among addicts than in the general population. Willis (1969*a*) examined the family history of 58 in-patient heroin addicts (42 males and 16 females) and noted that psychiatric disturbance, addiction to opiates and other drugs, alcoholism and criminal behaviour was more common in these families than in those of 100 control subjects; the parents of addicts were also more often absent from the home (Table 3.3). Similar family pathology (Table 3.4) was noted by Hawks *et al.* (1969) in their study of 74 methylamphetamine addicts (most of whom had also used heroin at some time).

Personality of Addicts

Drug addicts commonly show profound disorders of personality and Willis (1969a) found that all the patients he studied had inadequate, anti-social or other abnormal personalities. Their schooling tends to have been unsatisfactory, mainly because of a failure to demonstrate their intellectual potential and because of persistent truancy rather than the result of any lack of opportunity to do well (Willis, 1969a; Hawks *et al.*, 1969); there is no evidence that they are less intelligent than average (Bewley and Ben-Arie, 1968). They rarely have a stable work record and there is usually a history of

Table 3.3

FAMILY PATHOLOGY OF 58 BRITISH HEROIN ADDICTS
(Willis, 1969a)

	Parents	Sibs
	%	%
Psychiatric illness	33	3
Opiate or other addiction	5	5
Alcoholism	34	—
Criminal behaviour	7	3
Parents dead	24	—
Parents separated or divorced	33	—

Table 3.4

FAMILY PATHOLOGY OF 74 METHYLAMPHETAMINE ADDICTS
(Hawks *et al.*, 1969)

	Mothers	Fathers	Sibs
	%	%	%
Abuse of alcohol	3	18	7
Abuse of drugs	4	3	16
Criminal convictions	0	7	19
Psychiatric disorder	14	5	12
Dead	13	16	—
Absence from home*	8	32	—

* For more than two years before patient aged 16—excluding
cases due to death of a parent.

progressive social deterioration so that their social class tends to be lower than that of their parents (Bewley and Ben-Arie, 1968; Willis, 1969a). Psychiatric disturbance not attributable to the abuse of drugs is fairly common. Willis (1969a) and Hawks *et al.* (1969) noted a high incidence of childhood neurotic traits among their patients and reported that about 10 per cent had had psychiatric treatment for disorders other than addiction.

Abuse of drugs is very frequently associated with criminal or delinquent behaviour. Willis (1969a) reported that 76 per cent of the heroin addicts in his investigation had appeared before the courts, while in the studies of Kosviner *et al.* (1968), Bewley and Ben-Arie (1968) and Hawks *et al.* (1969) the corresponding rates were 54 per cent, 83 per cent and 65 per cent respectively.

D

These authors found that about half the prosecutions were in relation to offences not involving the use of drugs and that these sometimes were committed before any drug abuse, suggesting that addiction tends to occur in delinquent personalities. This view is supported by observations on delinquent populations. Scott and Willcox (1965) found evidence of amphetamine abuse in about 17 per cent of 612 adolescents admitted to two remand homes in London, while in a later comparable study on 972 similar subjects Cockett and Marks (1969) reported an incidence of 6·9 per cent. Backhouse and James (1969) interviewed 290 boys aged 14 to 16 years who had been sentenced to a detention centre in South-East England during 1967 and obtained a history of drug-taking—mainly amphetamine and cannabis and less often barbiturates, heroin or cocaine—in 12 per cent.

Sexual promiscuity is a fairly constant feature and homosexuality is not uncommon. Hawks *et al.* (1969) reported that of their female patients, half admitted to homosexual activities and 31 per cent to prostitution, while among their male patients, 19 per cent had had homosexual experiences and 5 per cent had been prostitutes. In Willis's series (1969*a*), homosexuality was admitted by 17 per cent of males and by 44 per cent of females.

The Development of Drug Dependence in the Individual

Various studies on British subjects have described the events leading to heroin addiction. Abuse of other drugs before starting to take heroin is the rule. Thus Kosviner *et al.* (1968) found that there had been prior experience of amphetamines or of cannabis by all of the 37 heroin users that they studied in an English provincial town. Use of these other drugs had begun at an average age of 15 or 16 years, i.e. one to two years before taking the first dose of heroin. Bewley and Ben-Arie (1968) made similar observations on 100 consecutive male heroin addicts and noted that before starting heroin, cannabis had been taken by 79, and oral amphetamines by 59. The degree to which the use of cannabis predisposes to heroin addiction is uncertain, but it seems likely that in only a small proportion of individuals is there a progression from one drug to another, since cannabis is certainly now very widely used in the United Kingdom, while heroin addiction remains relatively uncommon. The exact number of cannabis users is uncertain but Bewley (1966) has estimated that for every successful conviction following prosecution for drug offences involving cannabis there are probably 10-20 regular users who are not prosecuted and a further 10-20 persons who occasionally try the drug. If Bewley's estimate is correct there are now probably at least 30,000 to 60,000 regular users and an equal number of occasional users in the United Kingdom, since in 1968 there were 3071 convictions for cannabis offences (Spear, 1969).

Willis (1969*b*) questioned 58 British addicts and found that most started taking heroin either because they were curious about its effects or because they were depressed and hoped for relief. A few stated that they sought for an elevation of their mood above the normal and only one had apparently been persuaded by others to take the drug. Willis (1969b) also noted that about one-fifth of his subjects described their first experience of heroin as unpleasant, consistent with the personal observations of Oswald (1969) who noted no pleasurable consequences whatsoever. Intravenous administration from the start is most common but a small proportion of British addicts begin by sniffing the powdered drug or by giving it subcutaneously or intramuscularly. Following the first dose of heroin, some months usually elapse before it is taken every day, but a few start with daily injections (Willis 1969b).

Established heroin addicts usually use other drugs regularly. Thus of 100 studied by Bewley and Ben-Arie (1968), two-thirds took three or more drugs in addition to heroin and in only three cases was heroin the only drug used. Data from the studies by Bewley and Ben-Arie (1968) and by Willis (1969b) are given in Table 3.5. These figures are probably not representative of today's addicts, since there has been marked variation in the type of other drugs used over the years. Until about 1968 cocaine was very commonly

Table 3.5

USE OF DRUGS OTHER THAN HEROIN BY HEROIN ADDICTS

Drug	Bewley and Ben-Arie (1968)	Willis (1969b)
	%	%
Cannabis	83	98
Cocaine	67	81
Oral amphetamines	60	93
Lysergide (LSD)	15	38
Other opiates	38	41
Barbiturates	40	—

taken, but then the intravenous injection of methylamphetamine largely replaced cocaine among London addicts. More recently (Glatt, 1969), methylamphetamine has been less fashionable and the use of intravenous barbiturates has become more common. Other drugs sometimes used by heroin addicts include ephedrine, sedatives and tranquillizers, glue and solvents, methylphenidate, phenmetrazine and methadone (Hawks *et al.*, 1969) and trichlorethylene (Kosviner *et al.*, 1968). Tobacco smoking is more common and tends to be heavier among heroin addicts than in the general population (Bewley and Ben-Arie, 1968) while excessive use of alcohol was noted in 40 per cent of cases by Willis (1969b) and in 24 per cent of cases by Hawks *et al.* (1969).

The observable effects of heroin abuse have been described by Rathod, de Alarcón and Thomson (1967) who interviewed a sample of parents of addicts and a number of the addicts themselves. They found that recent injection of heroin produces a number of obvious changes lasting two or three hours; most commonly these include the appearance of a dreamy detached state, lack of concentration, refusal to eat proper meals, rubbing of the eyes, chin and nose and scratching of the arms and legs, and resentment at being disturbed. Changes noted by the parents when the effects of the heroin begin to wear off include irritability, restlessness, sweating, and less commonly yawning and running of the eyes and nose. With regular use of heroin, changes in the mode of life can be observed; the parents reported unexpected absences from home (presumably to obtain supplies of drugs), loss of interest in organized activities, impairment of appetite, deterioration in personal appearance, a tendency to spend long periods alone in the bedroom, and an increased use of the telephone. Rathod and his colleagues suggest that all these observations may facilitate the recognition, both by doctors and laymen, of heroin abuse.

United States heroin addicts tend to have similar characteristics to those in Great Britain, but there are some important differences. Willis (1969*a*, *b*) compared 50 New York addicts with 58 from the United Kingdom and noted that American addicts tended to have lower social backgrounds, to start taking heroin at an earlier age and to abuse amphetamines, cannabis and LSD more often than their British counterparts. Disturbances in the family and in early life, and the prevalence of delinquency and sexual deviation did not however differ significantly between the two groups.

REFERENCES

BACKHOUSE, C. I. and JAMES, I. P. (1969). The relationship and prevalence of smoking, drinking and drug taking in (delinquent) adolescent boys. *Brit. J. Addict.* **64**, 75-79.

BEWLEY, T. (1966). Recent changes in the pattern of drug abuse in the United Kingdom. *Bull. Narcot.* **18**, No. 4, 1-13.

BEWLEY, T. H. and BEN-ARIE, O. (1968). Morbidity and mortality from heroin dependence. 2. Study of 100 consecutive patients. *Brit. med. J.* **1**, 727-730.

COCKETT, R. and MARKS, V. (1969). Amphetamine taking among young offenders. *Brit. J. Psychiat.* **115**, 1203-1204.

GLATT, M. M. (1969). The changing British drug scene. *Lancet*, **2**, 429-430.

GLATT, M. M., PITTMAN, D. J., GILLESPIE, D. G. and HILLS, D. R. (1967). *The Drug Scene in Great Britain*. London.

HAWKS, D., MITCHESON, M., OGBORNE, A. and EDWARDS, G. (1969). Abuse of methylamphetamine. *Brit. med. J.* **2**, 715-721.

KOSVINER, A., MITCHESON, M. C., MYERS, K., OGBORNE, A., STIMSON, G. V., ZACUNE, J. and EDWARDS, G. (1968). Heroin use in a provincial town. *Lancet*, **1**, 1189-1192.

OSWALD, I. (1969). Personal View. *Brit. med. J.* **1**, 438.

RATHOD, N. H., DE ALARCÓN, R. and THOMSON, I. G. (1967). Signs of heroin usage detected by drug users and their parents. *Lancet*, **2**, 1411-1414.

SCOTT, P. and WILLCOX, D. R. C. (1965). Delinquency and the amphetamines. *Brit. J. Addict.* **61**, 9-27.

SPEAR, H. B. (1969). The growth of heroin addiction in the United Kingdom. *Brit. J. Addict.* **64**, 245-255.

WILLIS, J. H. (1969*a*). Drug dependence: some demographic and psychiatric aspects in U.K. and U.S. subjects. *Brit. J. Addict.* **64**, 135-146.

WILLIS, J. H. (1969*b*). The natural history of drug dependence: some comparative observations on United Kingdom and United States subjects. In *Scientific Basis of Drug Dependence* (Editor Steinberg, H.), pp. 301-321. London.

MORBIDITY AND MORTALITY OF HEROIN ADDICTION

Serious medical complications are common among heroin addicts and recent reviews include those by Cherubin (1967a), Louria, Hensle and Rose (1967), Sapira (1968) and Louria (1969). Table 3.6 lists the complications

Table 3.6

MEDICAL COMPLICATIONS ASSOCIATED WITH 100 CONSECUTIVE CASES OF
IIEROIN ADDICTION
(Bewley and Ben-Arie, 1968)

Septic complications		39
Septic injection sites and abscesses	23	
Pneumonia	6	
Septicaemia	3	
Flexion contractures after multiple abscesses	2	
Cellulitis	2	
Pyrexia of undetermined origin	2	
Syringe-transmitted syphilis	1	
Hepatitis		29
Definite (hospital information)	22	
Probable (information from other sources)	7	
Overdose of drugs		17
Other		12
Needle broken off and left in patient	4	
Tuberculosis	3	
Barbiturate withdrawal fits	2	
Cocaine rash	2	
Radial nerve palsy associated with self-injection	1	

seen in 100 consecutive cases admitted to a London hospital (Bewley and Ben-Arie, 1968) while Table 3.7 gives a diagnostic breakdown of 100 admissions with major medical complications to a New York hospital. The pattern is somewhat different in Great Britain from that in the United States,

Table 3.7

MEDICAL COMPLICATIONS IN 96 NEW YORK HEROIN ADDICTS
(100 admissions) (Louria *et al.*, 1967)

Overdosage	9
Endocarditis	8
Embolic pneumonia and lung abscess	3
Hepatitis	42
Tetanus	1
Pneumonia	14
Local sepsis at injection sites	21
Pyrogenic reactions	2

possibly because American addicts inject illicit heroin which has been adulterated with a diluent such as lactose, mannitol or quinine, whereas English addicts, at least until very recently, always use a prescribed pure preparation (tabs. diamorphine hydrochloride, B.P.C.).

Overdosage

Overdosage of heroin occurs for a number of reasons. Some cases arise when addicts fail to realize that their tolerance to the drug has markedly decreased following a period of abstinence in hospital or prison (James, 1967), and in the United States the heroin content of bought material varies widely and an unintentional overdose may result from the use of a particularly potent preparation (Louria *et al.*, 1967). The toxic effects include impairment of consciousness, depression of respiration and miosis, and treatment should include the administration of nalorphine (3-20 mg intramuscularly) and assistance of respiration.

In the United States a number of cases of acute pulmonary oedema have been reported. Steinberg and Karliner (1968) described 16 cases who developed respiratory depression and cyanosis, with radiological evidence of pulmonary oedema after an intravenous injection of heroin; 14 of their patients were comatose and two died. They advise treatment with nalorphine and oxygen, and, since half developed pneumonia, the administration of antibiotics. Other fatal cases have been reported by Helpern and Rho (1966) and by Cherubin (1967*a*). The pathogenesis is uncertain but suggested explanations include hypersensitivity (acute anaphylactic reaction), opiate induced apnoea, and the precipitation of cardiac failure by the injection of large amounts of adulterant (Sapira, 1968). Clinical recovery occurs within a few days but evidence of impaired lung function (reduction of vital capacity and of forced expiratory volume) may persist for some weeks (Karliner, Steinberg and Williams, 1969). Overdosage and pulmonary oedema are the commonest causes of death among American addicts (Siegel, Helpern and Ehrenreich, 1966) and accounted for 29 per cent of the fatalities in the British series reported by Bewley, Ben-Arie and James (1968).

Overdosage of non-narcotic drugs is sometimes seen and of 30 heroin addicts examined in a London hospital casualty department during one year, six were found to be suffering from barbiturate poisoning (Cameron, 1964).

Infections

Unhygienic techniques of injection are responsible for the infections and septic conditions which are commonly seen in heroin dependent subjects. The methods of British addicts (described by Briggs, McKerron, Souhami *et al.*, 1967, and by Bewley, Ben-Arie and Marks, 1968) are similar to those of American addicts (Louria *et al.*, 1967). The skin, needles and syringes are rarely sterilized or cleaned before injection, and although tap water is usually used to dissolve the heroin, sometimes saliva or water drawn from a lavatory pan is employed instead. Sharing of syringes and needles is very common, encouraging the transmission of disease from addict to addict.

Hepatitis

The association between dependence on parenteral heroin and hepatitis is strong. Of 100 London heroin addicts observed by Bewley, Ben-Arie and

Marks (1968) 29 gave a history of hepatitis, while Kosviner, Mitcheson, Myers *et al.* (1968) obtained evidence of previous hepatitis in 38 per cent of addicts in an English provincial town. In the United States, Levine and Payne (1960) noted a history of past hepatitis in 62 per cent of their cases, while epidemics among heroin addicts have been reported by Rosenstein (1967) and by Dismukes, Karchmer, Johnson and Dougherty (1968). Louria *et al.* (1967) found that in New York, hepatitis was the commonest medical complication among addicts necessitating admission to hospital and moreover that the majority of cases of hepatitis there were related to the parenteral abuse of drugs. New cases of heroin addiction can sometimes be detected by a survey of jaundice among young adults; in Crawley, Sussex, 20 per cent of cases first came to light in this way (de Alarcón and Rathod, 1968).

The hepatitis is of the homologous serum type, and is presumably transmitted through the sharing of unsterilized needles and syringes. Bewley, Ben-Arie and Marks (1968) found an association between such sharing and a history of jaundice, while Cohen and Dougherty (1968) have reported that transfusion of addicts' blood increases seventy-fold the risk of homologous serum hepatitis in the recipient. Syringe transmitted jaundice has also been reported among users of intravenous LSD (Materson and Barrett-Connor, 1967). As with the hepatitis occurring in non-addicts there is biochemical evidence of liver damage with markedly raised serum levels of conjugated bilirubin, aspartate aminotransferase (S.G.O.T.) and alanine aminotransferase (S.G.P.T.). Recovery is the rule and only one of the 42 patients observed by Louria *et al.* (1967) died of acute hepatic necrosis, although five patients had clinical and histological evidence of permanent liver damage.

Mild chronic liver dysfunction is not uncommon in heroin addicts, even in the absence of a history of jaundice. Sixty per cent of 284 London addicts studied by Bewley, Ben-Arie and Marks (1968) showed abnormalities of liver function, an incidence slightly lower than that found either by Potter, Cohen and Norris (1960) or by Levine and Payne (1960) in American studies, where it was 75 per cent and 67 per cent respectively. Sapira, Jasinski and Gorodetzky (1968) found that the longer the addict had been using parenteral routes the more likely was there to be evidence of liver disease. That the damage may be permanent is suggested by Kaplan's finding (1963) that 7 of 13 ex-addicts, all of whom had been in prison without access to drugs for at least six months, showed biochemical evidence of impaired liver function.

Histological changes in the liver indicative of permanent damage, particularly an increase of inflammatory cells and of fibrous tissue in the portal areas, have also been reported. Seventy-five per cent of a series of narcotic addicts dying suddenly showed such changes compared with 28 per cent of a control group (Norris and Potter, 1965) and Kaplan (1963) obtained biopsy evidence of liver damage in seven of his 13 ex-addict prisoners. These changes are reminiscent of those seen in chronic viral hepatitis, but malnutrition, hepatotoxic effects of contaminants in the injected material and co-existent alcoholism are alternative possibilities. Marks and Chapple (1967) have suggested that a direct hepatotoxic action of heroin or cocaine or of contaminants may be responsible, or, alternatively, an infection of the liver by organisms of low pathogenicity. A direct toxic effect of chronically administered heroin seems unlikely since neither animal studies (Brooks, Deneau, Potter *et al.*, 1963) nor long-term administration of morphine to human volunteers (Gorodetzky, Sapira, Jasinski and Martin, 1968) has produced any evidence of this. Barrett and Boyle (1968) have suggested that intravenous methylamphetamine may be hepatotoxic and they consider that its effects, which they call "hippie hepatitis", are distinct from those of chronic viral hepatitis.

Local Sepsis

Septic conditions (skin abscesses, cellulitis and thrombophlebitis) comprise the most common medical complication of parenteral abuse of heroin (Cherubin, 1967*a*; Bewley and Ben-Arie, 1968; Louria *et al.*, 1967). Bewley and Ben-Arie (1968) reported an incidence of 25 per cent in their series, and a further 2 per cent had flexion contractures following multiple abscesses (Table 3.6); Louria *et al.* (1967) reported 21 cases (Table 3.7) including three patients with an unusual picture of multiple deep necrotic skin lesions without marked purulent discharge at subcutaneous infection sites, presumably the effect of an adulterant. Among addicts who sniff their heroin, inflammation and perforation of the nasal septum may occur. Messinger (1962) found a 4·8 per cent incidence of septal perforation among 2185 American heroin addicts; in only seven cases could cocaine be implicated as a possible aetiological factor.

Septicaemia

Blood-stream spread of infection from local sepsis leading to bacterial or monilial endocarditis, septicaemia and septic pulmonary embolism occurs occasionally. Louria *et al.* (1967) reviewed 48 cases of endocarditis (including 8 in their own series of 100 consecutive admissions, Table 3.7) and observed that in addicts the condition differs in some ways from that seen in non-addicts. First, the responsible organisms are more commonly coagulase-positive *Staphylococcus aureus*, enterococcus or candida. Secondly, there is a very high mortality rate (69 per cent in the cases reviewed by Louria *et al.*, 1967) and thirdly, only a minority, about 25 per cent, have definite predisposing structural disease of the valves. Lastly, about one-third of cases involve the right side of the heart. Similar observations have been made in reviews by Sapira (1968) and by Cherubin, Baden, Kavaler *et al.* (1968).

Briggs *et al.* (1967) have reported eleven patients with septic pulmonary infarctions and multiple lung abscesses, presumably due to blood stream spread from septic injection sites. All were severely ill, presenting with fever and respiratory symptoms, but initially there were often only minor radiological changes in the lungs. Nine showed evidence of acute sepsis at injection sites and positive blood cultures were obtained in nine cases; two patients died. The commonest responsible organism was *Staphylococcus aureus*, and

Briggs and his colleagues advise treating patients suspected of having this complication with at least two anti-staphylococcal drugs such as benzyl-penicillin and cloxacillin in high dosage while awaiting the results of blood and sputum culture. Similar cases of staphylococcal embolic pneumonia have been reported in the United States (Louria et al., 1967; Sapira, 1968).

Other Infections

The incidence of venereal disease is high among addicts, presumably due to sexual promiscuity, although Bewley and Ben-Arie (1968) have reported a case of syringe-transmitted syphilis. Biological false-positive reactions for syphilis are however quite common (Harris and Andrei, 1967). These are characterized by positive reactions with serological tests using non-specific antigens (e.g. the Wassermann reaction) associated with negative reactions in tests using treponemal extracts (e.g. the *Treponema pallidum* immobiliza-tion test). The cause of these false-positive reactions in addicts is not known, but they do not seem to be related to liver damage. Cherubin and Millian (1968) have shown that the sera of narcotic addicts may give non-specific positive reactions with other tests such as the complement fixation tests for lymphogranuloma venereum and Q fever and these authors relate these findings to hyperglobulinaemia.

Tetanus is a not uncommon complication among addicts in New York, particularly when injections are given subcutaneously, and the mortality is high (Cherubin, 1967b; 1968), but no case has been reported in Great Britain. At one time, syringe-transmitted malaria was prevalent among addicts in the United States, but this complication has not been seen for many years (Helpern and Rho, 1966). Pulmonary tuberculosis is somewhat more common among addicts than in the general population, presumably due to their unhygienic way of life (Bewley and Ben-Arie, 1968; Sapira, 1968).

Other Complications

Various other physical complications of heroin abuse have been reported, mainly from the United States. First, the repeated intravenous injection of preparations containing inert substances may, through embolism, cause thrombosis of the small pulmonary vessels and subsequent pulmonary hypertension and right ventricular failure (Wendt, Puro, Shapiro et al., 1964; Sapira, 1968). Secondly, Richter and Rosenberg (1968) have reported four heroin addicts who developed acute transverse myelitis of the thoracic spinal cord within a few hours of a self-administered intravenous injection. Post-mortem examination of one case showed extensive necrosis of the cord and no evidence of a vascular cause, and the authors suggest that the condition might be a hypersensitivity reaction. Thirdly, asymptomatic pulmonary atelectasis has been reported by Gelfand, Hammer and Hevizy (1967) who noted linear shadows in the routine chest radiographs of 14 addicts. Lastly an increased incidence of bronchial asthma among heroin-dependent subjects has been observed by Sapira (1968).

Mortality

Between 1955 and 1966 there were 69 deaths among "non-therapeutic" heroin addicts in Great Britain, a mortality-rate of 27 per 1000 per annum, some 28 times the rate for the general population of the same age (James, 1967; Bewley, Ben-Arie and James, 1968). The causes of death are given in Table 3.8. Accidental overdoses accounted for 29·0 per cent of all deaths, and suicide for 23·2 per cent. Among male addicts the suicide rate was more than 50 times as great as in the general population.

Table 3.8

CAUSES OF DEATH AMONG "NON-THERAPEUTIC" HEROIN ADDICTS IN BRITAIN 1955-66
(Bewley, Ben-Arie and James, 1968)

Cause of death	Males	Females	Both sexes
			(%)
Suicide	14	2	23·2
Accidental narcotic overdose	13	3	} 29·0
Sudden death ("addiction")	4	0	
Violent death	5	1	
Septic conditions	12	3	} 47·8
Other "natural" causes	10	2	
Total	58	11	100·0

In New York City, the mortality rate is somewhat lower than in Great Britain, about 10 per 1000 per annum, and there are differences in the distribution of causes. In particular sudden death due to overdosage or acute pulmonary oedema is more common in New York where it accounts for almost half the fatalities (Table 3.9).

Table 3.9

CAUSES OF DEATH AMONG NEW YORK ADDICTS 1950-61
(Louria *et al.*, 1967)

Cause of death	Males	Females	Both sexes
			(%)
Overdosage and sudden death	644	118	48·0
Pyogenic infections	92	36	8·1
Tetanus	48	83	8·3
Hepatitis	25	5	1·9
Chronic narcotic addiction	175	38	13·4
Tuberculosis	26	8	2·1
Other causes	223	65	18·2
Total	1233	353	100·0

REFERENCES

BARRETT, P. V. D. and BOYLE, J. D. (1968). "Hippie hepatitis": the possible role of methamphetamine in chronic active hepatitis. *Gastroenterology*, **54**, 1219.

BEWLEY, T. H. and BEN-ARIE, O. (1968). Morbidity and mortality from heroin dependence. 2. Study of 100 consecutive inpatients. *Brit. med. J.* **1**, 727-730.

BEWLEY, T. H., BEN-ARIE, O. and JAMES, I. P. (1968). Morbidity and mortality from heroin dependence. 1. Survey of heroin addicts known to Home Office. *Brit. med. J.* **1**, 725-726.

BEWLEY, T. H., BEN-ARIE, O. and MARKS, V. (1968). Morbidity and mortality from heroin dependence. 3. Relation of hepatitis to self-injection techniques. *Brit. med. J.* **1**, 730-732.

BRIGGS, J. H., McKERRON, C. G., SOUHAMI, R. L., TAYLOR, D. J. E. and ANDREWS, H. (1967). Severe systemic infections complicating "mainline" heroin addiction. *Lancet*, **2**, 1227-1231.

BROOKS, F. B., DENEAU, G. A., POTTER, H. P., REINHOLD, J. G. and NORRIS, R. F. (1963). Liver function tests in morphine-addicted and in non-addicted rhesus monkeys. *Gastroenterology*, **44**, 287-290.

CAMERON, A. J. (1964). Heroin addicts in a casualty department. *Brit. med. J.* **1**, 594-598.

CHERUBIN, C. E. (1967a). The medical sequelae of narcotic addiction. *Ann. intern. Med.* **67**, 23-33.

CHERUBIN, C. E. (1967b). Urban tetanus. The epidemiologic aspects of tetanus in narcotic addicts in New York City. *Arch. environm. Hlth.* **14**, 802-808.

CHERUBIN, C. E. (1968). Clinical severity of tetanus in narcotic addicts in New York City. *Arch. intern. Med.* **121**, 156-158.

CHERUBIN, C. E., BADEN, M., KAVALER, F., LERNER, S. and CLINE, W. (1968). Infective endocarditis in narcotic addicts. *Ann. intern. Med.* **69**, 1091-1098.

CHERUBIN, C. E. and MILLIAN, S. J. (1968). Serologic investigations in narcotic addicts. I. Syphilis, lymphogranuloma venereum, herpes simplex, and Q fever. *Ann. intern. Med.* **69**, 739-742.

COHEN, S. N. and DOUGHERTY, W. J. (1968). Transfusion hepatitis arising from addict blood donors. *J. Amer. med. Ass.* **203**, 427-429.

DE ALARCÓN, R. and RATHOD, N. H. (1968). Prevalence and early detection of heroin abuse. *Brit. med. J.* **2**, 549-553.

DISMUKES, W. E., KARCHMER, A. W., JOHNSON, R. F. and DOUGHERTY, W. J. (1968). Viral hepatitis associated with illicit parenteral use of drugs. *J. Amer. med. Ass.* **206**, 1048-1052.

GELFAND, M. L., HAMMER, H. and HEVIZY, T. (1967). Asymptomatic pulmonary atelectasis in drug addicts. *Dis. Chest*, **52**, 782-787.

GORODETZKY, C. W., SAPIRA, J. D., JASINSKI, D. R. and MARTIN, W. R. (1968). Liver disease in narcotic addicts. I. The role of the drug. *Clin. Pharmacol. Ther.* **9**, 720-724.

HARRIS, W. D. M. and ANDREI, J. (1967). Serologic tests for syphilis among narcotic addicts. *N.Y. St. J. Med.* **67**, 2967-2974.

HELPERN, N. and RHO, Y-M. (1966). Deaths from narcotism in New York City. Incidence, circumstances, and postmortem findings. *N.Y. St. J. Med.* **66**, 2391-2408.

JAMES, I. P. (1967). Suicide and mortality amongst heroin addicts in Britain. *Brit. J. Addict.* **62**, 391-398.

KAPLAN, K. (1963). Chronic liver disease in narcotics addicts. *Amer. J. dig. Dis.* **8**, 402-410.

KARLINER, J. S., STEINBERG, A. D. and WILLIAMS, M. H. (1969). Lung function after pulmonary oedema associated with heroin overdose. *Arch. intern. Med.* **124**, 350-353.

KOSVINER, A., MITCHESON, M. C., MYERS, K., OGBORNE, A., STIMSON, G. V., ZACUNE, J. and EDWARDS, G. (1968). Heroin use in a provincial town. *Lancet*, **1**, 1189-1192.

LEVINE, R. A. and PAYNE, M. A. (1960). Homologous serum hepatitis in youthful heroin users. *Ann. intern. Med.* **53**, 164-178.

LOURIA, D. B. (1969). Medical complications of pleasure-giving drugs. *Arch. intern. Med.* **123**, 82-87.

LOURIA, D. B., HENSLE, T. and ROSE, J. (1967). The major medical complications of heroin addiction. *Ann. intern. Med.* **67**, 1-22.

MARKS, V. and CHAPPLE, P. A. L. (1967). Hepatic dysfunction in heroin and cocaine users. *Brit. J. Addict.* **62**, 189-195.

MATERSON, B. J. and BARRETT-CONNOR, E. (1967). L.S.D. "main-lining". A new hazard to health. *J. Amer. med. Ass.* **200**, 1126-1127.

MESSINGER, E. (1962). Narcotic septal perforations due to drug addiction. *J. Amer. med. Ass.* **179**, 964-965.

NORRIS, R. F. and POTTER, H. P. (1965). Hepatic inflammation in narcotic addicts. Viral hepatitis a possible cause. *Arch. environm. Hlth.* **11**, 662-668.

POTTER, H. P., COHEN, N. N. and NORRIS, R. F. (1960). Chronic hepatic dysfunction in heroin addicts. *J. Amer. med. Ass.* **174**, 2049-2051.

RICHTER, R. W. and ROSENBERG, R. N. (1968). Transverse myelitis associated with heroin addiction. *J. Amer. med. Ass.* **206**, 1255-1257.

ROSENSTEIN, B. J. (1967). Viral hepatitis in narcotics users. An outbreak in Rhode Island. *J. Amer. med. Ass.* **199**, 698-700.

SAPIRA, J. D. (1968). The narcotic addict as a medical patient. *Amer. J. Med.* **45**, 555-588.

SAPIRA, J. D., JASINSKI, D. R. and GORODETZKY, C. W. (1968). Liver disease in narcotic addicts. III. The role of the needle. *Clin. Pharmacol. Ther.* **9**, 725-739.

SIEGEL, H., HELPERN, M. and EHRENREICH, T. (1966). The diagnosis of death from intravenous narcotism. *J. forens. Sci.* **11**, 1-16.

STEINBERG, A. D. and KARLINER, J. S. (1968). The clinical spectrum of heroin pulmonary oedema. *Arch. intern. Med.* **122**, 122-127.

WENDT, V. E., PURO, H. E., SHAPIRO, J., MATHEWS, W. and WOLF, P. L. (1964). Angiothrombotic pulmonary hypertension in addicts. "Blue Velvet" addiction. *J. Amer. med. Ass.* **188**, 755-757.

NEW DRUG TREATMENTS OF MORPHINE-TYPE DEPENDENCE

High-Dosage Methadone (Dole-Nyswander)

Since 1964, Dole and Nyswander have been treating heroin addicts in the United States by administering methadone in amounts sufficient to block the effect of other narcotic drugs, and they and other workers have reported encouraging results (Dole and Nyswander 1965, 1966, 1968; Freedman, Fink, Sharoff and Zaks, 1967; Dole, Nyswander and Warner, 1968; Brill, 1968; Jaffe, Zaks and Washington, 1969; Dole, Robinson, Orraca *et al.*, 1969). Dole and Nyswander have selected their patients, restricting the treatment to those addicts in the age group 20 to 50 years who give a history of four years or more of heroin abuse and of several relapses after withdrawal treatment, who have no major medical complications and who have freely accepted the treatment. The patients are first admitted to hospital, although in recent years the treatment has been given sometimes to outpatients. The initial dose of methadone (given as a liquid by mouth) depends on how recently the patient has been taking heroin and ranges from 5 to 20 mg twice daily. It is then increased gradually over the course of four to six weeks to 80 to 120 mg per day; if the rate of increase is too little withdrawal symptoms will appear while if it is too great the patient will become sedated. After six weeks the patient is discharged taking one dose every morning and thereafter he attends the clinic to receive his methadone and to give a sample of urine for the detection of illicit drugs, daily at first but later at less frequent intervals. In successful cases the patient loses his craving for morphine-type drugs, but if he does experiment with heroin or other narcotics these have little or no effect and in particular do not produce the characteristic euphoria. The only observable side-effect is constipation leading sometimes to faecal impaction but this may be prevented by the use of laxatives.

By March 1968, Dole and Nyswander had started treatment of 871 patients, but in 10 per cent it was stopped because of psychopathic behaviour or continued abuse of non-narcotic drugs. Methadone has no effect on alcohol or barbiturate types of dependence and Freedman et al. (1967) have suggested that this treatment is contraindicated in patients who are addicted to non-narcotic drugs. A further 3 per cent attended the clinic so irregularly that treatment was stopped, but among those who continued, the majority found employment and became socially acceptable, the use of heroin virtually disappeared and the crime rate, particularly that associated with the use of drugs, fell by at least 90 per cent. Attempts to withdraw methadone from the more successful cases have generally led to re-addiction to heroin, so that in the present state of knowledge, treatment must be continued indefinitely.

The Dole-Nyswander regime has been criticized. First, it has been suggested that it is unethical to use replacement drugs except in amounts which are just sufficient to prevent withdrawal symptoms and that the dose of methadone given actually gratifies the patient's addiction and aggravates matters (Ausubel, 1966). Secondly, it seems likely that the treatment is not a solution to the heroin problem since probably only a small proportion of all heroin addicts would be willing to cooperate (Committee on Alcoholism and Drug Dependence, 1967). Glatt (1969) points out that in the United Kingdom where treatment with methadone has to compete with legally available heroin and where relatively few addicts would satisfy Dole and Nyswander's criteria of suitability, the possible usefulness of the regime may be even less than in the United States.

REFERENCES

AUSUBEL, D. P. (1966). The Dole-Nyswander treatment of heroin addiction. J. Amer. med. Ass. 195, 949-950.
BRILL, H. (1968). Progress report of evaluation of methadone maintenance treatment program as of March 31, 1968. J. Amer. med. Ass. 206, 2712-2714.
COMMITTEE ON ALCOHOLISM AND DRUG DEPENDENCE (1967). Management of narcotic drug dependence by high-dosage methadone HCl technique. Dole-Nyswander program. J. Amer. med. Ass. 201, 956-957.
DOLE, V. P. and NYSWANDER, M. (1965). A medical treatment for diacetylmorphine (heroin) addiction. J. Amer. med. Ass. 193, 646-650.

DOLE, V. P. and NYSWANDER, M. E. (1966). Rehabilitation of heroin addicts after blockade with methadone. *N.Y. St. J. Med.* **66**, 2011-2017.

DOLE, V. P. and NYSWANDER, M. E. (1968). The use of methadone for narcotic blockade. *Brit. J. Addict.* **63**, 55-57.

DOLE, V. P., NYSWANDER, M. E. and WARNER, A. (1968). Successful treatment of 750 criminal addicts. *J. Amer. med. Ass.* **206**, 2708-2711.

DOLE, V. P., ROBINSON, J. W., ORRACA, J., TOWNS, E., SEARCY, P. and CAINE, E. (1969). Methadone treatment of randomly selected criminal addicts. *New Engl. J. Med.* **280**, 1372-1375.

FREEDMAN, A. M., FINK, M., SHAROFF, R. and ZAKS, A. (1967). Cyclazocine and methadone in narcotic addiction. *J. Amer. med. Ass.* **202**, 191-194.

GLATT, M. M. (1969). Rehabilitation of the addict. *Brit. J. Addict.* **64**, 165-182.

JAFFE, J. H., ZAKS, M. S. and WASHINGTON, E. N. (1969). Experience with the use of methadone in a multi-modality program for the treatment of narcotic users. *Int. J. Addict.* **4**, 481-490.

Use of Narcotic Antagonists

In recent years cyclazocine and nalaxone have been used in the United States to prevent relapse in abstinent heroin addicts. These drugs, like nalorphine, antagonize the pharmacological effects of opiates including their euphoriant action, and if given repeatedly to subjects receiving narcotics they greatly reduce the development of physical dependence on the latter. When administered to established addicts they precipitate withdrawal symptoms (Martin, Gorodetzky and McLane, 1966; Jasinski, Martin and Haertzen, 1967; Martin, 1967; Martin and Gorodetzky, 1967).

Small doses of narcotic antagonists produce euphoria, exhilaration and sometimes tiredness and in larger amounts, inability to concentrate, irritability, racing of thoughts and, occasionally, psychotomimetic effects such as visual hallucinations and paranoid delusions. With repeated administration these subjective effects lessen and the dose can be increased but there is no such development of tolerance to their narcotic antagonist actions (Martin, 1967). Continued administration of these drugs leads to the development of physical dependence, and withdrawal then produces an abstinence syndrome characterized by lacrimation, rhinorrhoea, yawning, diarrhoea and fever, similar to but not so severe as that seen in morphine abstinence. A characteristic feature of the withdrawal syndrome is the experience of momentary strange feelings described by the patients as "light-headedness" or as "electric shocks" which occur particularly after drinking hot or cold fluids or while falling asleep. An important difference between narcotic withdrawal and narcotic-antagonist withdrawal is that the latter is not associated with any craving or drug-seeking behaviour. Naloxone appears to produce less physical dependence than either nalorphine or cyclazocine (Jasinski *et al.*, 1967; Fink, Zaks, Sharoff *et al.*, 1968). Cross-tolerance and cross-dependence between nalorphine and cyclazocine have been observed (Fraser and Rosenberg, 1966).

Treatment of opiate dependence with narcotic antagonists involves withdrawal of the narcotic followed, after some days, by prolonged administration of the antagonist. Nalorphine is unsuitable because it is effective only when given parenterally and furthermore it has such a short duration of action that to give continuous protection it needs to be administered every few hours. Both cyclazocine and naloxone are effective by mouth and have relatively long durations of action (at least 20 hours for cyclazocine and about 10 hours for naloxone) and these have been used; neither drug, however, is available at present in the United Kingdom.

Freedman and his colleagues have now treated 60 American men with cyclazocine, all of whom had been addicted to narcotics for more than two years. (Freedman, Fink, Sharoff and Zaks, 1967, 1968; Freedman and Fink, 1968) while Jaffe and Brill (1966) have obtained good results in 9 of 11 patients who have received the drug. The first phase of the treatment consists of withdrawal of the narcotic drug, usually by substituting methadone in gradually decreasing doses. Some days after withdrawal when there is no longer any physical dependence (this may be tested by noting the effects of administering a small dose of nalorphine) cyclazocine is introduced. Freedman suggests an initial daily dose of 0·2 mg increasing by 0·2 mg per day for 10 days and then by 0·4 mg per day for 5 days, so that the patient is then receiving 4·0 mg every morning. During this induction phase subjective side-effects of cyclazocine may occur (somnolence, irritability, hallucinations, etc.) indicating that the rate of increase is too great in relation to the speed at which tolerance is being developed. The actual dose of cyclazocine reached varies and has to be determined in each case by occasional testing with intravenous heroin 15 mg; the optimal dose is that which just completely abolishes the effects of the heroin.

When the dose of cyclazocine has been determined the patient can be discharged to outpatient care and he continues to take the drug every morning. Should he experiment with heroin he finds that it has no euphoriant effect and moreover that repeated administration does not lead to physical dependence. Of 58 discharged patients reported by Freedman, Fink et al. (1968), 27 had remained in regular treatment for at least two months but 31 had withdrawn. Common side-effects of chronic cyclazocine administration include elation, dizziness, headaches, restlessness and insomnia, all of which tend to subside with time, and constipation and increased libido which tend to persist. Less common are depression, abdominal pains, muscular twitches, paranoid ideation and visual hallucinations. Where these unwanted effects are prominent they are sometimes relieved by dividing the dose and giving it twice daily, but occasionally the drug must be discontinued.

The use of naloxone has been described by Fink et al. (1968) who have treated 7 male narcotic addicts. As with cyclazocine treatment, the narcotic is first withdrawn and then naloxone is given in an initial dose of 10 to 20 mg twice daily increasing gradually to about 100 mg twice daily, the actual dose depending on the response to testing with intravenous heroin.

REFERENCES

FINK, M., ZAKS, A., SHAROFF, R., MORA, A., BRUNER, A., LEVIT, S. and FREEDMAN, A. M. (1968). Naloxone in heroin dependence. *Clin. Pharmacol. Ther.* **9**, 568-577.

FRASER, H. F. and ROSENBERG, D. E. (1966). Comparative effects of I. Chronic administration of cyclazocine (ARC-II-C-3), II. Substitution of nalorphine for cyclazocine, and III Chronic administration of morphine. Pilot crossover study. *Int. J. Addict.* **1**, 86-98.

FREEDMAN, A. M. and FINK, M. (1968). Basic concepts and use of cyclazocine in the treatment of narcotic addiction. *Brit. J. Addict.* **63**, 59-69.

FREEDMAN, A. M., FINK, M., SHAROFF, R. and ZAKS, A. (1967). Cyclazocine and methadone in narcotic addiction. *J. Amer. med. Ass.* **202**, 191-194.

FREEDMAN, A. M., FINK, M., SHAROFF, R. and ZAKS, A. (1968). Clinical studies of cyclazocine in the treatment of narcotic addiction. *Amer. J. Psychiat.* **124**, 1499-1504.

JAFFE, J. H. and BRILL, L. (1966). Cyclazocine, a long acting narcotic antagonist: its voluntary acceptance as a treatment modality by narcotics abusers. *Int. J. Addict.* **1**, 99-123.

JASINSKI, D. R., MARTIN, W. R. and HAERTZEN, C. A. (1967). The human pharmacology and abuse potential of n-allylnoroxymorphone (naloxone). *J. Pharmacol. exp. Ther.* **157**, 420-426.

MARTIN, W. R. (1967). Opioid antagonists. *Pharmacol. Rev.* **19**, 463-521.

MARTIN, W. R. and GORODETZKY, C. W. (1967). Cyclazocine, an adjunct in the treatment of narcotic addiction. *Int. J. Addict.* **2**, 85-93.

MARTIN, W. R., GORODETZKY, C. W. and McLANE, T. K. (1966). An experimental study in the treatment of narcotic addicts with cyclazocine. *Clin. Pharmacol. Ther.* **7**, 455-465.

The Rationale of Methadone and Narcotic Antagonist Therapies

There are two theoretical grounds for using methadone and the narcotic antagonists in the treatment of narcotic addiction. In the first place they block the actions of self-administered narcotic drugs so that the addict obtains no satisfaction from their use and is not motivated to continue taking them. Hence the administration of these drugs paves the way for social rehabilitation. Methadone appears to have two advantages over cyclazocine or naloxone in facilitating this object. First it relieves drug craving whereas the narcotic antagonists do not, and secondly the development of strong physical dependence on methadone ensures that the patient will continue to take it, whereas cyclazocine can be stopped with little difficulty. These advantages are perhaps reflected in the greater patient cooperation apparently achieved with methadone, but this is obtained at a price, because it is dependent on the establishment of methadone addiction.

The second rationale for these agents is that they may positively help the addict to learn to live without narcotic drugs. Wikler (1965) has suggested that the continued use of narcotics and the tendency to become re-addicted after withdrawal may be determined to some extent by conditioning mechanisms. He points out that injections of narcotics relieve both anxiety and the distress of withdrawal symptoms, so that when anxiety arises in a person who has previously taken drugs he will tend to resort to them again. Furthermore, the repeated association between certain environmental cues such as addict friends, drug haunts, needles, syringes, etc. and subjective feelings such as craving and withdrawal discomfort may lead to conditioning such that the cues themselves will produce the feelings and make the subject take drugs even though there may be no physical need.

In theory, these conditioned responses could be extinguished by repeated exposure to drugs and associated cues, provided that gratification was prevented by blocking agents, but it would be unjustified to encourage patients on methadone or cyclazocine to run the risks of taking illicit drugs even though theory suggests that they should if the treatment is to be most effective.

That dependence on heroin may involve learnt behaviour receives support from a study by Thomson and Rathod (1968) who treated 13 drug-free heroin addicts by aversion therapy in which preparations for self-injection of heroin were repeatedly associated with apnoea induced by the administration of intravenous suxamethonium chloride; 10 patients completed the treatment of whom 9 had remained abstinent at the time of follow-up.

REFERENCES

THOMSON, I. G. and RATHOD, N. H. (1968). Aversion therapy for heroin dependence. *Lancet*, **2**, 382-384.
WIKLER, A. (1965). Conditioning factors in opiate addiction and relapse. In *Narcotics* (Editors Wilner, D. M. and Kassebaum, G. G.), pp. 85-100. New York.

CHAPTER 4

DELIRIUM TREMENS AND ALLIED CONDITIONS

*The Acute Neuropsychiatric Complications of Chronic Alcoholism.
Physical Dependence of Alcohol and Barbiturate Types. The Drug
Treatment of Alcohol Withdrawal*

THE ACUTE NEUROPSYCHIATRIC COMPLICATIONS
OF CHRONIC ALCOHOLISM

Effects of Alcohol on the Nervous System

ALCOHOL affects the nervous system in a number of different ways (Victor, 1966). First there is a direct toxic action leading to drunkenness, coma or alcoholic excitement ("pathological intoxication"). Secondly there are the effects of the vitamin deficiencies which accompany chronic alcoholism, including Wernicke's encephalopathy, which, although an acute neuropsychiatric complication, is considered in Chapter 8 and not here. Thirdly, there are a number of neurological diseases of uncertain aetiology which are associated with alcoholism, such as cortical cerebellar degeneration, Marchiafava-Bignami disease, central pontine myelinolysis and cerebral

Table 4.1

SYMPTOMS AND SIGNS OF ALCOHOL WITHDRAWAL

Motor	*Autonomic*
Limb tremor	Sweating
Truncal ataxia	Fever
Overactivity	Dilated pupils
Restlessness	Tachycardia
Muscle cramps	

Sleep	*Gastrointestinal*
Vivid dreams	Anorexia
Nightmares	Nausea
Insomnia	Vomiting
	Diarrhoea

Perceptual
Unstructured visual and auditory perceptions
Illusions and misinterpretations
Visual, auditory, gustatory, olfactory and haptic hallucinations
Pruritus

Confusion
Disorientation for time, place, person
Memory impairment

Other
Severe anxiety
Delusions
Epileptic seizures

104

atrophy (Mancall, 1961). Fourthly, there are those disturbances where the nervous system is indirectly affected, for example by alcohol-induced hypoglycaemia (Demoura, Correia and Madeira, 1967; Madison, 1968) or by hepatic encephalopathy due to alcoholic cirrhosis of the liver (Summerskill, Davidson, Sherlock and Steiner, 1956; Read, Sherlock, Laidlaw and Walker, 1967).

In addition to the above disorders, profound neuropsychiatric disturbances occur on withdrawing alcohol in persons who have been drinking excessively for long periods of time and this chapter is primarily concerned with such disturbances. Table 4.1 lists the symptoms and signs which have been noted during alcohol withdrawal. These tend to occur when the blood alcohol level is low and are sometimes improved by the ingestion of alcohol, in contrast to the acute effects of alcohol such as dysarthria, ataxia and impairment of consciousness, which are associated with high blood alcohol levels and which are aggravated by further drinking.

The phenomena in Table 4.1 tend to occur as four fairly distinct syndromes, namely alcoholic tremulousness, alcoholic hallucinosis, alcoholic epilepsy and delirium tremens. Here these four conditions will be considered separately even though, as is discussed later, they tend to merge into one another and to be atypical.

REFERENCES

DEMOURA, M. C., CORREIA, J. P. and MADEIRA, F. (1967). Clinical alcohol hypo-glycaemia. *Ann. intern. Med.* **66**, 893-905.

MADISON, L. L. (1968). Ethanol-induced hypoglycemia. *Advanc. metabol. Dis.* **3**, 85-109.

MANCALL, E. L. (1961). Some unusual neurologic diseases complicating chronic alcoholism. *Amer. J. clin. Nutr.* **9**, 404-413.

READ, A. E., SHERLOCK, S., LAIDLAW, J. and WALKER, J. G. (1967). The neuro-psychiatric syndromes associated with chronic liver disease and an extensive portal-systemic collateral circulation. *Quart. J. Med.* **36**, 135-150.

SUMMERSKILL, W. H. J., DAVIDSON, E. A., SHERLOCK, S. and STEINER, R. E. (1956). The neuropsychiatric syndrome associated with hepatic cirrhosis and an extensive portal collateral circulation. *Quart. J. Med.* **25**, 245-266.

VICTOR, M. (1966). Treatment of alcoholic intoxication and the withdrawal syndrome. A critical analysis of the use of drugs and other forms of therapy. *Psychosom. Med.* **28**, 636-650.

Alcoholic Tremulousness

The immediate effects of alcohol are so short lived that symptoms of withdrawal may occur after only a few hours' abstinence. With the development of even mild physical dependence withdrawal phenomena appear after the short period of abstinence during sleep. Thus alcoholics, on waking in the morning, particularly during a period of heavy drinking, may complain of unsteadiness and trembling of the limbs ("the shakes"), anxiety, weakness, nausea, vomiting and sweating, and may crave alcohol. Drinking produces complete though temporary relief but the symptoms are likely to recur the following day. Of 306 members of Alcoholics Anonymous studied by Edwards, Hensman, Hawker and Williamson (1966), 82 per cent had experienced severe morning shakes, while of 50 deteriorated ("Skid Row") alcoholics, 90 per cent had morning shakes, 92 per cent had morning nausea and 82 per cent morning sweats (Edwards, Hawker, Williamson and Hensman, 1966). Carrie (1965) studied 20 alcoholics without obvious clinical abnormality, all of whom had abstained from alcohol for at least 36 hours and he observed that the amplitude of the tremor of the outstretched fingers of these patients was much greater than that of non-alcoholic controls.

Morning anorexia, nausea and vomiting are usually attributed to alcoholic gastritis but it seems possible that they are true withdrawal phenomena of central origin since similar disturbances have been noted as part of the barbiturate abstinence syndrome, where there is no question of a responsible gastric lesion (Isbell, Altschul, Kornetsky et al., 1950).

Where physical dependence on alcohol is very strong, relative or absolute withdrawal is associated with more severe and more persistent tremulousness and gastrointestinal disturbance and with severe anxiety, insomnia and nightmares and occasionally with mild mental confusion and with fleeting illusions and auditory and visual hallucinations. These symptoms are most severe some 24 to 36 hours after the last drink and they generally subside within a few days. Insomnia and subjective feelings of anxiety may persist, however, for as long as two weeks and since these symptoms are relieved by alcohol the early discharge from hospital of tremulous patients carries a considerable risk of immediate relapse.

REFERENCES

CARRIE, J. R. G. (1965). Finger tremor in alcoholic patients. *J. Neurol. Neurosurg. Psychiat.* **28**, 529-532.

EDWARDS, G., HAWKER, A., WILLIAMSON, V. and HENSMAN, C. (1966). London's Skid Row. *Lancet*, **1**, 249-252.

EDWARDS, G., HENSMAN, C., HAWKER, A. and WILLIAMSON, V. (1966). Who goes to Alcoholics Anonymous? *Lancet*, **2**, 382-384.

ISBELL, H., ALTSCHUL, S., KORNETSKY, C. H., EISENMAN, A. J., FLANARY, H. G. and FRASER, H. F. (1950). Chronic barbiturate intoxication. An experimental study. *Arch. Neurol. Psychiat. (Chic.)* **64**, 1-28.

Alcoholic Hallucinosis

This condition is characterized by auditory hallucinations occurring in the absence of clouding of consciousness, confusion, or disorientation, after long-continued abuse of alcohol. Visual, olfactory and tactile hallucinations, tremulousness and epileptic fits sometimes occur and the condition may develop into typical delirium tremens (Victor and Adams, 1953; Victor and Hope, 1958: Gross, Halpert, Sabot and Polizos, 1963; Scott, 1967; Sabot, Gross and Halpert, 1968). In the majority of cases the onset of the illness is in the period immediately following cessation of drinking. Of 76 episodes reported by Victor and Hope (1958) only 15 began while the patient was still drinking, but three of these patients were reducing their alcoholic intake substantially at the time when they first experienced hallucinations. In the remaining cases the illness began after drinking had stopped, most frequently after 12-48 hours of complete abstinence (Table 4.2).

Table 4.2

RELATIONSHIP OF TIME OF ONSET OF ALCOHOLIC HALLUCINOSIS TO
CESSATION OF DRINKING
(Victor and Hope, 1958)

Time of onset	*No. of cases*
While drinking	15
After stopping drinking	
12-24 hours	17
1-2 days	15
2-3 days	6
3-4 days	6
4-7 days	9
Uncertain	8
Total	76

The phenomenology of alcoholic hallucinosis has been studied by Victor and Hope (1958), Gross, Halpert, Sabot and Polizos (1963), Saravay and Pardes (1967), Sabot *et al.* (1968) and by Scott, Davies and Malherbe (1969). The most common experience is of hallucinatory voices, perceived to be in external objective space and which are accepted by the patient as being real. Of 33 patients reported by Scott *et al.* (1969), 29 heard voices, while the others experienced hallucinatory noises and sounds. The patient shows an appropriate emotional response to the voices and if they are threatening he may try to escape or even attempt suicide. They are usually recognized as belonging to the patients' friends or family, but sometimes they are not familiar and rarely they are attributed to the Devil or God. In this respect they resemble the auditory hallucinations of schizophrenia (see Chapter 2). Multiple voices, particularly talking to one another about the patient in the third person, may be heard. Generally they are hostile, threatening, insulting, accusatory or otherwise unpleasant or disturbing, but sometimes they are benign or neutral in tone, calling the patient's name or producing casual conversation.

The auditory hallucinations are commonly associated with unstructured auditory perceptions, either simple phasic noises (e.g. brief loud sounds, clicks, or drilling or wooshing noises) or sustained tinnitus most commonly a buzzing noise, but sometimes humming, ringing, blowing or whistling (Gross, Halpert, Sabot and Polizos, 1963; Saravay and Pardes, 1967; Sabot *et al.*, 1968). These phenomena occur in 30 to 50 per cent of all patients with severe symptoms of alcohol withdrawal. They tend to be very intimately connected with the auditory hallucinations and Gross, Halpert, Sabot and Polizos (1963) have argued that the tinnitus is probably due to a disturbance of the cochlea or of its central connections and that it may be partly responsible for the hallucinations. Consistent with this view that the tinnitus is not itself an hallucination, Saravay and Pardes (1967) have suggested that the simple phasic noises heard by these patients arise from intermittent contractions of palatal and middle ear muscles.

Visual hallucinations, when they occur in alcoholic hallucinosis, are similar in character to those of delirium tremens. Sabot *et al.* (1968) have described the visual hallucinations of 44 alcoholic women. Animals—most commonly small creatures such as insects or mice crawling across the floor, but sometimes snakes, horses, cats or dogs—were seen by 23 patients, while 13 had hallucinations of human beings; occasionally the hallucination was of an inanimate object. These experiences have the characteristics of true hallucinations and are accepted by the patient as real. They are often terrifying, particularly when visual hallucinations of people are combined and integrated with auditory hallucinations of speech. Commonly associated with visual hallucinations are elementary visual disturbances such as intermittent blurring of sight and the perception in the field of vision of flashes of light, shadows, spots etc. (Saravay and Pardes, 1967; Sabot *et al.*, 1968).

Alcoholic hallucinosis is generally a benign transient illness lasting a few days but rarely some weeks or months and ending with acquisition of insight and no permanent sequelae. Of 76 episodes studied by Victor and Hope (1958), 14 lasted for less than one day and 64 (84 per cent) for less than one week; in four cases the condition immediately preceded delirium tremens. If drinking is resumed the hallucinosis sometimes persists indefinitely (Victor and Hope, 1958). The duration of the hallucinations was very much longer in the series of 33 cases reported by Scott *et al.* (1969); it was less than one week in only nine per cent of cases and more than eight weeks in 48 per cent, but these findings must be considered unusual.

Occasionally, as in four patients observed by Victor and Hope (1958) the hallucinations continue even though the patient does not drink and a picture clinically indistinguishable from schizophrenia emerges. Bleuler was impressed by the fact that in alcoholic hallucinosis the hallucinations were often similar in character to those of schizophrenia and he suggested that the condition might in fact be schizophrenia precipitated by chronic alcohol intoxication or withdrawal (Gross, Halpert and Sabot, 1963). But there is now good reason to believe that alcoholic hallucinosis and schizophrenia are quite distinct entities. Johanson (1961) and Scott (1967) have shown that the incidence of schizophrenia in the families of patients with alcoholic hallucinosis is no higher than that in the general population, while Victor and Hope (1958) noted that their four patients whose condition most strongly resembled schizophrenia differed from schizophrenics in having cyclothymic premorbid personalities and a late age of onset. The distinction between the two conditions is, however, not always clear and follow-up of 33 cases after some years by Scott *et al.* (1969) led these authors to suspect strongly that three of the patients were schizophrenic from the onset of their illnesses.

REFERENCES

GROSS, M. M., HALPERT, E. and SABOT, L. (1963). Some comment on Bleuler's concept of acute alcoholic hallucinosis. *Quart. J. Stud. Alcohol*, 24, 54-60.

GROSS, M. M., HALPERT, E., SABOT, L. and POLIZOS, P. (1963). Hearing disturbances and auditory hallucinations in the acute alcoholic psychoses. I Tinnitus: incidence and significance. *J. nerv. ment. Dis.* 137, 455-465.

JOHANSON, E. (1961). Acute hallucinosis, paranoic reactions and schizophreniform psychoses in alcoholic patients. *Acta Soc. med. upsal.* 66, 105-128.

SABOT, L. M., GROSS, M. M. and HALPERT, E. (1968). A study of acute alcoholic psychoses in women. *Brit. J. Addict.* 63, 29-49.

SARAVAY, S. M. and PARDES, H. (1967). Auditory elementary hallucinations in alcohol withdrawal psychosis. *Arch. gen. Psychiat.* 16, 652-658.

SCOTT, D. F. (1967). Alcoholic hallucinosis—an aetiological study. *Brit. J. Addict.* 62, 113-125.

SCOTT, D. F., DAVIES, D. L. and MALHERBE, M. E. L. (1969). Alcoholic hallucinosis. *Int. J. Addict.* 4, 319-330.

VICTOR, M. and ADAMS, R. D. (1953). The effect of alcohol on the nervous system. *Res. Publ. Ass. Res. nerv. ment. Dis.* 32, 526-573.

VICTOR, M. and HOPE, J. M. (1958). The phenomenon of auditory hallucinations in chronic alcoholism. A critical evaluation of the status of alcoholic hallucinosis. *J. nerv. ment. Dis.* 126, 451-481.

Alcoholic Epilepsy ("Rum Fits")

The prevalence of epilepsy in chronic alcoholism is about 10 to 12 per cent—much higher than in the general population—and the relationship between the two conditions has been studied by Rhinehart (1961), by Victor and Brausch (1967) and by Victor (1968). Of 241 alcoholics with epilepsy seen by Victor and his colleagues, there was evidence in 21 cases that either head injury or a focal cortical lesion was of aetiological importance and in a further seven cases a diagnosis of idiopathic epilepsy was made on the basis of generalized convulsions without discernible cause, with onset preceding abuse of alcohol. Even among those patients where drinking was clearly not entirely responsible for the fits, withdrawal of alcohol appeared to be of some aetiological importance since their seizures more commonly occurred in the period immediately after a bout of drinking than during periods of persistent sobriety. The remaining patients (the overwhelming majority) reported by Victor and Brausch (1967) and by Victor (1968) showed no evidence of brain damage but could not be categorized as idiopathic. Typically, they had been drinking excessive amounts of alcohol for many years before the first convulsion. Their fits—always grand mal in type—occurred immediately after a period of heavy drinking, usually within 13 to 36 hours of the last drink (Figure 4.1). Only a very small proportion of the fits occurred while the patient was intoxicated (i.e. within six hours of the last drink) and of those who had their fit within 6 to 12 hours of abstaining, a proportion had been passing though a period of relative abstinence. Victor and Brausch noted that the occurrence of multiple seizures (two to six in the course of a few hours) was slightly more common than single fits, and that some patients developed status epilepticus.

Rhinehart (1961) reported 19 patients with "rum fits", most commonly arising within 48 hours of withdrawal of alcohol. Eighteen had grand mal seizures while one had focal fits, and all except two of the patients had solitary convulsions. In 11 of the cases the fits occurred in association with delirium tremens and in six of these there was clear evidence that the delirium

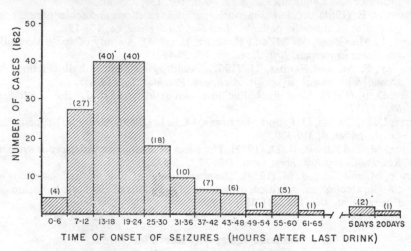

Figure 4.1 Onset of fits in relation to duration of alcoholic abstinence. (Victor and Brausch, 1967)

followed the convulsion. In the series of 241 patients described by Victor (1968) 75 (31 per cent) showed an association with delirium tremens, but the fit always came first although the interval between the two was sometimes extremely short.

The relationship between alcoholic epilepsy and delirium tremens has also been shown by other investigators (Table 4.3); the overall incidence of epilepsy in the seven studies listed is 19·5 per cent. Among the 30 cases where the two conditions were associated in Victor and Adam's (1953) series, the epilepsy preceded the delirium in all except one.

Table 4.3

INCIDENCE OF EPILEPTIC FITS IN DELIRIUM TREMENS

Authors	No. of cases of delirium tremens	Incidence of epilepsy (per cent)
Victor and Adams (1953)	101	30·0
Peck (1960)	20	30·0
Lundquist (1961)	74	20·3
Tavel et al. (1961)	289	17·6
Nielsen (1965)	42	11·9
Cutshall (1965)	205	17·1
Saravay and Pardes (1967)	29	20·6
Total	760	19·5

REFERENCES

CUTSHALL, B. J. (1965). The Saunders-Sutton syndrome: an analysis of delirium tremens. *Quart. J. Stud. Alcohol*, **26**, 423-448.
LUNDQUIST, G. (1961). Delirium tremens. *Acta psychiat. scand.* **36**, 443-466.
NIELSEN, J. (1965). Delirium tremens in Copenhagen. *Acta psychiat. scand.* Supplement 187, pp 1-92.
PECK, R. E. (1960). Delirium tremens at Meadowbrook hospital. *N. Y. St. J. Med.* **60**, 3409-3413.
RHINEHART, J. W. (1961). Factors determining "rum fits". *Amer. J. Psychiat.* **118**, 251-252.
SARAVAY, S. M. and PARDES, H. (1967). Auditory elementary hallucinations in alcohol withdrawal psychosis. *Arch. gen. Psychiat.* **16**, 652-658.
TAVEL, M. E., DAVIDSON, W. and BATTERTON, T. D. (1961). A critical analysis of mortality associated with delirium tremens. *Amer. J. med. Sci.* **242**, 18-29.
VICTOR, M. (1968). The pathophysiology of alcoholic epilepsy. *Res. Publ. Ass. Res. nerv. ment. Dis.* **46**, 431-454.
VICTOR, M. and ADAMS, R. D. (1953). The effect of alcohol on the nervous system. *Res. Publ. Ass. Res. Nerv. ment. Dis.* **32**, 526-573.
VICTOR, M. and BRAUSCH, C. (1967). The role of abstinence in the genesis of alcoholic epilepsy. *Epilepsia (Amst.)*, **8**, 1-20.

Delirium Tremens

Delirium tremens is characterized by:

1. *Severe confusion* with clouding of consciousness, disorientation in time and place and impairment of recent memory.

2. *Disorders of perception:* illusions and misinterpretations of sensory stimuli; unstructured perceptions and vivid hallucinations. (These are mainly visual, but in addition there may be auditory, gustatory, olfactory or haptic disturbances).

3. *Profound insomnia.*

4. *Autonomic disturbances:* profuse sweating, tachycardia, fever, dilatation of the pupils and hypertension.

5. *Psychomotor agitation.* Restlessness, shouting and extremely severe anxiety.

6. *Tremulousness* and truncal ataxia.

7. *Gastrointestinal disturbances:* anorexia, nausea, vomiting, diarrhoea.

8. *Delusions*, usually secondary to the hallucinations.

9. *Leucocytosis*, elevation of the erythocyte sedimentation rate and transient impairment of hepatic function.

10. *Dehydration* and electrolyte disturbances

In most cases the illness is preceded by acute alcoholic tremulousness, sometimes by alcoholic epilepsy and occasionally by alcoholic hallucinosis. Victor and Adams (1953) noted the time of onset in relation to the period of abstinence in 44 cases. Only two of their patients (4 per cent) developed the condition within 24 hours of the last drink, and in the majority the onset was after 48 to 96 hours of complete abstinence; in only seven patients (15 per cent) did the illness start more than 96 hours after stopping drinking. In a series of 42 patients reported by Nielsen (1965), however, 47 per cent were drinking right up to the onset of the delirium; in 26 per cent the period of abstinence was 2-3 days; in 19 per cent, 4-5 days; and in seven per cent, 7-8 days.

Delirium tremens characteristically begins at night and the condition persists for some days with nocturnal exacerbation of symptoms, often ending with a period of deep prolonged sleep from which the patient awakes free of symptoms and with little or no memory for the delirious period. The course of the illness is shown in Figure 4.2 which demonstrates the incidence of four

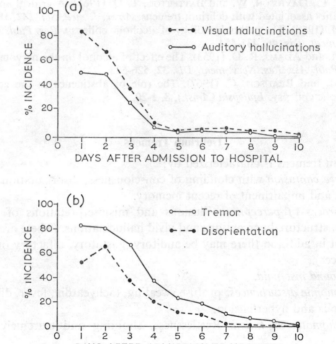

Figure 4.2 Course of major symptoms of delirium tremens after hospitalization among 42 patients. (Nielsen, 1965)
(a) Visual and auditory hallucinations
(b) Tremor and disorientation

major symptoms (tremor, disorientation and visual and auditory hallucinations) among the 42 patients reported by Nielsen (1965). Tremulousness tends to persist for a longer period than the other disturbances and Morgan (1968) noted that of eight alcoholic patients with hallucinations, tremulousness and truncal ataxia, the limb tremor lasted on average for more than seven days and the truncal ataxia for more than eight days. The average duration of the delirium was noted by Cutshall (1965) to be 3·4 days in his series of 205 cases and 3·8 days by Lundquist (1961) in his series of 74 patients, while Table 4.4 presents data on 69 cases reported by Victor and Adams (1953).

Table 4.4

DURATION OF DELIRIUM TREMENS IN 69 PATIENTS
(Victor and Adams, 1953)

Duration	No.	%
24 hours or less	10	14·5
25-48 hrs.	17	24·6
49-72 hrs.	30	43·5
73-96 hrs.	6	8·7
97 hours or more	6	8·7
Total	69	100·0

Fluid and Electrolyte Disturbances

Most clinicians emphasize that patients with delirium tremens are dehydrated and they stress the need for fluid replacement. Ethyl alcohol inhibits antidiuretic hormone and consequently induces a water diuresis (Roberts, 1963), but fluid loss from excessive sweating and from the gastrointestinal tract also contributes to the dehydration. Recent studies however have suggested that the presumption that alcoholics in withdrawal are always dehydrated may not be true. Indeed, Beard and Knott (1968) who measured the total body water, extracellular fluid volume and plasma volume of 30 chronic alcoholics during withdrawal noted isosmotic *overhydration* on admission to hospital and a decrease of body water content towards normal over the following few days. These patients, however, were not typical of chronic alcoholics in that they showed no clinical evidence of dehydration, malnutrition or gastrointestinal disturbance. Findings consistent with overhydration have also been observed by Shaw, Frizel, Camps and White (1969) who measured the brain water and electrolyte concentrations of alcoholic suicides.

Potassium deficiency is not uncommon during alcohol withdrawal and hypokalaemia was noted in 64 per cent of 50 patients by Vetter, Cohn and Reichgott (1967); in nine patients (18 per cent) the serum potassium level was below 2·6 mEq/l and in 23 patients (46 per cent) it was in the range 2·6-3·4 mEq/l. Potassium depletion is probably due partly to decreased intake and partly to increased gastrointestinal loss, but Vetter *et al.* (1967) found no evidence that it was responsible for the psychiatric manifestations, since the serum potassium level did not correlate with the presence or absence of hallucinations or delirium. Hypokalaemia during alcohol withdrawal has also been noted by Sereny, Rapoport and Husdan (1966).

Low concentrations of serum magnesium (below 1·75 mEq/l) have been reported in chronic alcoholics (Heaton, Pyrah, Beresford *et al.*, 1962; Fankushen, Raskin, Dimich and Wallach, 1964). The ingestion of ethyl alcohol increases the urinary loss of magnesium (Heaton *et al.*, 1962; Kalbfleisch, Lindeman, Ginn and Smith, 1963; Dick, Evans and Watson, 1969) and this seems to be the most important factor, but other determinants are malnutrition and impairment of absorption of magnesium from the gut.

In acute alcohol withdrawal more severe hypomagnesaemia is sometimes seen (Flink, Stutzman, Anderson *et al.*, 1954; Nielsen, 1963; Milner and Johnson, 1965) and the 24 hour exchangeable body magnesium may be low (Martin and Bauer, 1962) possibly due to increased loss of magnesium from the gut and in the sweat. Magnesium deficiency may cause fits, generalized tremulousness and mental changes similar to those seen in delirium tremens (Suter and Klingman, 1955; Flink, McCollister, Prasad, *et al.*, 1957) and it has been suggested that the administration of magnesium salts may accelerate recovery (Beroz, Conran and Blanchard, 1962). But it seems doubtful that the depletion is of aetiological importance since the serum level may rise to normal as the delirium subsides even where treatment has not included the administration of magnesium (Mendelson, Wexler, Kubzansky, *et al.*, 1959), while Victor (1968) cites two cases where delirium tremens developed after correction of the magnesium deficiency. Magnesium depletion may however be a cause of alcoholic epilepsy since the intravenous administration of magnesium sulphate appears to abolish the EEG abnormalities seen in patients with rum fits (Victor, 1968).

Although there is doubt about the relevance of magnesium depletion in delirium tremens, where a serious degree of hypomagnesaemia is found it would seem reasonable to give magnesium sulphate intramuscularly, one to two grammes every six hours as a 50 per cent solution (Flink *et al.*, 1957; Nielsen, 1965).

Other Complications

Physical illnesses, particularly infections and the effects of trauma commonly complicate delirium tremens. In 43 per cent of the 101 cases studied by Victor and Adams (1953) there was such an associated illness, while Tavel,

Table 4.5

PHYSICAL COMPLICATIONS AMONG 291 NON-FATAL CASES
OF DELIRIUM TREMENS
(Tavel *et al.*, 1961)

Complication	Incidence
Liver disease	18%
Pneumonia	15%
Fractures	5%
Pulmonary tuberculosis	4%

Davidson and Batterton (1961) found liver disease, pneumonia, fractures or pulmonary tuberculosis in a significant proportion of their series of 291 cases of non-fatal delirium tremens (Table 4.5).

There are a number of possible reasons for the association. First, delirium tremens occurs usually after many years of heavy drinking—in the series described by Cutshall (1965), the mean duration of alcohol abuse was 17·9 years—and many of these patients will therefore have physical disorders due, directly or indirectly, to the alcoholism. Secondly, injury (possibly occurring while drunk) or the development of a physical illness may lead to admission to hospital and to the withdrawal of alcohol. Of 1870 male patients admitted for operation to a New York hospital during a fourteen-month period, five were suffering from delirium tremens on admission and a further 33 developed the disorder while in hospital (Glicksman and Herbsman, 1968). These authors noted that delirium tremens was more common among patients admitted as an emergency. Thirdly, delirium tremens itself may predispose to infection, particularly pneumonia.

Table 4.6

MORTALITY IN DELIRIUM TREMENS

Authors	Deaths (per cent)
Victor and Adams (1953)	15·0
Lundquist (1961)	10·2
Tavel et al. (1961)	11·8
Cutshall (1965)	6·3

Mortality

Unlike the other manifestations of alcohol withdrawal, delirium tremens carries an appreciable mortality risk, highest during the first three or four days. Some representative data are given in Table 4.6. Tavel et al. (1961) reviewed 39 fatalities. In 21 of their cases death was due to some complicating condition such as intracranial trauma, lung abscess, pneumonia or other infection or injury, but in 18 cases death appeared to be due to the delirium tremens itself. Comparison with survivors showed that a fatal outcome was associated with pulmonary or liver disease and with hyperthermia (fever above 104° F.) in the absence of infection. These authors also found that epileptic fits tended to be associated with a fatal outcome, but Cutshall (1965) was unable to confirm this. Of 15 deaths reported by Victor and Adams (1953), nine appeared to be due to complicating illnesses, particularly pneumonia and liver disease, but in the remaining cases the delirium itself seemed to be responsible. Like Tavel et al. (1961), Victor and Adams (1953) noted that a fatal outcome was more likely in patients with complicating disease.

REFERENCES

BEARD, J. D. and KNOTT, D. H. (1968). Fluid and electrolyte balance during acute withdrawal in chronic alcoholic patients. *J. Amer. med. Ass.* 204, 135-139.
BEROZ, E., CONRAN, P. and BLANCHARD, R. W. (1962). Parenteral magnesium in the prophylaxis and treatment of delirium tremens. *Amer. J. Psychiat.* 118, 1042-1043.
CUTSHALL, B. J. (1965). The Saunders-Sutton syndrome; an analysis of delirium tremens. *Quart, J. Stud. Alcohol*, 26, 423-448.

DICK, M., EVANS, R. A. and WATSON, L. (1969). Effect of ethanol on magnesium excretion. *J. clin. Path.* **22**, 152-153.

FANKUSHEN, D., RASKIN, D., DIMICH, A. and WALLACH, S. (1964). The significance of hypomagnesemia in alcoholic patients. *Amer. J. Med.* **37**, 802-812.

FLINK, E. B., McCOLLISTER, R., PRASAD, A. S., MELBY, J. C. and DOE, R. P. (1957). Evidences for clinical magnesium deficiency. *Ann. intern. Med.* **47**, 956-968.

FLINK, E. B., STUTZMAN, F. L., ANDERSON, A. R., KONIG, T. and FRASER, R. (1954). Magnesium deficiency after prolonged parenteral fluid administration and after chronic alcoholism complicated by delirium tremens. *J. Lab. clin. Med.*, **43**, 169-183.

GLICKSMAN, L. and HERBSMAN, H. (1968). Delirium tremens in surgical patients. *Surgery*, **64**, 882-890.

HEATON, F. W., PYRAH, L. N., BERESFORD, C. C., BRYSON, R. W. and MARTIN, D. F. (1962). Hypomagnesaemia in chronic alcoholism. *Lancet*, **2**, 802-805.

KALBFLEISCH, J. M., LINDEMAN, R. D., GINN, H. E. and SMITH, W. O. (1963). Effects of ethanol administration on urinary excretion of magnesium and other electrolytes in alcoholic and normal subjects. *J. clin. Invest.* **42**, 1471-1475.

LUNDQUIST, G. (1961). Delirium tremens. *Acta psychiat. scand.* **36**, 443-466.

MARTIN, H. E. and BAUER, F. K. (1962). Magnesium 28 studies in the cirrhotic and alcoholic. *Proc. roy. Soc. Med.* **55**, 912-914.

MENDELSON, J., WEXLER, D., KUBZANSKY, P., LEIDERMAN, P. H. and SOLOMON, P. (1959). Serum magnesium in delirium tremens and alcoholic hallucinosis. *J. nerv. ment. Dis.* **128**, 352-357.

MILNER, G. and JOHNSON, J. (1965). Hypomagnesaemia with delirium tremens. Report of a case with fatal outcome. *Amer. J. Psychiat.* **122**, 701-702.

MORGAN, H. G. (1968). Acute neuropsychiatric complications of chronic alcoholism. *Brit. J. Psychiat.* **114**, 85-92.

NIELSEN, J. (1963). Magnesium metabolism in acute alcoholics. *Dan. med. Bull.* **10**, 225-233.

NIELSEN, J. (1965). Delirium tremens in Copenhagen. *Acta psychiat. scand.* Supplement 187, pp 1-92.

ROBERTS, K. E. (1963). Mechanism of dehydration following alcohol ingestion. *Arch. intern. Med.* **112**, 154-157.

SERENY, G., RAPOPORT, A., and HUSDAN, H. (1966). The effect of alcohol withdrawal on electrolyte and acid-base balance. *Metabolism*, **15**, 896-904.

SHAW, D. M., FRIZEL, D., CAMPS, F. E. and WHITE, S. (1969). Brain electrolytes in depressive and alcoholic suicides. *Brit. J. Psychiat.* **115**, 69-79.

SUTER, C. and KLINGMAN, W. O. (1955). Neurologic manifestations of magnesium depletion states. *Neurology (Minneap.),* **5**, 691-699.

TAVEL, M. E., DAVIDSON, W. and BATTERTON, T. D. (1961). A critical analysis of mortality associated with delirium tremens. *Amer. J. med. Sci.* **242**, 18-29.

VETTER, W. R., COHN, L. H. and REICHGOTT, M. (1967). Hypokalaemia and electrocardiographic abnormalities during acute alcohol withdrawal. *Arch. intern. Med.* **120**, 536-541.

VICTOR, M. (1968). The pathophysiology of alcoholic epilepsy. *Res. Publ. Ass. Res. nerv. ment. Dis.* **46**, 431-454.

VICTOR, M. and ADAMS, R. D. (1953). The effect of alcohol on the nervous system. *Res. Publ. Ass. Res. nerv. ment. Dis.* **32**, 526-573.

Thiamine Deficiency in Withdrawal States

Vitamin B deficiency, particularly of thiamine, is not uncommon in chronic alcoholism, and if very severe is responsible for the development of Wernicke's encephalopathy, polyneuritis, pellagra or alcoholic amblyopia (Victor and

Adams, 1961). The deficiency arises mainly from the anorexia associated with chronic alcoholism and from the replacement in the diet by alcohol of vitamin-containing foods, but in addition alcohol impairs the absorption of thiamine from the gut and interferes with its hepatic storage and utilization (Tomasulo, Kater and Iber, 1968). There is no evidence that the metabolism of alcohol involves increased utilization of thiamine; indeed, less may be required for the breakdown of alcohol than for the metabolism of carbo-hydrate (Butler and Sarett, 1948).

Using a microbiological method, Fennelly, Frank, Baker and Leevy (1964a) found that 44 per cent of a series of chronic alcoholics without peripheral neuropathy and 86·2 per cent of similar patients with neuropathy had reduced blood thiamine levels. Kershaw (1967) employing a similar direct method of assay studied 40 alcoholic patients during withdrawal and observed that the severer the symptoms the lower was the blood thiamine level (Table 4.7). The mean value for 12 patients with no withdrawal symptoms was 27·6 mμg/ml,

Table 4.7

RELATIONSHIP OF WHOLE BLOOD THIAMINE LEVELS TO THE INTENSITY OF
WITHDRAWAL SYMPTOMS IN ALCOHOLICS
(Kershaw, 1967)

Intensity of withdrawal symptoms	Number of subjects	Mean whole blood thiamine (mμg/ml)
Nil	12	27·6
Mild (slight tremor)	9	25·8
Moderate (tremor, anxiety and insomnia)	5	24·5
Severe (marked tremor, restlessness and nightmares)	5	20·2
Delirium tremens	9	17·6
Non-alcoholic controls	24	24·8

not significantly different from that found among a control group of 24 non-alcoholic subjects where the mean value was 24·8 mμg/ml. The lowest mean value (17·6 mμg/ml) was found in the group of nine patients with delirium tremens. Although this association suggests that the intensity of the withdrawal symptoms is dependent on the degree of thiamine deficiency, a more probable explanation is that both variables are dependent on the severity and duration of the alcoholism. Kershaw (1967) also estimated the blood nicotinic acid levels of 15 patients with delirium tremens and noted abnormally low concentrations in three cases.

Direct estimation of blood thiamine is a complicated and difficult procedure and indirect measures of thiamine deficiency are more commonly used. These are based on the fact that thiamine pyrophosphate is a co-enzyme in a number of biochemical reactions; in particular it catalyses the decarboxylation of pyruvic acid and is a co-factor to transketolase in the metabolism of pentose phosphate. In thiamine deficiency, pyruvic acid tends to accumulate in the tissues, but high fasting blood levels are only found in very severe depletion, as in Wernicke's encephalopathy (Victor, Altschule, Holliday, *et al.*, 1957). Where the deficiency is less pronounced high blood levels of pyruvic acid are only found consistently after the ingestion of carbohydrate.

Joiner, McCardle and Thompson (1950) have devised a test (commonly called the "pyruvate tolerance test") in which blood pyruvate is estimated in the fasting resting subject and at later intervals after the oral administration of two doses of 50 g glucose. Morgan (1968), using this test, studied the pyruvate metabolism of 17 chronic alcoholic patients with withdrawal symptoms. Pyruvate levels tended to be higher than normal especially after glucose loading and particularly in those patients with visual hallucinations or delirium tremens. Figure 4.3 gives Morgan's data on hallucinated and non-hallucinated patients and also gives the values obtained by Joiner *et al.* (1950) from 50 subjects without evidence of thiamine deficiency. Five of Morgan's eight hallucinated patients gave pyruvate curves typical of thiamine

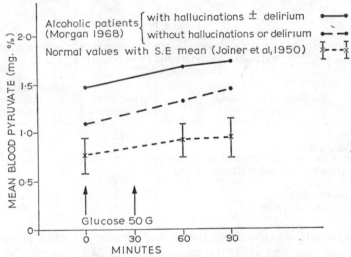

Figure 4.3 Blood pyruvate levels (fasting and after glucose loading) among alcoholics and non-thiamine deficient controls

deficiency while in nine subjects without visual hallucinations only one gave a result typical of thiamine deficiency. Biochemical factors other than thiamine deficiency affect the blood pyruvate level and high values are found in thyrotoxicosis, congestive cardiac failure, after exercise and in cases of peripheral neuropathy not due to thiamine deficiency (Joiner *et al.*, 1950).

In recent years attention has been paid to blood transketolase activity as an index of thiamine deficiency (Wolfe, Brin and Davidson, 1958; Dreyfus, 1962; Fennelly, Frank, Baker and Leevy, 1964a, 1967; Delaney, Lankford and Sullivan, 1966). This is an *in vitro* test carried out on a single sample of blood. Characteristic of thiamine deficiency is a reduction of transketolase activity which is increased by the addition of thiamine pyrophosphate to the substrate.

Estimations of blood transketolase activity in thiamine deficient subjects correlate well with direct measurement of blood thiamine concentration (Fennelly *et al.*, 1964*a*). In Wernicke's encephalopathy the activity is markedly reduced (Wolfe *et al.*, 1958; Dreyfus, 1962) and low values have been found by Fennelly *et al.* (1964*a*, 1967) in alcoholic peripheral neuropathy and by Delaney *et al.* (1966) in 26 of 70 chronic alcoholics. In patients with cirrhosis the interpretation of low blood transketolase activity may present some difficulty; here the administration of thiamine may not correct the abnormality suggesting that thiamine deficiency is not responsible (Fennelly *et al.*, 1964*b*, 1967). Apart from this difficulty, transketolase estimation seems a useful method of detecting thiamine depletion and it has practical advantages over pyruvate studies in that the patient needs no preparation and in that vitamin therapy can be started immediately after a single specimen of blood has been taken.

REFERENCES

BUTLER, R. E. and SARETT, H. P. (1948). The effect of isocaloric substitution of alcohol for dietary carbohydrate upon the excretion of B vitamins in man. *J. Nutr.* **35**, 539-548.

DELANEY, R. L., LANKFORD, H. G. and SULLIVAN, J. F. (1966). Thiamine, magnesium and plasma lactate abnormalities in alcoholic patients. *Proc. Soc. exp. Biol. (N.Y.)* **123**, 675-679.

DREYFUS, P. M. (1962). Clinical application of blood transketolase determinations. *New Engl. J. Med.* **267**, 596-598.

FENNELLY, J., FRANK, O., BAKER, H. and LEEVY, C. M. (1964*a*) Peripheral neuropathy of the alcoholic: I. Aetiological role of aneurin and other B-complex vitamins. *Brit. med. J.* **2**, 1290-1292.

FENNELLY, J., FRANK, O., BAKER, H. and LEEVY, C. M. (1964*b*). Transketolase activity in experimental thiamine deficiency and hepatic necrosis. *Proc. Soc. exp. Biol. (N.Y.)* **116**, 875-877.

FENNELLY, J., FRANK, O., BAKER, H. and LEEVY, C. M. (1967). Red blood cell-transketolase activity in malnourished alcoholics with cirrhosis. *Amer. J. clin. Nutr.* **20**, 946-949.

JOINER, C. L., McCARDLE, B. and THOMPSON, R. H. S. (1950). Blood pyruvate estimations in the diagnosis and treatment of polyneuritis. *Brain*, **73**, 431-452.

KERSHAW, P. W. (1967). Blood thiamine and nicotinic acid levels in alcoholism and confusional states. *Brit. J. Psychiat.* **113**, 387-393.

MORGAN, H. G. (1968). Acute neuropsychiatric complications of chronic alcoholism. *Brit. J. Psychiat.* **114**, 85-92.

TOMASULO, P. A., KATER, R. M. H. and IBER, F. L. (1968). Impairment of thiamine absorption in alcoholism. *Amer. J. clin. Nutr.* **21**, 1340-1344.

VICTOR, M. and ADAMS, R. D. (1961). On the aetiology of the alcoholic neurologic diseases with special reference to the role of nutrition. *Amer. J. clin. Nutr.* **9**, 379-396.

VICTOR, M., ALTSCHULE, M. D., HOLLIDAY, P. D., GONCZ, R-M., and COUNTY, A. (1957). Carbohydrate metabolism in brain disease. VIII. Carbohydrate metabolism in Wernicke's encephalopathy associated with alcoholism. *Arch. intern. Med.* **99**, 28-39.

WOLFE, S. J., BRIN, M. and DAVIDSON, C. S. (1958). The effect of thiamine deficiency on human erythrocyte metabolism. *J. clin. Invest.* **37**, 1476-1484.

E

The Relationship Between the Various Syndromes

While the condition of many patients can be diagnosed confidently as alcoholic tremulousness, alcoholic hallucinosis, alcoholic epilepsy or delirium tremens, intermediate forms are frequently seen. As has already been noted, alcoholic tremulousness may be associated with mild confusion and fleeting hallucinations; auditory hallucinosis is associated with other disturbances such as tremulousness, visual hallucinations, delusions not derived from the hallucinations, and fits in about two-thirds of cases; delirium tremens is preceded by epilepsy in up to 30 per cent of cases and less frequently by auditory hallucinosis; and Bartholomew (1967) has pointed out that in the individual case the clinical picture may vary considerably over short periods of time. Furthermore, Victor (1966) has described atypical delirious hallucin-atory states which differ from delirium tremens in that they (a) are rarely preceded by epilepsy (b) are characterized by the predominance of one type of symptom (e.g. confusion or delusions) and (c) are never fatal.

Table 4.8

CLASSIFICATION OF ALCOHOL WITHDRAWAL STATES
(Victor and Adams, 1953)

Syndrome	No.	%
Acute alcoholic tremulousness	92	60·1
Tremor and transient hallucinosis	30	19·6
Acute auditory hallucinosis	6	3·9
Typical delirium tremens	14	9·1
Atypical delirious hallucinatory states	11	7·2
Total	153	100·0

Using more or less traditional nomenclature, Victor and Adams (1953) classified 153 patients in alcohol withdrawal as in Table 4.8. Of these, 32 had epileptic fits during the course of the illness. Gross, Halpert, Sabot and Polizos (1963) and Sabot, Gross and Halpert (1968) have reported two series of acute alcoholic psychoses (of male and female patients respectively). Their classification and the distribution of their cases is given in Table 4.9. In the nomenclature of these authors "mixed psychoses" make up the majority of the illnesses. These are not typical of either alcoholic hallucinosis or delirium tremens, as, for example, where auditory hallucinations are associated with marked confusion, or where both visual and auditory hallucinations are very prominent, or where visual hallucinations occur without notable clouding of consciousness. Other clinicians would probably categorize these "mixed" illnesses in other ways.

The symptoms of alcohol withdrawal tend to occur in a particular sequence, i.e. tremulousness, fits, hallucinosis and delirium tremens, and hence these conditions may be viewed as points along a continuum rather than as distinct clinical entities. Gross, Halpert and Sabot (1967) have proposed such a diagnostic continuum on which every patient may be placed in terms of the degree of clouding of the sensorium and the intensity of the hallucinatory experiences. In the mildest cases there is neither obvious impairment of consciousness nor hallucinations, while in the most severe (as in delirium tremens) both types of disturbance are very prominent.

There is now much evidence that the intensity and type of symptoms are very closely related to the degree of physical dependence which, in turn, is related to the duration and severity of alcohol abuse. First, morning tremulousness occurs much earlier in the course of alcoholism than delirium tremens (see Table 8.4, p. 264). Secondly, the longer the period of continuous drinking before withdrawal, the more severe the symptoms. Morgan (1968)

Table 4.9

CLASSIFICATION OF ALCOHOL WITHDRAWAL

Syndrome	Males (Gross et al., 1963)	Females (Sabot et al., 1968)	Both sexes No.	%
Pre-delirium tremens	20	11	31	18·1
Auditory hallucinosis	15	7	22	12·9
Delirium tremens	20	5	25	14·6
Mixed states	51	42	93	54·4
Total	106	65	171	100·0

found that of nine patients who had been drinking continuously for six months or more before admission to hospital, eight experienced hallucinations and three were delirious; truncal ataxia was noted in seven of these patients and the average duration of limb tremor after admission was more than four days. In contrast, of eight patients who had been drinking continuously for less than six months, none experienced hallucinations or demonstrated delirium or truncal ataxia and the average duration of limb tremor was less than two days. Thirdly, Scott (1967) obtained evidence that delirium tremens is associated with a greater intake of alcohol than is hallucinosis. He compared the drinking habits of 26 patients with alcoholic hallucinosis with those of 26 matched cases of delirium tremens and noted that while the former preferred beer and the latter preferred spirits, the actual consumption of beer was greater among patients with delirium tremens than among patients with hallucinosis.

REFERENCES

BARTHOLOMEW, A. A. (1967). Alcoholic hallucinosis and myocardial change: a preliminary study. *Med. J. Aust.* **2**, 1109-1110.

GROSS, M. M., HALPERT, E. and SABOT, L. (1967). Toward a revised classification of the acute alcoholic psychoses. *J. nerv. ment. Dis.* **145**, 500-508.

GROSS, M. M., HALPERT, E., SABOT, L. and POLIZOS, P. (1963). Hearing disturbances and auditory hallucinations in the acute alcoholic psychoses. I. Tinnitus: incidence and significance. *J. nerv. ment. Dis.* **137**, 455-465.

MORGAN, H. G. (1968). Acute neuropsychiatric complications of chronic alcoholism. *Brit. J. Psychiat.* **114**, 85-92.

SABOT, L. M., GROSS, M. M. and HALPERT, E. (1968). A study of acute alcoholic psychoses in women. *Brit. J. Addict.* **63**, 29-49.

SCOTT, D. F. (1967). Alcoholic hallucinosis—an aetiological study. *Brit. J. Addict.*
    62, 113-125.
VICTOR, M. (1966). Treatment of alcoholic intoxication and the withdrawal syn-
    drome. A critical analysis of the use of drugs and other forms of therapy.
    Psychosom. Med. **28**, 636-650.
VICTOR, M. and ADAMS, R. D. (1953). The effect of alcohol on the nervous system.
    Res. Publ. Ass. Res. nerv. ment. Dis. **32**, 526-573.

The Role of Withdrawal

Alcoholic abstinence often appears to be important in the aetiology of the conditions discussed here, and which have therefore been referred to as withdrawal syndromes. The experimental production of tremulousness, fits, hallucinosis and delirium by Isbell, Fraser, Wikler *et al.* (1955) and by Mendelson and La Dou (1964) strongly supports this contention. Isbell *et al.* (1955) administered alcohol by mouth to 10 healthy volunteers in a daily dose of between 250 and 500 ml for varying periods of time. In four subjects, the alcohol was discontinued after periods ranging from 7 to 34 days and these then developed tremulousness, nausea, sweating and insomnia of brief duration. The other six subjects continued taking alcohol in large amounts for 48-87 days and on sudden withdrawal, all became tremulous and weak with vomiting, diarrhoea, hyperreflexia and fever. Two of these subjects had transient hallucinosis, three became frankly delirious and two had epileptic seizures. Mendelson and La Dou (1964) carried out a similar study on 10 chronic alcoholics to whom they gave increasing doses of 86 proof whisky up to a maximum of 40 fluid ounces (1136 ml) per day for 24 days. On sudden withdrawal tremor was noted in nine patients, three became disorientated and five had visual and one had auditory hallucinations.

Various authors have however pointed out that sometimes delirium tremens seems to occur in the absence of any withdrawal. Thus almost half of the 42 cases reported by Nielsen (1965) developed delirium tremens while still drinking, while among the 74 patients reported by Lundquist (1961) and among the 187 cases of Figurelli (1958) a history of abrupt withdrawal before the onset of the delirium was obtained in only a small proportion (25 per cent and 7·5 per cent respectively). It is possible that a mere reduction of alcohol intake is sufficient to precipitate delirium tremens but some clinicians (e.g. Figurelli, 1958 and Lundquist, 1961) have argued that the infections, head trauma and other injuries that so frequently precede the condition may be very important aetiologically. Furthermore, it has been suggested that in some instances the patient appears to stop drinking because of nausea and a distaste for alcohol and that these symptoms may be the first sign of the development of the disorder (Batchelor, 1969). Nielsen (1965) has also argued against the withdrawal theory, pointing out that in Denmark the incidence of delirium tremens fell suddenly in March 1917, from about 70 to about 10 cases per month at a time when, because of war conditions, spirits became very scarce and expensive, and relative or absolute withdrawal must have been very common.

There is also some doubt as to the relevance of abstinence to alcoholic hallucinosis. In 15 of 76 cases reported by Victor and Hope (1958) the hallucinosis began while the patient was still drinking and in only three of these 15 was there a history of a substantial reduction in alcohol intake immediately before its onset. Moreover, Morgan (1968) gives details of three patients whose visual hallucinations began while actually increasing their alcohol intake. Morgan noted that these three patients showed abnormalities of pyruvate metabolism, which in two were characteristic of thiamine deficiency, and he suggests that hallucinosis sometimes arises because of such deficiency, sometimes because of alcohol withdrawal and sometimes from a combination of both. While it is right at the present time to mention these doubts concerning the aetiology of the alcoholic "withdrawal" syndromes, the weight of evidence indicates that abstinence, either relative or absolute, is very often an extremely important cause.

REFERENCES

BATCHELOR, I. R. C. (1969). *Henderson and Gillespie's Textbook of Psychiatry.* Tenth Edition. London.

FIGURELLI, F. A. (1958). Delirium tremens. Reduction of mortality and morbidity with promazine. *J. Amer. med. Ass.* **166**, 747-750.

ISBELL, H., FRASER, H. F., WIKLER, A., BELEVILLE, R. E. and EISENMAN, A. J. (1955). An experimental study of the aetiology of "rum fits". *Quart. J. Stud. Alcohol*, **16**, 1-33.

LUNDQUIST, G. (1961). Delirium tremens. *Acta psychiat. scand.* **36**, 443-466.

MENDELSON, J. H. and LA DOU, J. (1964). Experimentally induced chronic intoxication and withdrawal in alcoholics: Part 2, Psychophysiological findings. *Quart. J. Stud. Alcohol*, Supplement 2, pp. 14-39.

MORGAN, H. G. (1968). Acute neuropsychiatric complications of chronic alcoholism. *Brit. J. Psychiat.* **114**, 85-92.

NIELSEN, J. (1965). Delirium tremens in Copenhagen. *Acta psychiat. scand.* Supplement 187, pp. 1-92.

VICTOR, M. and HOPE, J. M. (1958). The phenomenon of auditory hallucinations in chronic alcoholism. A critical evaluation of the status of alcoholic hallucinosis. *J. nerv. ment. Dis.* **126**, 451-481.

PHYSICAL DEPENDENCE OF ALCOHOL AND BARBITURATE TYPES

Although delirium tremens is most prevalent among alcoholics, similar conditions, often indistinguishable from those observed in alcoholism, have been reported among subjects who have become physically dependent on barbiturates and other sedative drugs.

Barbiturates

Fraser, Shaver, Maxwell and Isbell (1953) described 19 barbiturate addicts who had been taking 0·8-2·2 g barbiturate daily. On withdrawal, 12 developed a psychosis closely resembling alcoholic delirium tremens, and of these 11 had epileptic fits during the withdrawal period; another patient had withdrawal fits only and in three patients the symptoms were less severe and consisted mainly of anxiety and weakness. Similar examples of a delirium tremens-like state following withdrawal of drugs from barbiturate dependent patients have been reported by Isbell (1950) and by James (1963), while withdrawal fits have been noted by Kalinowsky (1942) and by Gardner (1967). The experimental production of physical dependence on barbiturates and the effect of withdrawal have been investigated by Isbell, Altschul, Kornetsky et al. (1950), by Fraser, Wilker, Essig and Isbell (1958) and by Oswald and Priest (1965). Isbell et al (1950) administered barbiturates to five volunteers for periods ranging from 92-144 days in doses of up to 3·8 g daily. On sudden withdrawal of the drug, all developed weakness, tremor, anxiety, nausea and vomiting; four had grand mal convulsions and in four the condition developed into a delirium tremens-like state, with auditory and visual hallucinations, confusion, disorientation and profound insomnia. Fraser et al. (1958) studied the effects of sudden withdrawal in 50 volunteers who had been taking various doses of secobarbital or pentobarbital continuously for periods ranging from 32 to 365 days. Of 20 subjects receiving 0·4 g daily or less for 90 days only one developed withdrawal symptoms (insomnia, tremor, anxiety, etc.). After moderately high doses (0·6-0·8 g/day) taken for up to two months the majority of subjects developed withdrawal symptoms, but only one had a convulsion and none became delirious. Withdrawal from more prolonged higher dosage (0·9-2·2 g daily for 32-144 days) invariably led to more severe abstinence symptoms and of 18 subjects on this dose 14 had convulsions and 12 became delirious.

Relatively low doses taken for short periods of time may however also lead to withdrawal symptoms. Oswald and Priest (1965) gave two volunteers amylobarbitone sodium 400 mg nightly for nine nights followed by 600 mg nightly for a further nine nights and then withdrew the drug; both subjects complained of insomnia and nightmares during the following two weeks. Nightmares during withdrawal from barbiturates have also been reported by Kales and Jacobson (1967).

Other Sedatives

Withdrawal psychoses closely resembling delirium tremens have been observed among patients dependent on other sedative drugs:

Chloral hydrate	Margetts (1950); James (1963); Robinson (1966)
Paraldehyde	Kalinowsky (1942)
Meprobamate ("*Miltown*", "*Equanil*")	Haizlip and Ewing (1958), Swanson and Okada (1963)
Carbromal ("*Adalin*")	James (1963)

Ethchlorvynol (*"Arvynol"*, *"Serenesil"*, *"Placidyl"*)	Hudson and Walker (1961); Aycrigg (1964); Wood and Flippin (1965); Abuzahra and Rossdale (1968); Blumenthal and Reinhart (1964); Garetz (1969)
Methaqualone (*"Mandrax"*, *"Melsed"*, *"Quaalude"*)	Ewart and Priest (1967)
Ethinamate (*"Valmidate"*)	Ellinwood, Ewing and Hoaken, (1962)
Methyprylone (*"Noludar"*)	Berger (1961)
Glutethimide (*"Doriden"*)	Johnson and Van Buren (1962)

In addition, oxazepam ("Serenid-D", "Rondar", "Serax") withdrawal was a possible cause of the mental disturbance in a patient reported by Selig (1966) and seizures following withdrawal of chlordiazepoxide ("Librium") and diazepam ("Valium") have been observed (Hollister, Motzenbecker and Degan, 1961; Aivazian, 1964).

Effects of Alcohol and Sedatives on Sleep

The similarity between alcohol and barbiturate withdrawal syndromes suggests a common mechanism. A further similarity which throws light on the nature of some of the withdrawal phenomena concerns the effect of these drugs on sleep.

Observations on normal subjects have shown that there are two types of sleep, namely rapid eye movement (REM) sleep (also known as paradoxical or hindbrain sleep) and non-rapid eye movement (NREM) sleep, (also known as orthodox or forebrain sleep). REM sleep is characterized by low voltage EEG waves at 4-10 cycles/sec, rapid jerky movements of the eyeballs and irregularities of heart rate and respiration; on waking a subject from this type of sleep he tends to report that he has been dreaming. NREM sleep is characterized by slow waves and sleep spindles in the EEG, immobility of the eyeballs and regularity of respiration and pulse; on waking from this type of sleep, subjects tend to report that they have been thinking rather than dreaming. In normal circumstances the initial sleep period is always of NREM type but after about one hour, sleep starts to alternate between the two types so that during an average night there are about five or six periods of REM sleep, each of about 20 minutes, and REM sleep makes up 20 to 25 per cent of the total (Oswald, 1968).

The effect of barbiturates and of barbiturate withdrawal on the pattern of sleep is shown in Figure 4.4 which sets out the results of an experiment by Oswald and Priest (1965). Two volunteers were given amylobarbitone sodium on 18 consecutive nights. Initially on a nightly dose of 400 mg the proportion of REM sleep fell very considerably but with the development of tolerance this effect lessened so that by the end of the first week the amount of REM sleep was much the same as on the base line nights before the drug was

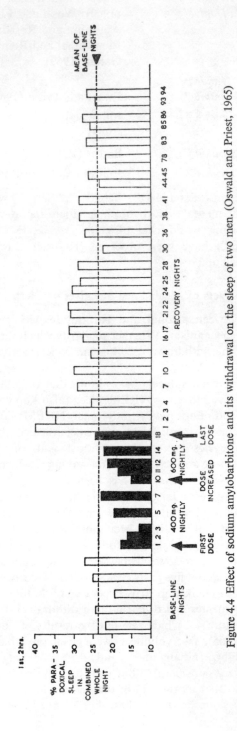

Figure 4.4 Effect of sodium amylobarbitone and its withdrawal on the sleep of two men. (Oswald and Priest, 1965)

started. The dose was increased on the tenth night of the investigation to 600 mg and again there was a transient reduction in the proportion of REM. On withdrawing the drug on the nineteenth night of the investigation a rebound was noted with an abnormally high amount of REM sleep and this persisted for several weeks after the last dose. During the period immediately after withdrawal both subjects slept badly and complained of nightmares. Evans, Lewis, Gibb and Cheetham (1968) have made similar observations on the effects of barbiturates, and nitrazepam ("Mogadon") and other sedative drugs have been shown to have comparable actions (Oswald and Priest, 1965; Oswald, Evans and Lewis, 1969).

There is good evidence that the administration of alcohol and its withdrawal affect sleep similarly. It has been shown that alcohol decreases the proportion of REM sleep and that with continued administration this effect declines (Gresham, Webb and Williams, 1963; Yules, Freedman and Chandler, 1966; Knowles, Laverty and Kuechler, 1968; Greenberg and Pearlman, 1967). The investigation of chronic alcoholics during withdrawal has shown a gross excess of REM sleep amounting to as much as 100 per cent of the total sleeping time in the period immediately before the onset of delirium tremens (Greenberg and Pearlman, 1967; Evans and Lewis, 1968a; Gross and Goodenough, 1968). Two current hypotheses link these observations with some of the clinical phenomena of alcohol and barbiturate abstinence. The first is a suggestion by Greenberg and Pearlman (1967) that prolonged suppression of central nervous system function by alcohol leads to pharmacological denervation with subsequent supersensitivity of central receptors similar to that postulated to account for the tolerance and withdrawal phenomena of opiate dependence (see Chapter 3) and that this supersensitivity is responsible for the greatly enhanced REM activity seen during alcohol withdrawal. Secondly, Evans and Lewis (1968b) have postulated that REM activity may be so intense during withdrawal that it spills over into waking life and is responsible there for the delirium of abstinent states. Whether or not these hypotheses are correct is uncertain, but there does seem to be support for the view that disturbances in the mechanisms responsible for REM sleep may also be responsible for the nightmares and delirium of abstinent states.

REFERENCES

ABUZAHRA, H. T. and ROSSDALE, M. (1968). Ethchlorvynol withdrawal symptoms. *Brit. med. J.* 2, 433-434.

AIVAZIAN, G. H. (1964). Clinical evaluation of diazepam. *Dis. nerv. Syst.* 25, 491-496.

AYCRIGG, J. B. (1964). Two cases of withdrawal from ethchlorvynol. *Amer. J. Psychiat.* 120, 1201-1203.

BERGER, H. (1961). Addiction to methyprylon. Report of case of 24-year-old nurse with possible synergism with phenothiazine. *J. Amer. med. Ass.* 177, 63-65.

BLUMENTHAL, M. D. and REINHART, M. J. (1964). Psychosis and convulsions following withdrawal from ethchlorvynol. *J. Amer. med. Ass.* 190, 154-155.

ELLINWOOD, E. H., EWING, J. A. and HOAKEN, P. C. S. (1962). Habituation to ethinamate. *J. Amer. med. Ass.* **266**, 185-186.

EVANS, J. I. and LEWIS, S. A. (1968a). Sleep studies in early delirium and during drug withdrawal in normal subjects and the effect of phenothiazines on such states. *Electroenceph. clin. Neurophysiol.* **25**, 507-509.

EVANS, J. I. and LEWIS, S. A. (1968b). Drug withdrawal state. An EEG sleep study. *Arch. gen. Psychiat.* **19**, 631-634.

EVANS, J. I., LEWIS, S. A., GIBB, I. A. M. and CHEETHAM, M. (1968). Sleep and barbiturates: some experiments and observations. *Brit. med. J.* **4**, 291-293.

EWART, R. B. L. and PRIEST, R. G. (1967). Methaqualone addiction and delirium tremens. *Brit. med. J.* **3**, 92-93.

FRASER, H. F., SHAVER, M. R., MAXWELL, E. S. and ISBELL, H. (1953). Death due to withdrawal of barbiturates. *Ann. intern. Med.* **38**, 1319-1325.

FRASER, H. F., WIKLER, A., ESSIG, C. F. and ISBELL, H. (1958). Degree of physical dependence induced by secobarbital or pentobarbital. *J. Amer. med. Ass.* **166**, 126-129.

GARDNER, A. J. (1967). Withdrawal fits in barbiturate addicts. *Lancet*, **2**, 337-338.

GARETZ, F. D. (1969). Ethchlorvynol (Placidyl). *Minn. Med.* **52**, 1131-1133.

GREENBERG, R. and PEARLMAN, C. (1967). Delirium tremens and dreaming. *Amer. J. Psychiat.* **124**, 133-142.

GRESHAM, S. C., WEBB, W. B. and WILLIAMS, R. L. (1963). Alcohol and caffeine: effect on inferred visual dreaming. *Science*, **140**, 1226-1227.

GROSS, M. M. and GOODENOUGH, D. R. (1968). Sleep disturbance in the acute alcoholic psychoses. *Psychiat. Res. Rep. Amer. psychiat. Ass.* **24**, 132-147.

HAIZLIP, T. H. and EWING, J. A. (1958). Meprobamate addiction. A controlled clinical study. *New Engl. J. Med.* **258**, 1181-1186.

HOLLISTER, L. E., MOTZENBECKER, F. P. and DEGAN, R. O. (1961). Withdrawal reactions from chlordiazepoxide ("Librium") *Psychopharmacologia (Berl.)*, **2**, 63-68.

HUDSON, H. S. and WALKER, H. I. (1961). Withdrawal symptoms following ethchlorvynol (Placidyl) dependence. *Amer. J. Psychiat.* **118**, 361.

ISBELL, H. (1950). Addiction to barbiturates and the barbiturate abstinence syndrome. *Ann. intern. Med.* **33**, 108-121.

ISBELL, H., ALTSCHUL, S., KORNETSKY, C. H., EISENMAN, A. J., FLANARY, H. G. and FRASER, H. F. (1950). Chronic barbiturate intoxication. An experimental study. *Arch. Neurol. Psychiat. (Chic.)* **64**, 1-28.

JAMES, I. P. (1963). Drug-withdrawal psychoses. *Amer. J. Psychiat.* **119**, 880-881.

JOHNSON, F. A. and VAN BUREN, H. C. (1962). Abstinence syndrome following glutethimide intoxication. *J. Amer. med. Ass.* **180**, 1024-1027.

KALES, A. and JACOBSON, A. (1967). Mental activity during sleep: recall studies, somnambulism, and effects of rapid eye movement deprivation and drugs. *Exp. Neurol.* Supplement 4, pp. 81-91.

KALINOWSKY, L. B. (1942). Convulsions in non-epileptic patients on withdrawal of barbiturates, alcohol and other drugs. *Arch. Neurol. Psychiat. (Chic.)* **48**, 946-956.

KNOWLES, J. B., LAVERTY, S. G. and KUECHLER, H. A. (1968). Effects of alcohol on REM sleep. *Quart. J. Stud. Alcohol*, **29**, 342-349.

MARGETTS, E. L. (1950). Chloral delirium. *Psychiat. Quart.* **24**, 278-299.

OSWALD, I. (1968). Drugs and sleep. *Pharmacol. Rev.* **20**, 273-303.

OSWALD, I., EVANS, J. I. and LEWIS, S. A. (1969). Addictive drugs cause suppression of paradoxical sleep with withdrawal rebound. In *Scientific Basis of Drug Dependence*. (Editor, Steinberg, H.), pp. 243-257, London.

OSWALD, I. and PRIEST, R. G. (1965). Five weeks to escape the sleeping pill habit. *Brit. med. J.* **2**, 1093-1099.

ROBINSON, J. T. (1966). A case of chloral hydrate addiction. *Int. J. soc. Psychiat.* **12**, 66-71.

SELIG, J. W. (1966). A possible oxazepam abstinence syndrome. *J. Amer. med. Ass.* **198**, 951-952.

SWANSON, L. A. and OKADA, T. (1963). Death after withdrawal of meprobamate. *J. Amer. med. Ass.* **184**, 780-781.

WOOD, H. P. and FLIPPIN, H. F. (1965). "Delirium tremens" following withdrawal of ethchlorvinol. *Amer. J. Psychiat.* **121**, 1127-1129.

YULES, R. B., FREEDMAN, D. X. and CHANDLER, K. A. (1966). The effect of ethyl alcohol on man's electroencephalographic sleep cycle. *Electroenceph. clin. Neurophysiol.* **20**, 109-111.

THE DRUG TREATMENT OF ALCOHOL WITHDRAWAL

The general management of patients with delirium tremens and related conditions is more or less agreed. Hallucinated and confused patients should be nursed in well-lit rooms and every effort should be made to allay their anxiety and apprehension. Most clinicians, as a routine, give large doses of Vitamin B complex (e.g. high potency "Parentrovite" Bencard, intravenously) and some advocate the routine administration of anticonvulsant drugs. Obviously, treatment must be given to any co-existing infection or injury, and where dehydration or electrolyte disturbances exist, these should be corrected, by intravenous infusion if necessary. Knott and Beard (1968) suggest that if there is any evidence of overhydration diuretics should be given.

Apart from these general measures, most patients are given drugs to control the symptoms, to hasten recovery, and to prevent the development of delirium tremens. On the basis that the symptoms are abstinence phenomena analogous to those which occur in opiate withdrawal, it might be expected that the administration of alcohol would be the best treatment. Indeed, Gessner (1965) has advocated that patients with delirium tremens should be given alcohol until signs of toxicity appear and that then it should be withdrawn very gradually. But in practice alcohol is relatively ineffective, either in prevention or treatment, even when given in doses equivalent to 600 mls of absolute alcohol per day (Golbert, Sanz, Rose and Leitschuh, 1967; Nichols, 1967). The poor response may be related to the very short duration of action of alcohol and to the difficulty in administering the very large and possibly dangerous amounts which are probably needed. For these reasons other drugs are to be preferred, particularly those with sedative actions which show cross-tolerance with alcohol (Fraser, Wikler, Isbell and Johnson, 1957). Of these drugs paraldehyde has been strongly recommended by Victor (1966) and by Gross (1967) and it certainly has a theoretical advantage over other drugs in that after depolymerization to acetaldehyde, it shares the same metabolic pathways as alcohol. But paraldehyde has to be given in large doses (up to 10 ml, four hourly) and it is unpleasant to take. Intramuscular administration is painful and since it irritates the stomach, giving it by mouth may aggravate any vomiting; Gross (1967) however has found that aluminium hydroxide gel ("Aludrox") given before each dose of oral paraldehyde improves its tolerance. A number of controlled studies of paraldehyde have been reported and are discussed below.

Other drugs commonly used—their efficacy is discussed below—are chlordiazepoxide and phenothiazine derivatives such as chlorpromazine. The use of chlordiazepoxide is theoretically sound: it has pharmacological effects similar to those of alcohol and in high dosage (200 mg or more daily) it might be expected to relieve the withdrawal symptoms. Phenothiazines, however, have no affinity to the alcohol-barbiturate group of drugs and there is no demonstrable cross-tolerance between them. Indeed, Essig and Fraser (1966) have shown, in animal studies, that chlorpromazine does not prevent experimentally-produced barbiturate-withdrawal convulsions. A possible theoretical basis for the use of phenothiazines has however been suggested by Evans and Lewis (1968a, b) who noted that chlorpromazine decreases the amount of REM sleep and that it prevents the "overswing" during alcohol and barbiturate withdrawal. These effects of chlorpromazine are identical to those of sedative drugs except that withdrawal of chlorpromazine is not followed by a period of excessive REM sleep. In theory then, chlorpromazine might have an advantage over sedatives in the treatment of drug withdrawal states.

Paraldehyde

Many investigators have found that paraldehyde is more effective than other drugs in the prevention and treatment of delirium tremens (e.g. Friedhoff and Zitrin, 1959; Thomas and Freedman, 1964; Golbert et al., 1967; Muller, 1969). Particularly notable is the study by Golbert et al. (1967) who compared four different drug treatments of 49 non-delirious patients with symptoms of alcohol withdrawal (Table 4.10). Of 12 patients treated by large doses of paraldehyde and chloral hydrate only one became delirious and in that case

Table 4.10

COMPLICATIONS OF ALCOHOLIC TREMULOUSNESS AND HALLUCINOSIS
WITH DIFFERENT TREATMENTS
(Golbert *et al.*, 1967)

Treatment (daily dose)	Number of patients	Delirium tremens	Complications Fits	Death
1. Alcohol (200-600 ml)	12	5	1	0
2. Chlordiazepoxide (0·6-3·2 g)	12	6	0	0
3. Promazine (0·6-3·6 g)	13	7	1	2
4. Paraldehyde (60-120 ml) + Chloral hydrate (2·0-6·0 g)	12	1	0	0

there was the possibility that the delirium was due to a pulmonary infection. In contrast, delirium tremens occurred in about one-half of the 37 patients treated by alcohol, chlordiazepoxide or promazine while two had fits and two died. Golbert *et al.* (1967) also treated 11 patients with delirium tremens by paraldehyde and chloral and noted that the hallucinations stopped within 24 hours in every case and that complications were infrequent, while of 12 similar delirious patients treated with promazine, two died and in five cases there was such general deterioration that the treatment was changed to paraldehyde and chloral.

Chlordiazepoxide

The efficacy of chlordiazepoxide is less certain than that of paraldehyde. Kaim, Klett and Rothfeld (1969) allocated 537 patients undergoing alcohol withdrawal to five different treatments: (*a*) chlordiazepoxide—up to 200 mg/day; (*b*) chlorpromazine—up to 400 mg/day; (*c*) hydroxyzine—up to 400 mg/day; (*d*) thiamine—up to 400 mg/day; and (*e*) placebo. Judging by the number of patients who developed fits or delirium tremens, chlordiazepoxide gave the best results and chlorpromazine the worst. Rosenfeld and Bizzoco (1961) found chlordiazepoxide to be more effective than placebo and Sereny and Kalant (1965) found it better than either promazine or placebo, but Koutsky and Sletten (1963) found no difference between the effects of intramuscular chlordiazepoxide (300 mg/day) and of saline.

Phenothiazines

Some of the studies where phenothiazines have been compared with other drugs have already been discussed. There is little evidence to suggest that any one preparation is more effective than any other. Laties, Lasagna, Gross, *et al.* (1958) found no significant difference between chlorpromazine and promazine, but Motto (1968) found that perphenazine seemed to give better results than chlorpromazine, promazine or mepazine. The most commonly used derivatives are chlorpromazine (200-800 mg daily) promazine (300-1200 mg daily) and thioridazine (150-200 mg daily). While not as effective overall as paraldehyde in the treatment of alcohol withdrawal, phenothiazines do seem to control the gastrointestinal disturbances and the excitement and agitation (Motto, 1968) and in milder conditions they may be particularly useful and indeed produce better results than paraldehyde (Thomas and Freedman, 1964). A disadvantage of these drugs is their tendency to cause epileptic fits and their administration during alcohol withdrawal may precipitate a convulsion (Fazekas, Shea, Ehrmantraut and Alman, 1957).

Chlormethiazole

Chlormethiazole edisylate ("Heminevrin") is a derivative of the thiazole moiety of thiamine (Figure 4·5). It is an hypnotic with anticonvulsant and muscle-relaxant properties and is most commonly used in the treatment of alcohol withdrawal. It is available as tablets and capsules (0·5 g) and as an 0·8 per cent sterile solution for injection. In most cases of delirium tremens or tremulous states the patient will take an oral preparation; initially the dose is 5-6 g daily in divided doses, and this is reduced gradually and after six days withdrawn. Where oral administration is not possible, the 0·8 per cent solution is given intravenously—higher concentrations tend to cause thrombophlebitis and intravascular haemolysis—either rapidly (e.g. 3-4 g over 1-2 hours) or more slowly (e.g. 8 g over 24 hours). With the intravenous route the patient becomes sedated rapidly and usually falls asleep, and in many cases is very much improved when he wakens some hours later (Laxenaire, Tridon and Poire, 1966; Sattes, 1966; Gershon, 1968) and treatment can be then continued orally.

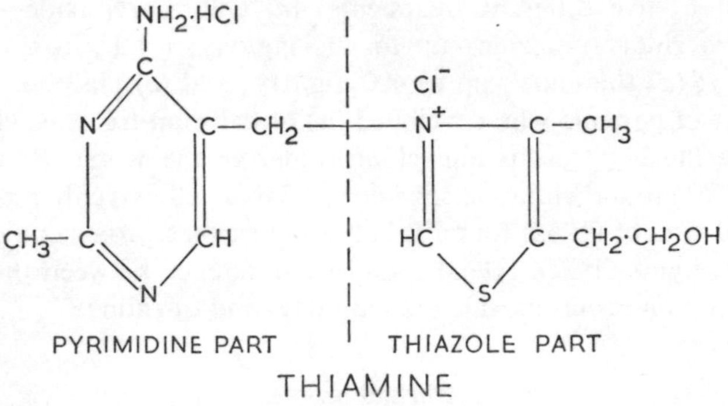

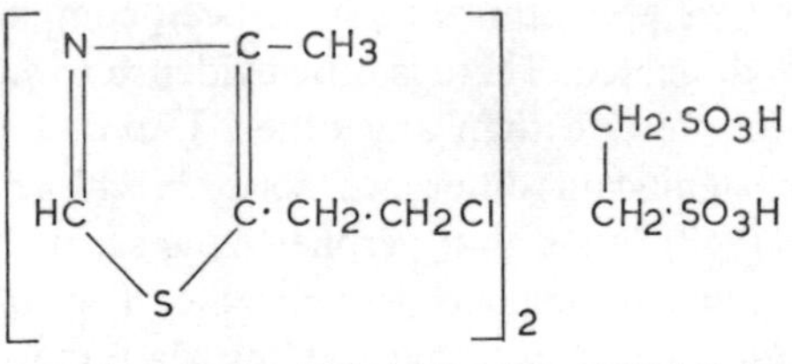

Figure 4.5 Structures of thiamine and of chlormethiazole edisylate

Three double-blind controlled trials of oral chlormethiazole have been reported. Glatt, George and Frisch, (1965, 1966) treated 49 alcoholic patients undergoing withdrawal with chlormethiazole and 48 similar patients with placebo tablets, and they found that chlormethiazole treatment produced significantly better results than placebo, both overall and as regards improvement in the individual symptoms. However, using similar dosages of chlormethiazole, Harfst, Greene and Lassalle (1967) found that amylobarbitone produced just as good results while Madden, Jones and Frisch (1969) noted no significant difference between the effects of chlormethiazole and trifluoperazine on alcohol withdrawal.

The side effects of chlormethiazole have been reviewed by Svedin (1966). Most common is a tingling sensation in the nose with sneezing which occurs almost immediately after the start of an intravenous infusion or 15-20 minutes after oral ingestion; Glatt *et al.* (1965, 1966) noted the occurrence of this sneeze reflex in almost one quarter of their patients. Less common is bronchorrhoea, but Madden *et al.* (1969) have pointed out the dangers of this in patients with bronchitis or bronchiectasis, or indeed with any respiratory infection. Anorexia, nausea and vomiting, urticaria and erythematous skin reactions and, less commonly, hypotension have been reported. In addition, chlormethiazole may produce physical dependence (Lundquist, 1966); indeed, Madden *et al.* (1969) have reported a patient who had a convulsion when the drug was stopped. Because of this risk of dependence, Glatt *et al.* (1965, 1966) warn against continuing treatment with chlormethiazole for more than six days.

REFERENCES

ESSIG, C. F. and FRASER, H. F. (1966). Failure of chlorpromazine to prevent barbiturate-withdrawal convulsions. *Clin. Pharmacol. Ther.* **7**, 466-469.

EVANS, J. I. and LEWIS, S. A. (1968a). Sleep studies in early delirium and during drug withdrawal in normal subjects and the effect of phenothiazines on such states. *Electroenceph. clin. Neurophysiol.* **25**, 508-509.

EVANS, J. I. and LEWIS, S. A. (1968b). Drug withdrawal state. An EEG sleep study. *Arch. gen. Psychiat.* **19**, 631-634.

FAZEKAS, J. F., SHEA, J. G., EHRMANTRAUT, W. R. and ALMAN, R. W. (1957). Convulsant action of phenothiazine derivatives. *J. Amer. med. Ass.* **165**, 1241-1245.

FRASER, H. F., WIKLER, A., ISBELL, H. and JOHNSON, N. K. (1957). Partial equivalence of chronic alcohol and barbiturate intoxication. *Quart. J. Stud. Alcohol*, **18**, 541-551.

FRIEDHOFF, A. J. and ZITRIN, A. (1959). A comparison of the effects of paraldehyde and chlorpromazine in delirium tremens. *N.Y. St. J. Med.* **59**, 1060-1063.

GERSHON, S. (1968). A review of the use of a thiazole derivative (hemineurin) in delirium tremens and allied conditions. *Psychiat. Res. Rep. Amer. psychiat. Ass.* **24**, 166-173.

GESSNER, P. K. (1965). Alcohol withdrawal. *J. Amer. med. Ass.* **193**, 77-78.

GLATT, M. M., GEORGE, H. R. and FRISCH, E. P. (1965). Controlled trial of chlormethiazole in treatment of the alcohol withdrawal phase. *Brit. med. J.* **2**, 401-404.

GLATT, M. M., GEORGE, H. R. and FRISCH, E. P. (1966). Evaluation of chlormethiazole in treatment for alcohol withdrawal syndrome. Results of a controlled trial. *Acta psychiat. scand.* Supplement 192, pp. 121-137.

GOLBERT, T. M., SANZ, C. J., ROSE, H. D. and LEITSCHUH, T. H. (1967). Comparative evaluation of treatments of alcohol withdrawal states. *J. Amer. med. Ass.* **201**, 99-102.

GROSS, M. M. (1967). Management of acute alcohol withdrawal states. *Quart. J. Stud. Alcohol*, **28**, 655-666.

HARFST, M. J., GREENE, J. G. and LASSALLE, F. G. (1967). Controlled trial comparing amobarbital and clomethiazole in alcohol withdrawal symptoms. *Quart. J. Stud. Alcohol*, **28**, 641-648.

KAIM, S. C., KLETT, C. J. and ROTHFELD, B. (1969). Treatment of the acute alcohol withdrawal state: a comparison of four drugs. *Amer. J. Psychiat.* **125**, 1640-1646.

KNOTT, D. H. and BEARD, J. D. (1968). A new approach to the treatment of acute withdrawal from alcohol. *Psychosomatics*, **9**, 311-313.

KOUTSKY, C. D. and SLETTEN, I. W. (1963). Chlordiazepoxide in alcohol withdrawal—intramuscular effects. *Minn. Med.* **46**, 354-357.

LATIES, V. G., LASAGNA, L., GROSS, G. M., HITCHMAN, I. L. and FLORES, J. (1958). A controlled trial of chlorpromazine and promazine in the management of delirium tremens. *Quart. J. Stud. Alcohol*, **19**, 238-243.

LAXENAIRE, M., TRIDON, P. and POIRE, P. (1966). Effect of chlormethiazole in treatment of delirium tremens and status epilepticus. *Acta psychiat. scand.* Supplement 192, pp. 87-110.

LUNDQUIST, G. (1966). The risk of dependence on chlormethiazole. *Acta psychiat. scand.* Supplement 192, pp. 203-204.

MADDEN, J. S., JONES, D. and FRISCH, E. P. (1969). Chlormethiazole and trifluoperazine in alcohol withdrawal. *Brit. J. Psychiat.* **115**, 1191-1192.

MOTTO, J. A. (1968). Acute alcohol-withdrawal syndromes; a controlled study of phenothiazine effectiveness. *Quart. J. Stud. Alcohol*, **29**, 917-930.

MULLER, D. J. (1969). A comparison of three approaches to alcohol-withdrawal states. *Sth. med. J. (Bgham, Ala.)*, **62**, 495-496.

NICHOLS, M. M. (1967). Acute alcohol withdrawal syndrome in a newborn. *Amer. J. Dis. Child.* **113**, 714-715.

ROSENFELD, J. E. and BIZZOCO, D. H. (1961). A controlled study of alcohol withdrawal. *Quart. J. Stud. Alcohol*, Supplement 1, pp. 77-84.

SATTES, H. (1966). Treatment of delirium tremens with chlormethiazole. *Acta psychiat. scand.* Supplement 192, pp. 139-143.

SERENY, G. and KALANT, H. (1965). Comparative clinical evaluation of chlordiazepoxide and promazine in treatment of alcohol-withdrawal syndrome. *Brit. med. J.* **1**, 92-97.

SVEDIN, C-O. (1966). Side effects in chlormethiazole therapy. *Acta psychiat. scand.* Supplement 192, pp. 199-201.

THOMAS, D. W. and FREEDMAN, D. X. (1964). Treatment of the alcoholic withdrawal syndrome. Comparison of promazine and paraldehyde. *J. Amer. med. Ass.* **188**, 316-318.

VICTOR, M. (1966). Treatment of alcoholic intoxication and the withdrawal syndrome. A critical analysis of the use of drugs and other forms of therapy. *Psychosom. Med.* **28**, 636-650.

CHAPTER 5

ANXIETY AND PHOBIC STATES

The Sympathetic Nervous System and Anxiety. Psychophysiological Aspects of Anxiety. Phobic States. Behaviour Therapy of Phobic Disorders.

THE SYMPATHETIC NERVOUS SYSTEM AND ANXIETY

Clinical Features of Anxiety

ANXIETY state or neurosis is characterized by unreasonable feelings of fear, tension or panic or of an expectancy that something unpleasant is going to happen; when very severe the patient may feel that death is imminent. Almost invariably there are physical symptoms, such as palpitations, abdominal sensations ("butterflies" or a feeling of emptiness), tremulousness, difficulty in breathing, paraesthesiae, chest discomfort or pain, dizziness or faintness, diarrhoea, frequency of micturition, headache, blurring of vision, sweating, dryness of the mouth and difficulty in swallowing. Other symptoms include insomnia, nightmares, difficulty in concentration, poor memory and depression (Hamilton, 1959).

Walker (1959) studied the clinical features and prognosis of 111 patients with anxiety neurosis where anxiety was the cardinal symptom and not an incidental aspect of some other disorder; phobic patients (whose unreasonable anxiety occurs only in relation to certain feared situations) were excluded from the study. He found that anxiety neurosis was an illness of young people; all except one patient were in the age group 20 to 35 years. Twenty-four of the patients in this series experienced their symptoms mainly or wholly in discrete attacks, unrelated to any obvious external circumstance. The illness of these patients almost invariably began suddenly and at full intensity. Typically the individual attacks occurred about twice daily with sudden onset, dying away gradually and in between the attacks the patients were relatively well apart from a common tendency to have symptoms of mild depression. Walker noted that the prognosis of these patients was always good and significantly better than that of patients with other types of anxiety (Table 5.1).

The term anxiety also denotes a normal reaction to a dangerous or potentially dangerous situation and there is some controversy as to whether or not this reaction is qualitatively distinct from anxiety state or neurosis. Adherents to the view that there is no distinction maintain that the latter is an exaggeration of the normal reaction, possibly the result of a stimulus which in most persons would not give rise to intense emotional disturbance. The opposite view is that anxiety state is an entity intrinsically different and possibly aetiologically distinct from the normal. Hamilton (1969) compared the

135

symptoms of 42 patients suffering from anxiety states with those of 53 patients with skin disorders who appeared to be very anxious. He noted quantitative differences only in the symptomatology of the two groups,

Table 5.1

MODE OF ONSET, PROGRESSION AND PROGNOSIS OF 111 PATIENTS WITH
ANXIETY STATE
(*Walker*, 1959)

Prognosis	*Complete recovery*			*No recovery*			*Partial recovery*		
Mode of onset*	G	R	I	G	R	I	G	R	I
Type of Progression Constant tension Unprecipitated exacerbation						13	6	4	
Episodic tension Precipitated	4			12			3	5	
Episodic tension Unprecipitated		1	23						
Fluctuating Tension				13			17	10	

* G = gradual; R = rapid; I = instantaneous

suggesting that anxiety state is not a distinct entity. Most psychiatrists appear to hold this view and information obtained from the study of normal subjects in anxiety-producing situations has been freely applied to anxiety states and has increased our understanding of this condition.

REFERENCES

HAMILTON, M. (1959). The assessment of anxiety states by rating. *Brit. J. med. Psychol.* **32**, 50-55.

HAMILTON, M. (1969). Diagnosis and rating of anxiety. In *Studies of Anxiety* (Editor, Lader, M. H.) British Journal of Psychiatry Special Publication No. 3. Ashford.

WALKER, L. (1959). The prognosis for affective illness with overt anxiety. *J. Neurol. Neurosurg. Psychiat.* **22**, 338-341.

Peripheral Mechanisms in Anxiety

Undoubtedly the experience of emotion is associated with and largely dependent upon physiological activity within the central nervous system and Smythies (1969) has recently reviewed existing knowledge which emphasizes the role of the amygdala, hypothalamus and other brain structures in relation to anxiety. Moreover, many of the drugs now known to be effective in the treatment of anxiety, such as the barbiturates, the benzodiazepines (e.g. chlordiazepoxide and diazepam) and meprobamate have important central actions and little or no effect on peripheral structures (Shepherd, Lader and

Rodnight, 1968). Nevertheless, most, if not all, of the physical symptoms of anxiety are the direct result of discharge of the autonomic nervous system (particularly of the sympathetic), and of increased secretion of catecholamines by the adrenal medulla. Lately much attention has been paid to these peripheral manifestations, and there has been a revival of the controversy of 50 years ago, between James and Lange on the one hand and Cannon on the other, as to the relationship between the physical and mental manifestations. The James-Lange theory proposes that "the feeling of the bodily changes as they occur is the emotion" (Lange and James, 1922), that is, that the peripheral changes actually cause or elicit the mental experience, while Cannon's hypothesis (Cannon, 1927) postulates that the bodily changes and the emotion have a common origin within the brain. Cannon criticized the view of James and Lange on various grounds, such as that the total separation of the viscera from the central nervous system does not alter emotional behaviour and that the artificial induction of the visceral changes (for example by the administration of sympathomimetic amines) does not produce the emotion. However, more recent studies, discussed below, suggest that peripheral stimulation does sometimes produce anxiety and that the hypothesis of James and Lange may be of value today.

Physical Effects of Sympathomimetic Drugs

The intimate relationship between sympathetic activity and anxiety has been demonstrated by a number of studies which have shown an increased urinary output of catecholamines (particularly adrenaline) in anxious subjects (Breggin, 1964; Levi, 1969) and also by other observations that many of the physical changes noted in anxiety can be reproduced by the administration of sympathomimetic amines to normal subjects. Hawkins, Monroe, Sandifer and Vernon (1960) gave adrenaline by continuous intravenous infusion (1 to 20 microgrammes per minute) to normal individuals and they observed pallor of the skin, tremor of the hands and lips, quavering of the voice, increased sweating, tachycardia and difficulty in breathing, similar to the manifestations of anxiety. These symptoms appear to be more readily produced by adrenaline than by noradrenaline (Breggin, 1964) and Marshall and Schnieden (1966) have shown that intravenous adrenaline but not noradrenaline significantly increases the tremor of anxious subjects.

Some of the biochemical changes which occur in anxiety are also similar to those seen after the administration of catecholamines. First, patients with anxiety states show, after exercise, a greater than normal rise in blood lactic acid concentration (Jones and Mellersh, 1946) while in normal subjects noradrenaline stimulates the production of lactic acid (Innes and Mickerson, 1965); secondly emotional arousal in normal subjects is associated with a rapid elevation of the free fatty acid concentration in the blood (Gottschalk, Cleghorn, Glesser and Iacono, 1965; Pinter, Peterfy, Cleghorn and Pattee, 1967) similar to that observed after the administration of adrenaline (Pinter and Pattee, 1967).

Mental Effects of Sympathomimetic Drugs

Although Cannon (1927) maintained that adrenaline did not cause emotional arousal, Breggin (1964) has re-examined the literature and has concluded that in certain circumstances it does produce the mental pheno-mena of anxiety in addition to the physical changes. Thus Wearn and Sturgis (1919) noted that adrenaline increased both the mental and physical distress of patients with "irritable heart syndrome", a condition now more commonly known as "effort syndrome", "neurocirculatory asthenia" or "hyperkinetic heart syndrome", and characterized by complaints of palpitations, chest discomfort, decreased exercise tolerance and anxiety in the absence of organic heart disease. Breggin (1964) suggests that the administration of parenteral adrenaline is likely to produce the subjective experience of anxiety in two circumstances: first, where the experimental conditions are themselves likely to cause anxiety and secondly, where the subject has previously experienced recurrent anxiety associated with symptoms of sympathetic overactivity. Breggin concludes that the peripheral manifestations may be both a consequence of central nervous system activity, as Cannon postulated, and a cause of emotion, as hypothesized by James and Lange. Thus, although the mental state may initiate the sympathetic activity, the latter may generate more mental disturbance if there has been a previously learnt association between the subjective and autonomic symptoms. If this view is correct, acute anxiety reactions may be self perpetuating and may be terminated by interfering with either the central or the peripheral processes.

Evidence that peripheral stimulation is important in anxiety has been adduced by Frohlich and his colleagues (Frohlich, Dustan and Page, 1966; Frohlich, Tarazi and Dustan, 1969) who studied the effects of intravenous isoprenaline (isoproterenol) hydrochloride on (a) 14 patients complaining of disturbing palpitations, chest discomfort and anxiety without evidence of an organic basis for their symptoms, (b) 13 patients with essential hypertension and (c) 25 normotensive volunteers. Isoprenaline (1 to 3 microgrammes per minute) had a much greater effect on the heart rate and cardiac output of the patients in the first group than in the other patients. Moreover, 9 patients in the first group developed severe anxiety, but neither the administration of saline to these individuals nor the infusion of isoprenaline to the hypertensive or normotensive controls had any obvious effect on the mental state. Frohlich and his colleagues also showed that the three groups did not differ in their blood pressure or heart rate responses to sympathetic stimulation induced by the cold pressor test or by change in posture, and they concluded that the abnormal response to isoprenaline was due to hypersensitivity of the beta-adrenergic receptors. (Adrenergic receptors are discussed below in the next section.) They also concluded that isoprenaline-induced anxiety is secondary to peripheral stimulation and that the condition of their first group of patients could best be described as "hyperdynamic beta-adrenergic circulatory state", an entity distinct from anxiety neurosis where any cardiac symptoms are due to excessive sympathetic discharge. Some support for this contention is given by an observation of theirs (Frohlich et al., 1969) that ordinarily anxious subjects do not show any increased sensitivity of the beta receptors. Davis (1969) however has pointed out that isoprenaline crosses the blood-brain barrier and excites the central nervous system and he suggests that it is the central actions rather than the peripheral ones which were responsible for the emotional arousal in Frohlich's patients. This mechanism however cannot be the explanation for anxiety induced by adrenaline which does not cross the blood-brain barrier.

Pitts and McClure (1967) have observed that the excessive production of catecholamines in anxiety states leads to increased formation of lactate and they hypothesize that it is the lactate which is directly responsible for the symptoms. In a double-blind study, they noted the effects of intravenous infusion of solutions of (a) sodium lactate, (b) sodium lactate and calcium chloride and (c) glucose-saline, given in random order to 14 patients with severe anxiety neurosis and to 10 normal subjects. In 13 of the 14 patients, the administration of 500 mM sodium lactate (10 ml per kilogramme body weight) over a 20-minute period produced severe anxiety, beginning within one to two minutes from the start of the infusion, with symptoms very similar to those which the patients had experienced previously during spontaneous attacks. Following completion of the infusion, the symptoms decreased rapidly, but feelings of exhaustion and of more than usual anxiety often persisted for up to 72 hours. Infusions of calcium chloride (20 mM) with the lactate produced less anxiety—in only one patient did it precipitate an attack—while glucose-saline had no obvious effect. Two of the 10 normal subjects experienced anxiety with the lactate but none were adversely affected by the calcium chloride-lactate or glucose-saline solutions. Pitts and McClure concluded that the precipitation of anxiety by lactate and its prevention by the concomitant administration of calcium indicates that lactate acts by complexing ionized calcium, thus reducing the amount of calcium available in the interstitial fluid at nerve endings with consequent impairment of normal neurotransmission. They also suggest that anxiety follows stress because the latter increases adrenaline release, the adrenaline leading to increased lactate production; their findings are thus linked with existing knowledge of adrenergic mechanisms in anxiety. Fink, Taylor and Volavka (1969) have repeated the study of Pitts and McClure and have confirmed their findings. All five of their anxious patients developed an acute anxiety reaction starting 8 to 12 minutes after the beginning of the lactate infusion and remaining severe for 15 to 30 minutes. For 2 to 7 days afterwards their patients experienced irritability, dysphoria, tension, fatigue and weakness. The response to lactate-calcium was less intense and glucose-saline was without effect. Only one of their four control subjects experienced anxiety with lactate and none responded adversely to lactate-calcium or glucose-saline infusions.

The explanation for these findings, put forward by Pitts and McClure, has been criticized. Lassers and Nimmo (1969) have calculated that the dose of lactate administered is not sufficient to depress the ionized calcium level in the interstitial fluid below normal. Grosz and Farmer (1969) also criticize, on various other grounds, the view that a reduction in ionized calcium concentration is responsible, although they agree that the administration of lactate does precipitate anxiety in susceptible individuals.

REFERENCES

BREGGIN, P. B. (1964). The psychophysiology of anxiety. *J. nerv. ment. Dis.* **139**, 558-568.

CANNON, W. B. (1927). The James-Lange theory of emotions: a critical examination and an alternative theory. *Amer. J. Psychol.* **39**, 106-124.

DAVIS, J. N. (1969). Increased β-receptor responsiveness. Central or peripheral? *Arch. intern. Med.* **123**, 101-102.

FINK, M., TAYLOR, M. A. and VOLAVKA, J. (1969). Anxiety precipitated by lactate. *New Engl. J. Med.* **281**, 1429.

FROHLICH, E. D., DUSTAN, H. P. and PAGE, I. H. (1966). Hyperdynamic beta-adrenergic circulatory state. *Arch. intern. Med.* **117**, 614-619.

FROHLICH, E. D., TARAZI, R. C. and DUSTAN, H. P. (1969). Hyperdynamic β-adrenergic circulatory state. Increased β-receptor responsiveness. *Arch. intern. Med.* **123**, 1-7.

GOTTSCHALK, L. A., CLEGHORN, J. M., GLESER, G. C. and IACONO, J. M. (1965). Studies of relationships of emotions to plasma lipids. *Psychosom. Med.* **27**, 102-111.

GROSZ, H. J. and FARMER, B. B. (1969). Blood lactate in the development of anxiety symptoms. *Arch. gen. Psychiat.* **21**, 611-619.

HAWKINS, D. R., MONROE, J. T., SANDIFER, M. G. and VERNON, C. R. (1960). Psychological and physiological responses to continuous epinephrine infusion—an approach to the study of the affect, anxiety. *Psychiat. Res. Rep. Amer. psychiat. Ass.* **12**, 40-50.

INNES, I. R. and MICKERSON, M. (1965). Drugs acting on postganglionic adrenergic nerve endings and structures innervated by them. (Sympathomimetic drugs.) In *The Pharmacological Basis of Therapeutics* (Editors, Goodman, L. S. and GILMAN, A.) 3rd Edition. New York.

JONES, M. and MELLERSH, V. (1946). A comparison of the exercise response in anxiety states and normal controls. *Psychosom. Med.* **8**, 180-187.

LANGE, C. G. and JAMES, W. (1922). *The Emotions.* Baltimore.

LASSERS, B. W. and NIMMO, I. A. (1969). Plasma lactate and interstitial calcium. *New Engl. J. Med.* **281**, 221.

LEVI, L. (1969). Neuro-endocrinology of anxiety. In *Studies of Anxiety* (Editor Lader, M. H.). British Journal of Psychiatry Special Publication No. 3. Ashford, Kent.

MARSHALL, J. and SCHNIEDEN, H. (1966). Effect of adrenaline, noradrenaline, atropine and nicotine on some types of human tremor. *J. Neurol. Neurosurg. Psychiat.* **29**, 214-218.

PINTER, E. J. and PATTEE, C. J. (1967). Effect of β-adrenergic blockade on resting and stimulated fat mobilization. *J. clin. Endocr.* **27**, 1441-1450.

PINTER, E. J., PETERFY, G., CLEGHORN, J. M. and PATTEE, C. J. (1967). The influence of emotional stress on fat mobilization: the role of endogenous catecholamines and the β-adrenergic receptors. *Amer. J. med. Sci.* **254**, 634-651.

PITTS, F. N. and McCLURE, J. N. (1967). Lactate metabolism in anxiety neurosis. *New Engl. J. Med.* **277**, 1329-1336.

SHEPHERD, M., LADER, M. and RODNIGHT, R. (1968). *Clinical Psychopharmacology.* London.

SMYTHIES, J. R. (1969). The neurophysiology of anxiety. In *Studies of Anxiety* (Editor Lader, M. H.). British Journal of Psychiatry Special Publication No. 3. Ashford, Kent.

WEARN, J. T. and STURGIS, C. C. (1919). Studies on epinephrin. I. Effects of the injection of epinephrin in soldiers with "irritable heart". *Arch. intern. Med.* 24, 247-268.

Effect of Adrenergic Blockade in Anxiety

Adrenergic Receptors

Ahlquist (1948) studied the effects of a number of different sympathomimetic amines on the heart, circulation, intestine, iris and ureter of experimental animals and deduced that there were two types of receptors (alpha and beta) at peripheral sympathetic sites which responded to stimulation by adrenaline. Pure alpha-receptor stimulating drugs such as phenylephrine produce only certain of the effects of adrenaline, namely vasoconstriction of the arterioles (with a consequent rise in arterial blood pressure), dilatation of the pupils and relaxation of the smooth muscle of the intestine. These effects are blocked by alpha-adrenergic-receptor blocking drugs such as the ergot alkaloids, phenoxybenzamine, phentolamine and thymoxamine.

Pure beta-receptor stimulating drugs such as isoprenaline, orciprenaline and noradrenaline increase the rate and force of the heart beat, dilate the arterioles (particularly those in skeletal muscle) and relax bronchial, intestinal and bladder smooth muscle. These responses are prevented by beta-adrenergic receptor blocking drugs such as pronethalol (now withdrawn from clinical use because of its carcinogenic effect in mice) and propranolol (Epstein and Braunwald, 1966; Shanks, 1966; Lucchesi and Whitsitt, 1969; Fitzgerald, 1969). The biochemical effects of catecholamines may also depend on the stimulation of the beta-receptors. Thus there is good evidence that both the increase in concentration of plasma free-fatty-acids following the administration of adrenaline and the hyperglycaemic response to insulin are mediated through these receptors since they are both blocked by propranolol (Abramson, Arky and Woeber, 1966; Pinter and Pattee, 1967). A useful review of the clinical pharmacology of beta-receptor-blocking drugs has been published by Dollery, Paterson and Conolly (1969).

Beta-Receptor Blockade in Anxiety

Peripheral manifestations of anxiety that are due to beta-adrenergic stimulation are blocked by specific receptor antagonists. Thus propranolol and other beta-blockers slow the heart rate and prevent palpitations in anxious subjects (Turner, Granville-Grossman and Smart, 1965; Nordenfelt, 1965; Besterman and Friedlander, 1965; Frohlich, Dustan and Page, 1966; Bollinger, Gander, Pylkkänen and Forster, 1966; Granville-Grossman and Turner, 1966; Marsden, Gimlette, McAllister *et al.*, 1968; Nordenfelt, Persson and Redfors, 1968; Frohlich, Tarazi and Dustan, 1969a; Imhoff,

Blatter, Fucella and Turri, 1969). A similar effect has been noted with guanethidine, the adrenergic-neuronal blocking actions of which are used in the treatment of hypertension. Brill, Welch, Condon and Jones (1965) showed that its administration to patients with sinus tachycardia led to complete relief of symptoms in doses (10 to 20 mg daily) not large enough to produce significant hypotension.

Patients with effort syndrome often show minor electrocardiographic abnormalities, particularly in the erect posture. These changes (depression of the S-T segment and low voltage, diphasic or inverted T waves in leads II, III, aVF and V_3-V_7) are corrected by beta adrenergic blocking agents (Nordenfelt, 1965; Furberg, 1967; Nordenfelt et al., 1968; Noskowicz and Chrzanowski, 1968). Effort syndrome is also characterized by increased cardiac output and beta-blockers also correct this (Frohlich et al., 1966, 1969a; Schweitzer, Pivoňka and Gregorová, 1968).

Propranolol also affects other peripheral manifestations of anxiety. Marsden et al. (1968) observed that it decreased the amplitude of muscle tremor and prolonged the achilles reflex time, suggesting that the tremor and brisk tendon jerks of anxiety are mediated through the beta-receptors. Pinter, Peterfy, Cleghorn and Pattee (1967) found that propranolol significantly diminished the mobilization of free fatty acids in response to anxiety.

The mental symptoms of anxiety are also sometimes favourably influenced by beta-adrenergic blockade. Nordenfelt (1965) described three patients whose nervousness and functional palpitations improved with propranolol. The administration of H 56/28, another beta-adrenergic blocking drug, to 14 patients with nervous heart complaints improved their nervousness and depression as well as their somatic symptoms (Nordenfelt et al., 1968). Frohlich et al. (1966, 1969a) reported that the mental symptoms of their patients with "hyperdynamic beta-adrenergic circulatory state" responded to propranolol, as did the panic induced in these patients by isoprenaline infusion. Granville-Grossman and Turner (1966) carried out a double-blind cross-over trial of oral propranolol (20 mg four times daily) and placebo on psychiatric outpatients with anxiety states and noted a significantly better overall response to the drug, mainly due to the relief, by propranolol, of autonomic symptoms. Wheatley (1969) reported a double-blind trial carried out by general practitioners on 105 patients with acute or chronic anxiety of at least one week's duration. Fifty-one patients received propranolol 30 mg three times daily and the remainder received chlordiazepoxide 10 mg three times daily. Frequent assessments over six weeks showed no difference in overall improvement between the two treatment groups, but patients receiving chlordiazepoxide fared significantly better as regards depression and sleep disturbance, while propranolol produced significantly fewer side-effects.

Mode of Action of Propranolol in Anxiety

The major effects of propranolol are at peripheral adrenergic synapses, and the relief of mental symptoms by this drug may be due to beta-adrenergic blockade as Frohlich *et al.* (1966, 1969*a*) have proposed. This mechanism may also account for the improvement in the mental state of patients with thyrotoxicosis who have been treated by propranolol (see Chapter 7). But an alternative possibility has been pointed out by Granville-Grossman and Turner (1966, 1967) and by Davis (1969). Propranolol readily penetrates the central nervous system (Laverty and Taylor, 1968) where at high concentration, it has sedative and anticonvulsant actions (Leszkovszky and Tardos, 1965) similar to those of barbiturates. Hence the relief of anxiety by propranolol may be comparable to the effect of amylobarbitone sodium, which Wing and Lader (1965) demonstrated to have a more pronounced effect on the physical symptoms than on the mental distress. The central actions of propranolol may however be irrelevant since de Risio and Murmann (1967), in an uncontrolled trial, have shown that INPEA, a beta-adrenergic blocking agent without sedative effect, relieves both the peripheral and mental manifestations of anxiety. Thus, experience with these blocking drugs seems to support the James-Lange theory of anxiety or Breggin's modification of it.

Untoward Effects of Propranolol

The beta-adrenergic blocking actions of propranolol may have serious and sometimes dangerous effects. The removal of the sympathetic drive to the heart decreases the force of cardiac contraction and hence may precipitate cardiac failure (Conway, Seymour and Gelson, 1968); propranolol should therefore be used very cautiously in patients with a history of cardiac decompensation. Beta-blockade may cause coronary vasoconstriction (Parratt and Grayson, 1966) and although it has been used with good effect in cases of angina pectoris (Gillam and Prichard, 1965) the psychiatrist should be careful in prescribing propranolol for patients with myocardial ischaemia. Other untoward effects on the cardiovascular system are hypotension, bradycardia and partial heart block.

Propranolol is contraindicated in patients with bronchial asthma, because in these patients it causes a marked reduction in ventilatory function and may precipitate bronchospasm (McNeill and Ingram, 1966; Richardson and Sterling, 1969). Propranolol also interferes with the glycogenolytic effect of catecholamines liberated in response to hypoglycaemia and it therefore tends to potentiate the actions of insulin or oral hypoglycaemic drugs, the dose of which might need to be reduced (Kotler, Berman and Rubenstein, 1966). Propranolol may also interfere with the recognition of hypoglycaemia because it prevents the tachycardia and sweating. In the presence of peripheral arterial insufficiency or Raynaud's phenomenon, it should be used cautiously; Frohlich, Tarazi and Dustan (1969*b*) have described two patients with "hyperdynamic beta-adrenergic circulatory state" who, after several weeks' treatment with propranolol 120 to 240 mg daily, developed cyanosis, coldness and pain in their limbs, and, in one case, impending gangrene of a foot. These vascular changes regressed on stopping the drug.

Other side-effects of a non-specific nature have been reviewed by Stephen (1966) and include light-headedness, erythematous rashes, non-thrombocytopenic purpura, and of particular interest to the psychiatrist, visual hallucinations. Hinshelwood (1969) has described a patient who received propranolol for the treatment of angina and who was admitted to a psychiatric hospital with vivid visual and tactile hallucinations and delusions secondary to these abnormal experiences. On withdrawal of the drug the mental state became normal, but the hallucinations recurred when it was reintroduced. Tinnitus has been described as a side-effect of propranolol by Mostyn (1969).

REFERENCES

ABRAMSON, E. A., ARKY, R. A. and WOEBER, K. A. (1966). Effects of propranolol on the hormonal and metabolic responses to insulin induced hypoglycaemia. *Lancet*, **2**, 1386-1389.

AHLQUIST, R. P. (1948). A study of the adrenotropic receptors. *Amer. J. Physiol.* **153**, 586-600.

BESTERMAN, E. M. M. and FRIEDLANDER, D. H. (1965). Clinical experiences with propranolol. *Postgrad. med. J.* **41**, 526-535.

BOLLINGER, A., GANDER, M., PYLKKÄNEN, P. O. and FORSTER, G. (1966). Treatment of the hyperkinetic heart syndrome with propranolol. *Cardiologia (Basel)*, **49**, Supplement II, pp. 68-82.

BRILL, I. C., WELCH, J. D., CONDON, R. J. and JONES, F. C. (1965). Sinus tachycardia. Possible control with guanethidine (Ismelin). *Arch. intern. Med.* **115**, 674-679.

CONWAY, N., SEYMOUR, J. and GELSON, A. (1968). Cardiac failure in patients with valvular heart disease after use of propranolol to control atrial fibrillation. *Brit. med. J.* **2**, 213-214.

DAVIS, J. N. (1969). Increased β-receptor responsiveness. Central or peripheral? *Arch. intern. Med.* **123**, 101-102.

DE RISIO, C. and MURMANN, W. (1967). Anxiety and the pulse. *Brit. med. J.* **2**, 373.

DOLLERY, C. T., PATERSON, J. W. and CONOLLY, M. E. (1969). Clinical pharmacology of beta-receptor-blocking drugs. *Clin. Pharmacol. Ther.* **10**, 765-799.

EPSTEIN, S. E. and BRAUNWALD, E. (1966). Beta-adrenergic receptor blocking drugs. Mechanisms of action and clinical applications. *New Engl. J. Med.* **275**, 1106-1112; 1175-1183.

FITZGERALD, J. D. (1969). Perspectives in adrenergic beta-receptor blockade. *Clin. Pharmacol. Ther.* **10**, 292-306.

FROHLICH, E. D., DUSTAN, H. P. and PAGE, I. H. (1966). Hyperdynamic beta-adrenergic circulatory state. *Arch. intern. Med.* **117**, 614-619.

FROHLICH, E. D., TARAZI, R. C. and DUSTAN, H. P. (1969a). Hyperdynamic β-adrenergic circulatory state. Increased β-receptor responsiveness. *Arch. intern. Med.* **123**, 1-7.

FROHLICH, E. D., TARAZI, R. C. and DUSTAN, H. P. (1969b). Peripheral artery insufficiency. A complication of beta-adrenergic blocking therapy. *J. Amer. med. Ass.* **208**, 2471-2472.

FURBERG, C. (1967). Adrenergic beta blockade and electrocardiographical ST-T changes. *Acta med. scand.* **181**, 21-32.

GILLAM, P. M. S. and PRICHARD, B. N. C. (1965). Use of propranolol in angina pectoris. *Brit. med. J.* **2**, 337-339.

GRANVILLE-GROSSMAN, K. L. and TURNER, P. (1966). The effect of propranolol on anxiety. *Lancet*, **1**, 788-790.

GRANVILLE-GROSSMAN, K. L. and TURNER, P. (1967). Anxiety and the pulse. *Brit. med. J.* 1, 49.

HINSHELWOOD, R. D. (1969). Hallucinations and propranolol. *Brit. med. J.* 2, 445.

IMHOF, P. R., BLATTER, K., FUCELLA, L. M. and TURRI, M. (1969). Beta-blockade and emotional tachycardia: radiotelemetric investigations in ski jumpers. *J. appl. Physiol.* 27, 366-369.

KOTLER, M. N., BERMAN, L. and RUBENSTEIN, A. H. (1966). Hypoglycaemia precipitated by propranolol. *Lancet*, 2, 1389-1390.

LAVERTY, R. and TAYLOR, K. M. (1968). Propranolol uptake into the central nervous system and the effect on rat behaviour and amine metabolism. *J. Pharm. Pharmacol.* 20, 605-609.

LESZKOVSZKY, G. and TARDOS, L. (1965). Some effects of propranolol on the central nervous system. *J. Pharm. Pharmacol.* 17, 518-519.

LUCCHESI, B. R. and WHITSITT, L. S. (1969). The pharmacology of beta-adrenergic blocking agents. *Progr. cardiovasc. Dis.* 11, 410-430.

MARSDEN, C. D., GIMLETTE, T. M. D., McALLISTER, R. G., OWEN, D. A. L. and MILLER, T. N. (1968). Effect of β-adrenergic blockade on finger tremor and achilles reflex time in anxious and thyrotoxic patients. *Acta endocr. (Kbh.)* 57, 353-362.

McNEILL, R. S. and INGRAM, C. G. (1966). Effect of propranolol on ventilatory function. *Amer. J. Cardiol.* 18, 473-475.

MOSTYN, R. H. L. (1969). Tinnitus and propranolol. *Brit. med. J.* 2, 766.

NORDENFELT, I., PERSSON, S. and REDFORS, A. (1968). Effect of a new adrenergic β-blocking agent, H 56/28, on nervous heart complaints. *Acta med. scand.* 184, 456-471.

NORDENFELT, O. (1965). Orthostatic ECG changes and the adrenergic beta-receptor blocking agent, propranolol (Inderal). *Acta med. scand.* 178, 393-401.

NOSKOWICZ, T. and CHRZANOWSKI, W. (1968). The influence of propranolol on functional alterations of the electrocardiogram. *Cardiologia (Basel)*, 52, 324-329.

PARRATT, J. R. and GRAYSON, J. (1966). Myocardial vascular reactivity after beta-adrenergic blockade. *Lancet*, 1, 338-340.

PINTER, E. J. and PATTEE, C. J. (1967). Effect of β-adrenergic blockade on resting and stimulated fat mobilization. *J. clin. Endocr.* 27, 1441-1450.

PINTER, E. J., PETERFY, G., CLEGHORN, J. M. and PATTEE, C. J. (1967). The influence of emotional stress on fat mobilization: the role of endogenous catecholamines and the β-adrenergic receptors. *Amer. J. med. Sci.* 254, 634-651.

RICHARDSON, P. S. and STERLING, G. M. (1969). Effects of β-adrenergic receptor blockade on airway conductance and lung volume in normal and asthmatic subjects. *Brit. med. J.* 3, 143-145.

SCHWEITZER, P., PIVOŇKA, M. and GREGOROVÁ, J. (1968). The hemodynamic effects of beta-adrenergic blockade in patients with neurocirculatory asthenia. *Cardiologia (Basel)*, 52, 246-251.

SHANKS, R. G. (1966). The pharmacology of beta sympathetic blockade. *Amer. J. Cardiol.* 18, 308-316.

STEPHEN, S. A. (1966). Unwanted effects of propranolol. *Amer. J. Cardiol.* 18, 463-472.

TURNER, P., GRANVILLE-GROSSMAN, K. L. and SMART, J. V. (1965). Effect of adrenergic receptor blockade on the tachycardia of thyrotoxicosis and anxiety state. *Lancet*, 2, 1316-1318.

WHEATLEY, D. (1969). Comparative effects of propranolol and chlordiazepoxide in anxiety states. *Brit. J. Psychiat.* 115, 1411-1412.

WING, L. and LADER, M. H. (1965). Physiological and clinical effects of amylobarbitone sodium therapy in patients with anxiety states. *J. Neurol. Neurosurg. Psychiat.* 28, 78-87.

PSYCHOPHYSIOLOGICAL ASPECTS OF ANXIETY

A number of physiological functions, particularly those mediated through the autonomic system, vary with the state of mental alertness or "arousal". Arousal is progressively lowered as a normally alert subject becomes drowsy, falls asleep and becomes more deeply unconscious, while levels of arousal above the normal are associated with an increase in emotional activity and very high levels are experienced as anxiety, terror or indeed any other strong emotion. It must be emphasized however that emotions are subjective experiences which cannot be studied directly except by introspection. Hence objective physiological observations which appear to give some indication of the level of arousal cannot contribute to an understanding of how people feel nor throw any light on their descriptive or dynamic psychopathology. The physiological indicators of arousal have been reviewed recently by Lader (1969). Increasing levels are associated with increases in heart rate, forearm blood flow, electrical activity of the muscles and electrical conductance of the palmar skin and with a decrease in finger pulse volume. Two of these measures, namely palmar skin conductance and forearm blood flow have been studied intensively in recent years in relation to anxiety and these are discussed below.

Palmar Skin Conductance

The electrical conductance (which is the reciprocal of the resistance and is measured in mhos) of the skin of the palms of the hands and of the soles of the feet is a sensitive indicator of emotional change. A wide variety of stimuli such as noise and smells, as well as signals which evoke emotions will cause a sudden increase in skin conductance lasting for a few seconds after the stimulus has ceased. This phenomenon, the Psychogalvanic Reflex (PGR) is known also as the "galvanic skin response" or "electrodermal response". The peripheral mechanism by which the PGR may be produced has been discussed by Montagu and Coles (1966). Three theories have been proposed to account for the electrical changes:

(a) that they are due to muscular activity beneath the skin at the site of the electrode;

(b) that they are secondary to changes in vasomotor tone in the blood vessels of the skin and

(c) that they are related to changes in sweat gland activity.

The evidence now favours very strongly the last of these three hypotheses. Lader and Montagu (1962) showed that atropine introduced into the palmar skin by iontophoresis abolished the PGR, presumably because of paralysis by the atropine of the cholinergically innervated sweat glands. Paralysis of the adrenergically innervated skin blood vessels by bretylium tosylate similarly introduced had no such effect.

Verghese (1968) has also brought forward evidence that the PGR is dependent on a cholinergic sympathetic mechanism. He studied a patient who had undergone a therapeutic bilateral cervical sympathectomy and demonstrated that, in order to elicit the PGR, normal sympathetic innervation was essential. In his patient, the PGR could be obtained from the feet (where the sympathetic nervous system was intact) but not from the hands (where it was not). Furthermore, he showed that cholinergic receptors were involved: infusion of acetylcholine into the brachial artery increased the conductance markedly whereas intra-arterial adrenaline or noradrenaline had much less effect.

The independence of the PGR and vasomotor responses has been demonstrated by Furedy and Gagnon (1969) while a direct association between changes in sweating and skin conductance has been shown by Adams and Vaughan (1965). It is also of relevance to the hypothesis that the PGR is a reflection of sweat gland activity that, at normal room temperature, sweating of the palms of the hands and of the soles of the feet is determined only by the emotional state and has no heat-regulating function (Kuno, 1956.)

Most of the electrical resistance of the skin is in the stratum corneum. The other skin structures and the interior of the body have negligible resistance in comparison, so that when a current is passed between two surface electrodes the resistance measured is the sum of the resistances of the two areas of stratum corneum under the electrodes. (It is not, as might be supposed, the resistance of the surface of the skin between the electrodes.) The sweat ducts perforate the stratum corneum and when they contain sweat, current passes more readily; hence the more sweat glands that are active, the greater the conductance (Montagu and Coles, 1966; Lader and Wing, 1966).

REFERENCES

Adams, T. and Vaughan, J. A. (1965). Human eccrine sweat gland activity and palmar electrical skin resistance. *J. appl. Physiol.* **20**, 980-983.

Furedy, J. J. and Gagnon, Y. (1969). Relationships between and sensitivities of the galvanic skin reflex and two indices of peripheral vasoconstriction in man. *J. Neurol. Neurosurg. Psychiat.* **32**, 197-201.

Kuno, Y. (1956). *Human Perspiration.* Springfield, Illinois.

Lader, M. H. (1969). Psychophysiological aspects of anxiety. In *Studies of Anxiety* (Editor Lader, M. H.). British Journal of Psychiatry Special Publication No. 3. Ashford.

Lader, M. H. and Montagu, J D. (1962). The psychogalvanic reflex: a pharmacological study of the peripheral mechanism. *J. Neurol. Neurosurg Psychiat.* **25**, 126-133.

Lader, M. H. and Wing, L. (1966). *Physiological Measures, Sedative Drugs and Morbid Anxiety.* London.

Montagu, J. D. and Coles, E. M. (1966). Mechanism and measurement of the galvanic skin response. *Psychol. Bull.* **65**. 261-279.

Verghese, A. (1968). Some observations on the psychogalvanic reflex. *Brit. J. Psychiat.* **114**, 639-642.

Palmar Skin Conductance in Psychiatric Disorders

In general, the palmar skin conductance under resting conditions is greater in anxious subjects than in normal individuals, but absolute measures of this background skin conductance are of relatively little value in indicating the level of arousal, since they are dependent to some extent on other variables such as the electrical qualities of the individual's skin. Lader (1964, 1967, 1969a) has however shown that both the frequency of spontaneous fluctuations in skin conductance and the habituation rate of the PGR are closely dependent on level of arousal.

Spontaneous Fluctuations in Skin Conductance

Under resting conditions the skin conductance shows occasional momentary fluctuations independent of any obvious external stimulus. In normal subjects these spontaneous fluctuations occur infrequently—perhaps two or three times every minute—but in anxious patients the interval between them is much decreased. Lader (1967) studied 90 patients with anxiety or phobic conditions and showed a significantly positive correlation ($r = +0.58$; $p < 0.001$) between the frequency of spontaneous fluctuations and ratings of overt anxiety made by the investigator at the time of the recording. He also found that the number of spontaneous fluctuations correlated significantly with the degree of anxiety rated by the patient and with the frequency of past panic attacks.

Habituation of the PGR

The repeated application of a stimulus which evokes a PGR leads to a gradual diminution in the response. The rate at which this habituation occurs has been studied in normal subjects and in patients with anxiety, phobic conditions and other psychiatric disorders. Lader's technique (Lader, 1964, Lader and Wing, 1966) is to apply non-polarizing skin electrodes, one to the palmar surface of the thumb and the other to an area of the arm prepared by mild surface abrasion, and to pass a current of constant intensity between the two. The potential difference between the electrodes is recorded continuously and this, by Ohm's law, is at any time proportional to the resistance. After a period of rest (10 to 12 minutes), 20 auditory stimuli are presented to the subject at approximately one-minute intervals (the exact intervals varying randomly from 45 to 80 seconds). The stimuli are pure tones of 1000 cycles per second, of 100-decibel intensity and of one second duration and may be produced quite satisfactorily from a tape recording. The size of each PGR is measured as the change in log conductance (i.e. the difference between the logarithm of the skin conductance at the height of the PGR and the logarithm of the background conductance). Change in log conductance is an indication of the ratio of the two conductances.

Lader (1964) showed that the change in log conductance with successive stimuli decreases exponentially, indicating that there is a linear relationship between the logarithm of the stimulus number and the size of the PGR. The slope of this line gives the rate of habituation and is significantly greater in normal controls than in patients with anxiety states (Figure 5.1). In a study of 90 patients with anxiety or phobic conditions and 75 normal subjects, Lader

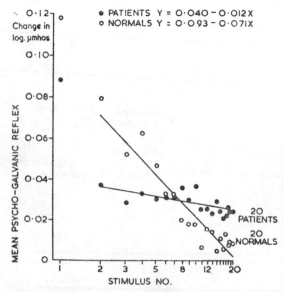

Figure 5.1 Habituation regression lines of the psycho-galvanic reflex relating to 20 patients with anxiety states and 20 normal subjects. (Lader and Wing, 1964)

(1967) found that habituation of the PGR was negatively correlated with ratings of anxiety, both overt and subjective, and with the frequency of spontaneous fluctuations. Thus slow habituation of the PGR and frequent spontaneous fluctuations both seem to be associated with anxiety or increased arousal, and the inverse linear relationship between these two physiological measures is demonstrated in Figure 5.2.

Included in Figure 5.2 are data on habituation and spontaneous fluctuation obtained by Lader and Sartorius (1968) on 10 patients with conversion hysteria (i.e. patients with neurological symptoms and signs without any demonstrable organic basis). Spontaneous fluctuations were significantly more frequent in these patients' recordings than in those of patients with anxiety or phobic states and even greater than in those of normal controls. There was also a tendency, though not statistically significant, for the hysterics to increase the size of the PGR as the stimuli were repeated, i.e. to show negative habituation. Although overt anxiety was not very obvious in these patients—consistent with the view that hysterics often demonstrate "belle indifference"—their self-ratings showed a high level of anxiety. The importance of this finding that hysterics seem to be grossly over-aroused cannot yet be assessed.

Lader and Wing (1969) have investigated 35 patients with a primary diagnosis of moderate or severe depression. Seventeen of the patients, categorized as predominantly agitated showed low habituation rates and very frequent spontaneous fluctuations, similar to the tracings of patients with severe

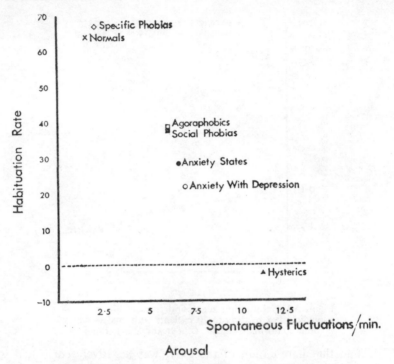

Figure 5.2 Relationship between habituation rate of PGR and frequency of spontaneous fluctuations in skin conductance. (Lader 1969a)

anxiety. Thirteen retarded depressives, however, showed significantly fewer spontaneous fluctuations than normal controls; most responded only slightly to the auditory stimuli and hence it was not possible to calculate habituation rates, although it seems likely that they were very high.

Some interesting observations on skin conductance have also been made in relationship to depersonalization and derealization. Lader and Wing (1964) reported an anxious woman whose habituation was being measured and who during the test procedure showed a sudden marked decrease in the number of spontaneous fluctuations in background conductance associated with a subjective experience of the phenomena of derealization which subsided at the end of the test. A further patient, described by Lader (1969a) complained of symptoms of depersonalization and her skin resistance at that time was very high and showed no spontaneous fluctuations. Recovery occurred after some weeks and she reverted to her usual anxious state; her skin resistance was then much lower and numerous spontaneous fluctuations were observed.

Effect of Drugs on Palmar Skin Conductance

Sedative Drugs

Lader (1964) observed that in normal subjects cyclobarbitone accelerated habituation of the PGR and decreased the number of spontaneous fluctuations, and that these effects were more notable with high doses. In a further series of experiments, Wing and Lader (1965) used a double-blind balanced cross-over procedure to observe the effects of amylobarbitone sodium 65 mg three times daily and placebo on 20 anxious patients. They noted a significant increase in habituation rate and a significant decrease in the number of spontaneous fluctuations during drug treatment and the symptoms of these patients lessened. They also showed that chlordiazepoxide has effects similar to amylobarbitone sodium, both on the symptoms of anxiety and on the skin conductance measures of arousal, and by means of an elegant comparative bioassay demonstrated that 65 mg (1 grain) of amylobarbitone sodium was equivalent to approximately 9 mg of chlordiazepoxide (Lader and Wing, 1965). Lader (1967) observed that sedatives such as chlordiazepoxide, meprobamate and the barbiturates appear to be most effective in those phobic or anxious patients who show the most general anxiety and whose skin conductance measures suggest the greatest arousal and he put forward the view that sedatives might be effective in these conditions because they diminish the level of arousal.

Stimulant Drugs

Lader (1969b) compared the effects of amphetamine sulphate, caffeine citrate and placebo on normal volunteers. Both drugs produced significant increases in the alertness reported by the subjects and both drugs significantly slowed the rate of habituation of the PGR and increased the frequency of spontaneous fluctuations. One of the 10 subjects however showed a paradoxical response to amphetamine in that although the habituation rate decreased and the number of spontaneous fluctuations increased, he became drowsy. Comparative bioassay showed that 10 mg of amphetamine sulphate was equivalent to about 600 mg of caffeine citrate (i.e. to about three average cups of coffee).

REFERENCES

LADER, M. H. (1964). The effect of cyclobarbitone on the habituation of the psycho-galvanic reflex. *Brain*, **87**, 321-340.

LADER, M. H. (1967). Palmar skin conductance measures in anxiety and phobic states. *J. psychosom. Res.* **11**, 271-281.

LADER, M. H. (1969a). Psychophysiological aspects of anxiety. In *Studies of Anxiety* (Editor Lader, M. H.). British Journal of Psychiatry Special Publication No. 3. Ashford.

LADER, M. H. (1969b). Comparison of amphetamine sulphate and caffeine citrate in man. *Psychopharmacologia (Berl.)*, **14**, 83-94.

LADER, M. H. and SARTORIUS, N. (1968). Anxiety in patients with hysterical conversion symptoms. *J. Neurol. Neurosurg. Psychiat.* **31**, 490-495.

F

LADER, M. H. and WING, L. (1964). Habituation of the psycho-galvanic reflex in patients with anxiety states and in normal subjects. *J. Neurol. Neurosurg. Psychiat.* **27**, 210-218.

LADER, M. H. and WING, L. (1965). Comparative bioassay of chlordiazepoxide and amylobarbitone sodium therapies in patients with anxiety states using physiological and clinical measures. *J. Neurol. Neurosurg. Psychiat.* **28**, 414-425.

LADER, M. H. and WING, L. (1966). *Physiological Measures, Sedative Drugs and Morbid Anxiety.* London.

LADER, M. H. and WING, L. (1969). Physiological measures in agitated and retarded depressed patients. *J. psychiat. Res.* **7**, 89-100.

WING, L. and LADER, M. H. (1965). Physiological and clinical effects of amylobarbitone sodium therapy in patients with anxiety states. *J. Neurol. Neurosurg. Psychiat.* **28**, 78-87.

Peripheral Blood Flow

Arousal is associated with a redistribution of blood in the body; the visceral and skin vessels constrict while those in the muscles dilate, and these changes have obvious value in preparing the organism for intensive muscular activity. The visceral vessels are difficult to study, but the vasomotor tone of the skin vessels may be measured by plethysmographic determination of the pulse volume of the finger, since blood flow in the digits is almost entirely through the skin. Ackner (1956) showed that the finger pulse-volume was much reduced in anxious patients compared with other psychiatric patients free of anxiety or with normal controls and that the administration of quinalbarbitone sodium to induce sleep increased it.

Forearm blood-flow is mainly through the muscles and this has been investigated extensively in recent years in relation to psychiatric conditions. The technique involves applying tourniquets, arterial at the wrist and venous at the elbow, and measuring the initial rate of swelling of the forearm. Two methods have been used to measure the rate of swelling: (a) by immersing the forearm in a water jacket and determining the rate at which the water is displaced (described by Kelly, 1967) and (b) by applying a mercury-in-rubber strain gauge around the forearm; as the forearm swells the gauge stretches and the electrical resistance of the mercury falls (Harper, Gurney, Savage and Roth, 1965; Brierley, 1969; Bloch and Davies, 1969). Measures by these two methods correlate well with one another, but using the strain gauge may have some advantages over the other method, in that it is more portable and more quickly applied (Brierley, 1969). As a measure of arousal, however, forearm blood flow has an important limitation in that it can be measured only intermittently. Readings can be taken only at intervals of one minute or more, whereas other measures such as skin conductance can be recorded continuously.

Forearm blood flow is increased by muscular exercise, alcohol and by certain drugs, including chlorpromazine. It is also altered by anaemia, thyrotoxicosis and other high cardiac-output states, and by other conditions including hypothyroidism (Kelly, 1967). Hence deductions about the level of arousal should be made only from measurements on resting subjects who are not under the influence of drugs and who have no disease which might interfere with the investigation.

Forearm Blood Flow in Psychiatric Disorders

Kelly (1966) studied 20 patients with severe chronic anxiety, 40 patients with various psychoneuroses without prominent anxiety, and 40 normal (non-psychiatric) controls. Under resting ("basal") conditions forearm blood flow (measured as millilitres per minute per 100 millilitres of forearm tissue) of the anxious patients was more than twice that of the other two groups. Stressing the subjects by asking them to subtract 17 serially from 393, and to give their answers in time with a metronome beating every two seconds, while being harassed and criticized continuously, increased the forearm blood flow. Furthermore, clinical improvement in anxiety (occurring spontaneously, as a result of treatment with amylobarbitone sodium, diazepam or chlordiazepoxide, or as a consequence of modified leucotomy) is associated with a decrease in forearm blood flow (Kelly, 1966; Kelly, Walter and Sargant, 1966; Rosenberg and Buttsworth, 1969; Kelly, Brown and Shaffer, 1969).

Kelly and Walter (1968, 1969) have studied further series of patients suffering from a variety of psychiatric conditions (including anxiety and agitated depression) together with a series of controls (Table 5.2). The

Table 5.2

"BASAL" FOREARM BLOOD FLOW AND SELF-RATINGS OF ANXIETY IN
NORMAL CONTROLS AND VARIOUS PATIENT GROUPS
(*Kelly and Walter*, 1968)

Diagnostic category	Number of patients	Mean "basal" forearm blood flow ml/100 ml/min	Mean self-rating of anxiety*
Chronic anxiety	41	4·45	3·98
Agitated depression	15	3·54	4·87
Schizophrenia	20	3·31	4·44
Obsessional neurosis	20	2·65	3·80
Phobic state	32	2·26	3·06
Hysteria	9	2·20	2·56
Non-agitated depression	43	2·13	3·55
Personality disorder	15	1·90	3·40
Depersonalization	8	1·84	4·25
Normal controls	60	2·21	1·64

* High scores indicate severe anxiety

anxious patients had the highest "basal" forearm blood flow, and this measure correlated significantly both with ratings of anxiety by the patients and with scores on the Taylor Scale of Manifest Anxiety. High rates of blood flow were also found in patients with agitated depression, as might be expected; schizophrenics also showed high values consistent with other evidence that schizophrenics are over-aroused (Venables, 1968). Patients with phobias had flow rates close to the normal, and these findings are consistent with those of Harper *et al.* (1965). Kelly (see Table 5.4) found that agoraphobics had slightly higher forearm blood flow rates than did other phobics or normal controls, but the difference was not statistically significant.

Kelly and his colleagues have put forward the view that "basal" forearm blood flow is a measure of anxiety particularly of the "free floating" kind, but this may be unwarranted. Gelder and Mathews (1968) studied the changes in forearm blood flow among 19 phobic patients; first, when anxiety was induced by getting the patients to visualize in their imagination phobic scenes and secondly, when they were subjected to stressful mental arithmetic. Forearm blood flow was greatest during the periods of stressful mental arithmetic, but the patients themselves reported little in the way of anxiety then. Visualization of feared scenes produced more modest increases in blood flow but subjective anxiety was very great, suggesting that forearm blood flow is not just an indicator of anxiety but possibly of other emotional states as well.

Somewhat contrary to the experience of Kelly and his colleagues, Bloch and Davies (1969) found no significant difference in "basal" forearm blood flow between anxious and non-anxious patients; there were however only 10 subjects in each group and there was a tendency for the anxious patients to give higher values.

Brierley (1969) has shown that loud noise increases forearm blood flow and that in normal subjects repeated stimulation leads to an exponential decline in response (i.e. habituation occurs). Agoraphobic patients, however, (whose "basal" forearm blood flow was somewhat higher than that of normal subjects) showed significantly less habituation.

REFERENCES

ACKNER, B. (1956). The relationship between anxiety and the level of peripheral vasomotor activity. An experimental study. *J. psychosom. Res.* 1, 21-48.

BLOCH, S. and DAVIES, B. (1969). Forearm blood-flow in anxious and non-anxious patients. *Aust. N.Z. J. Psychiat.* 3, 86-88.

BRIERLEY, H. (1969). The habituation of forearm muscle blood flow in phobic subjects. *J. Neurol. Neurosurg. Psychiat.* 32, 15-20.

GELDER, M. G. and MATHEWS, A. M. (1968). Forearm blood flow and phobic anxiety. *Brit. J. Psychiat.* 114, 1371-1376.

HARPER, M., GURNEY, C., SAVAGE, R. D. and ROTH, M. (1965). Forearm blood flow in normal subjects and patients with phobic anxiety states. *Brit. J. Psychiat.* 111, 723-731.

KELLY, D. H. W. (1966). Measurement of anxiety by forearm blood flow. *Brit. J. Psychiat.* 112, 789-798.

KELLY, D. H. W. (1967). The technique of forearm plethysmography for assessing anxiety. *J. psychosom. Res.* 10, 373-382.

KELLY, D., BROWN, C. C. and SHAFFER, J. W. (1969). A controlled physiological, clinical and psychological evaluation of chlordiazepoxide. *Brit. J. Psychiat.* 115, 1387-1392.

KELLY, D. H. W. and WALTER, C. J. S. (1968). The relationship between clinical diagnosis and anxiety, assessed by forearm blood flow and other measurements. *Brit. J. Psychiat.* 114, 611-626.

KELLY, D. and WALTER, C. J. S. (1969). A clinical and physiological relationship between anxiety and depression. *Brit. J. Psychiat.* **115**, 401-406.

KELLY, D. H. W., WALTER, C. J. S. and SARGANT, W. (1966). Modified leucotomy assessed by forearm blood flow and other measurements. *Brit. J. Psychiat.* **112**, 871-881.

ROSENBERG, C. M. and BUTTSWORTH, F. J. (1969). Effects of diazepam on anxiety as measured by forearm blood flow. *Aust. N.Z. J. Psychiat.* **3**, 89-91.

VENABLES, P. H. (1968). Experimental psychological studies of chronic schizophrenia. In *Studies in Psychiatry* (Editors Shepherd, M. and Davies, D. L.). London.

Eyelid Conditioning

The acquisition and extinction of conditioned eyelid responses in phobic patients has been studied by Martin, Marks and Gelder (1969). They used an apparatus, described by Martin (1963) consisting of specially constructed goggles on which is mounted a tube through which a puff of air (the un-conditioned stimulus—UCS) can be directed on to the cornea. The eyeblink response is detected by means of a photoelectric cell also mounted on the goggles. The conditioned stimulus (CS), a sound of pure tone delivered through headphones, precedes the puff of air by 440 m sec. Repeated presentation of the CS followed by the UCS leads to conditioning, i.e. an eyeblink occurring after the CS but before the UCS. Eyeblinks voluntarily made to avoid the puff also occur during this period but they have different characteristics and can be distinguished from conditional responses. For example, voluntary eyeblinks shut the eye completely and persist until after the UCS, whereas conditioned responses are usually partial and when the UCS is delivered the eyes have already started to open (Spence and Ross, 1959).

Martin *et al.* (1969) studied 62 phobic patients—19 with specific animal phobias, 28 with agoraphobia and 15 with social phobias. Each patient received 30 acquisition trials (CS+UCS) followed by 10 extinction trials (CS alone) and the number of conditioned eyeblinks during acquisition and during extinction were noted. The animal phobics showed rapid conditioning and slow extinction, while the agoraphobics tended to condition slowly. Patients with social phobias showed no particular conditioning characteristics. These findings suggest that animal phobias (but not other phobic conditions) arise as a consequence of the conditioning characteristics of the patient and Martin and her colleagues favour the view that these phobias result from failure to extinguish the relatively common normal fear of animals present in childhood.

Martin *et al.* (1969) also found a significant correlation between eyelid conditioning and the response to treatment and particularly to desensitization therapy; the best responses were among those who conditioned most rapidly.

REFERENCES

MARTIN, I. (1963). Eyelid conditioning and concomitant GSR activity. *Behav. Res. Ther.* **1**, 255-265.

MARTIN, I., MARKS, I. M. and GELDER, M. (1969). Conditioned eyelid responses in phobic patients. *Behav. Res. Ther.* **7**, 115-124.
SPENCE, K. W. and ROSS, L. E. (1959). A methodological study of the form and latency of eyelid responses in conditioning. *J. exp. Psychol.* **58**, 376-381.

PHOBIC STATES

Classification of Phobic States

Marks (1969), in his excellent monograph on *Fears and Phobias*, defines phobia as a special form of fear which

(*a*) is out of proportion to the demands of the situation

(*b*) cannot be explained or reasoned away

(*c*) is beyond voluntary control

(*d*) leads to avoidance of the feared situation.

Many adults have mild fears such as of snakes (even if harmless), spiders, mice, darkness, heights or lifts, but these normal fears do not lead to total avoidance of the situation. Specific fears, such as of strangers, of being left alone, of darkness or of snakes or dogs are even more common among children, but their frequency and intensity diminish markedly with increasing age and they may be considered as normal phenomena.

Marks distinguishes normal fears from phobias. This distinction seems to be a valid one as there is some evidence that at least some normal fears (e.g. of heights and snakes) occur regularly in many different animal species and that they may have an innate basis.

A further distinction may be made between phobic symptoms—which may occur as relatively minor features of various psychiatric illnesses, particularly in affective disorders, but sometimes in obsessive compulsive neurosis, schizophrenia and personality disorder—and phobic states, where the phobias themselves constitute the illness and other symptoms, if any, are of much less importance.

Marks (1969) classifies phobic states as in Table 5.3 which also gives the relative distribution of the different types in two unselected series, one at the Maudsley Hospital (Marks, 1969) and one collected by Snaith (1968).

Table 5.3

PHOBIAS IN ADULTS

	Relative incidence (%)	
	Marks (1969)	Snaith (1968)
Class I Phobias of external stimuli		
1. Agoraphobia	60	56
2. Social phobias	8	29
3. Animal phobias	3	2
4. Miscellaneous specific phobias	14	10
Class II Phobias of internal stimuli		
5. Illness phobias	15	2
6. Obsessive phobias	(Classified separately under obsessive compulsive neurosis)	

Marks distinguishes phobias of external stimuli (Class I) from phobias of internal stimuli (Class II). Class II phobias, about which less is known, are classified as illness phobias—where the sufferers fear illness such as cancer or venereal disease, or death or injury, and which merge with hypochondriacal conditions—and obsessive phobias. Obsessive phobias, which commonly take the form of a fear of contamination or fear of harming oneself or others, may dominate the clinical picture of obsessive compulsive neurosis. They differ from other phobias in that there is no direct fear of an object or situation, but only of the possible consequences. Thus an obsessive may fear that he might be contaminated by contact with dogs or that he might harm someone if a knife came into his possession, yet he does not fear dogs or knives as such. Obsessive phobias are usually classified under obsessive compulsive neurosis.

On the basis of the symptomatology and natural history, of the results of psychological testing and of psychophysiological investigations, and of the response to treatment, Marks has distinguished four types of Class I phobias and these are discussed in detail below. In particular Agoraphobia and Animal Phobias appear to be two distinct entities. Social Phobias (fears of certain social situations) and Miscellaneous Specific Phobias (e.g. fear of thunder, heights, darkness etc.) have also been delineated, but there is some doubt whether these are entities as distinct as the other two types.

Clinical Features of Phobic States

Agoraphobia

The clinical features of agoraphobia (sometimes known as phobic anxiety) have been well described in recent years by Gelder and Marks (1966), Snaith (1968), Roth (1969) and Marks (1969). Selected series of agoraphobics have been reported by Roberts (1964) who confined his study to 38 "housebound housewives" (agoraphobic married women who were unable to leave their homes unaccompanied) and by Roth (1959) who reported 135 cases of agoraphobia with prominent depersonalization ("phobic anxiety-depersonalization syndrome").

Symptomatology

The most prominent fear expressed by agoraphobics is that of going away from home or other shelter (Snaith, 1968). They are afraid of going into open spaces or on to the street, and they fear entering public places such as shops, crowds, trains, buses, theatres, cinemas or churches. Because of these fears they experience great difficulty in working, shopping or pursuing their leisure interests. When in the feared situation they are liable to experience intense anxiety or panic, the manifestations of which include light-headedness or faintness, general weakness and unsteadiness, as well as the more usual physical symptoms of anxiety; depersonalization and derealization may also occur. These panic attacks are relieved within minutes of leaving the feared situation, although they may not subside completely until the patient returns home. They are less likely to occur when the patient is accompanied, especially if by her husband or a close friend, and many sufferers feel more secure when out of doors if they can push a perambulator, a shopping basket on wheels or a bicycle. Agoraphobics who experience panic attacks in churches, theatres or cinemas may take care, when in these situations, to seat themselves near the aisle so that they can leave quickly if necessary. Hairdressing and barber shops pose a special problem for some of these patients because of the difficulty in leaving should panic occur, and many agoraphobics avoid them completely. When at home they feel less fearful though some are afraid of being alone.

Agoraphobics usually, if not always, show psychiatric symptoms other than their phobias. Anxiety, even when not in a feared situation, is extremely common, and Snaith (1968) has shown that "free-floating" anxiety and feelings of tension without apparent reason are very much more common and more severe among agoraphobics than in patients with other phobias. Indeed, Snaith (1968) and Lader and Mathews (1968) have suggested that agoraphobic fears are the direct product of the anxiety itself. Certainly, the severity of the agoraphobia tends to vary with the level of anxiety and if the anxiety subsides the phobias may remit.

Depersonalization or derealization—an unpleasant feeling of strangeness or unreality in the patient (or in his surroundings), which is recognized by the subject to be an abnormal phenomenon and which is associated with a lack of emotional feeling (Ackner, 1954)—occur commonly in agoraphobics. Forty-eight per cent of Snaith's (1968) series of 27 agoraphobics had experienced depersonalization compared with only 14 per cent of 21 patients with other phobias. Depersonalization is often precipitated by a bout of panic in a feared situation—in which case it is likely to be short-lived—or it may occur independently of anxiety and persist for long periods of time.

Frigidity is not uncommon in female agoraphobics: it was noted in 53 per cent of cases by Roberts (1964), in 55 per cent by Marks and Gelder (1965) and in three-quarters of the patients studied by Gelder and Marks (1966). However, frigidity usually precedes the onset of the phobias and may therefore be independent of them. Only a small proportion of agoraphobic men complain of impotence or premature ejaculation (Marks, 1969).

Mild depression, often related to the severity of the phobias, and minor obsessions and compulsions are not uncommon. Personality problems, expressing themselves particularly as difficulties in relationships with other people and in an inability to express aggressive feelings also occur frequently. Occasionally specific phobias, for example of thunder, may co-exist with agoraphobia, but they are not characteristic of the condition (Roberts, 1964; Snaith, 1968).

Natural History and Course

The prevalence of agoraphobia in the general adult population has been estimated at 0·63 per cent by Agras, Sylvester and Oliveau (1969), but most sufferers are not disabled by the condition. About two per cent of all psychiatric patients are agoraphobic and in most series about two-thirds are female. Most commonly, the illness starts between the ages of 18 and 35 years and the onset is rarely before puberty or after the age of 40; the mean age at onset of a series of Maudsley Hospital patients was 24 years (Marks, 1969). This is in marked contrast to the early age of onset of animal phobias, which is almost always before the age of eight years (Marks and Gelder, 1966).

The onset of agoraphobia is often quite sudden, and marked by an acute panic attack sometimes associated with symptoms of depersonalization. Snaith (1968) noted that in two-thirds of his agoraphobic patients, there was a sudden onset, while Mendel and Klein (1969) have described 25 cases where the condition began after an acute anxiety attack. Twenty-eight of Roberts' (1964) series of 38 patients remembered vividly the onset and 23 of these gave a history of mental strain immediately preceding the first panic attack. For example, one patient's illness started while travelling to visit her sick child in hospital and another began on receiving a letter informing her of her husband's infidelity; a number had their first symptoms during or shortly after an organic illness. In Roth's series (1959) precipitation by calamitous circumstances was often striking and in 83 per cent of his 135 patients the illness was consequent upon distressing events such as the death or serious illness in a close relative or friend, illness or acute danger to the patient herself, acute domestic or marital distress, or childbirth.

Following the initial panic attack the patient begins to experience fear of the situation in which it occurred and with further bouts of anxiety, the fears become generalized. In those patients where the illness does not start suddenly, it may take months or years to develop and occasionally the disorder may appear to be merely an exaggeration of the premorbid personality, which tends to be anxious, shy and dependent. Roberts (1964) noted that his patients tended to have anxious meticulous personalities, and half gave a history of well marked neurotic traits (usually phobic) in childhood. The high incidence of frigidity before the onset of the phobias also points to a disturbance in the premorbid personality.

Once agoraphobia has developed the condition tends to fluctuate in severity. Snaith (1968) noted complete remission, with a return to a normal state of mind, in 37 per cent of cases. These remissions were often unrelated to treatment or to any other observable circumstance but could last for weeks, months or years. (This is in contrast to phobias other than agoraphobia where similar remission occurred in only five per cent of Snaith's series.)

Prognosis

Roberts (1964) followed up 38 married agoraphobic women for $1\frac{1}{2}$ to 16 years after discharge from in-patient treatment. On admission to hospital all had been unable to leave their homes unaccompanied, and some were unable to go out at all, but on discharge, after treatment by supportive psychotherapy and encouragement to go out, 84 per cent had improved. At follow-up however only 24 per cent showed complete recovery with absolute freedom from phobic symptoms; 24 per cent were still housebound while 53 per cent showed some improvement compared with their initial condition in that, although still fearful, they were able to leave the house unaccompanied. The condition at follow up was related, to a statistically significant degree, to age at onset and to type of onset; the prognosis was better in patients whose illnesses began gradually after the age of 34 years. There was a tendency also (though statistically insignificant) for less severely phobic patients to do better. The outcome of treatment with behaviour therapy and the factors determining response in the individual patient are discussed later in this chapter.

Physiological and Psychological Measures

Agoraphobics, like patients with anxiety states, tend to score high on questionnaire tests of neuroticism and to be introverted. They also tend to have many neurotic symptoms as evidenced by their high scores on the Cornell Medical Index (Marks, 1969). Psychophysiological investigations (described earlier in this chapter) indicate a high level of arousal; the skin conductance shows frequent spontaneous fluctuations and the PGR habituates slowly. "Basal" forearm blood flow rates tend to be increased, though not to a degree which is significantly different from normal, and the rate of acquisition of eyeblink conditioned responses is normal. These findings, together with some of the clinical characteristics of agoraphobia, are summarized in Table 5.4.

Table 5.4

CLINICAL AND PSYCHOPHYSIOLOGICAL DATA. NORMAL SUBJECTS, ANXIETY NEUROTICS AND PHOBICS. MEAN VALUES.
(Marks, 1969)

	Anxiety states	Agora-phobia	Social phobia	Animal phobia	Normal subjects
Per cent women	50	75	60	95	50
Age at onset (years)	25	24	19	4*	-
Age at treatment (years)	36	32	27	30	-
Overt anxiety (0-6 scale)	2·6	2·0	2·0	0·4	0
Spontaneous fluctuations in skin conductance	36	32	33	12	6
Habituation rate of PGR	29	39	39	68	64
"Basal" forearm blood flow (ml/min/100 ml)	4·8*	2·9	2·6	2·2	2·0
Eyeblink conditioning	11	15	19	21**	14

* differs significantly from other groups
** differs significantly from all other groups except social phobia

Animal Phobias

Marks (1969) has reviewed 23 patients with animal phobias seen at the Maudsley Hospital. Ten feared birds (particularly pigeons) or feathers; six had spider phobias, two had dog phobias, and, in one case each, the phobia was of cats, worms and frogs. When in the feared situation animal phobics become anxious and even terror stricken, and they may go to extraordinary lengths to avoid it. In general the phobias are isolated and the patients are otherwise free of psychiatric disturbance although nightmares of the feared animal sometimes occur. Only four patients (all with bird phobias) in Marks' series had other important fears; two had social phobias and two were agoraphobic. Other specific animal phobias reported in the literature include phobias of moths, wasps and bees, but phobias of birds and of spiders appear to be the most common in psychiatric practice. Animal phobias probably represent the severest examples of the fear of animals which commonly occur in the adult population, but which, unlike phobias, are not disabling.

Marks (1969) found that patients with animal phobias were often fearful in childhood, but tended to come from stable and happy families. Forty per cent were frigid, however, and only 30 per cent appeared to have a satisfactory sexual life. Unlike agoraphobia, animal phobias almost always start before puberty. Of 18 patients described by Marks and Gelder (1966) all except one developed their phobia before the age of eight years and none started in adult life. Moreover, once the phobia is established it persists and its intensity does not vary in the same way as agoraphobia. Because of the early onset, the origins are not usually known, but sometimes there is a history of a sudden onset in relation to a specific event. Animal phobias are extremely common among children of both sexes, but most recover spontaneously. Marks (1969) suggests that those presenting to psychiatrists in adult life represent childhood phobias that have failed to improve. But adults with animal phobias are relatively rare and almost all of them are women (only one patient of the 23 described by Marks, 1969, was a man). Why a very small proportion of phobic girls do not improve is not known, but it may be due to a greater tolerance, by society, of fears among girls than among boys.

Psychological and Physiological Measures

Since animal phobics are generally free of other psychiatric symptoms (particularly of "free-floating" anxiety), it is not surprising that they score normally on questionnaire tests of Neuroticism and Extroversion, and that they score low on check-lists of symptoms. Consistent with these findings, the level of arousal, as measured by the frequency of spontaneous fluctuations in the skin resistance, the rate of habituation of the PGR and the forearm blood flow, is normal. These patients however show very rapid acquisition and slow extinction of eyeblink conditioned responses, and it may be that this abnormality determines the initial production of the phobia and its persistence. Table 5.4 summarizes some of the clinical characteristics of animal phobias, together with the results of psychological and physiological investigations.

Social Phobias

Patients with these phobias complain of a fear of being criticized in certain social situations which they therefore tend to avoid (Taylor, 1966; Marks,

1969; Roth, 1969). Of 14 patients with social phobias studied by Snaith (1968) the fear was of crowded places (in 4 subjects) of eating in public (3 subjects) and of being watched at work, of speaking in public, of persons in authority, of social situations, of making mistakes at work, of written examinations and of lecture halls (one patient in each category). Other social situations which are sometimes feared include playing games, speaking to strangers, and sitting on a bus or train in the view of others. Patients with social phobias often fear that they will show that they are afraid, for example by trembling, blushing, sweating, or vomiting, and they may feel it reasonable that others should criticize them for doing so.

Marks (1969) described a series of 23 social phobics, of whom nearly half gave a history of depression and 22 per cent of anxiety outside the feared situation. Two patients (nine per cent) had other phobias in addition to the social ones. The distribution of ages at onset was mainly in the range of 15 to 30 years. In most cases the illness started gradually, but some patients could relate the onset to a clear-cut incident which in itself was not unduly embarrassing. In other cases the illness appeared to develop after puberty as a gradual intensification of social sensitivity present since early childhood. Half of Marks' patients were anxious or shy in early life and there was some suggestion of a higher than normal incidence of broken homes. More than one-third of the female patients were frigid. Once established the illness tends to run a fairly continuous course without fluctuation.

In many ways, (e.g. as regards premorbid personality, age at onset and presence of other symptoms) the social phobias resemble agoraphobia, and psychological tests show a similar tendency to neuroticism and introversion in the two conditions. Skin resistance and forearm blood flow studies are also similar, but the rate of acquiring conditioned eyeblink responses is somewhat higher in social phobics than in agoraphobics and the results of desensitization treatment are better. These findings are summarized in Table 5.4.

Miscellaneous Specific Phobias

In this category are included monosymptomatic phobias of heights, of various natural phenomena such as darkness, thunder, lightning, high winds, storms and of doctors and dentists (Marks, 1969). Like animal phobias the fears are discrete and are not usually associated with other psychiatric symptoms. Moreover, once established, they do not show any spontaneous fluctuation in severity but, like animal phobias, respond to desensitization therapy. What little information is available from physiological tests suggests that they show normal levels of arousal (Lader, 1967; Marks, 1969). Apart from the symptomatology, two features distinguish them from animal phobias; first, they are distributed approximately equally between the sexes, and secondly, they may arise at any time between early childhood and old age.

REFERENCES

ACKNER, B. (1954). Depersonalization. I Aetiology and phenomenology. *J. ment. Sci.* **100**, 838-853.

AGRAS, S., SYLVESTER, D. and OLIVEAU, D. (1969). The epidemiology of common fears and phobias. *Comprehens. Psychiat.* **10**, 151-156.

GELDER, M. G. and MARKS, I. M. (1966). Severe agoraphobia: a controlled prospective trial of behaviour therapy. *Brit. J. Psychiat.* **112**, 309-319.

LADER, M. H. (1967). Palmar skin conductance measures in anxiety and phobic states. *J. psychosom. Res.* **11**, 271-281.

LADER, M. H. and MATHEWS, A. M. (1968). A physiological model of phobic anxiety and desensitization. *Behav. Res. Ther.* **6**, 411-421.

MARKS, I. M. (1969). *Fears and Phobias.* London.

MARKS, I. M. and GELDER, M. G. (1965). A controlled retrospective study of behaviour therapy in phobic patients. *Brit. J. Psychiat.* **111**, 561-573.

MARKS, I. M. and GELDER, M. G. (1966). Different ages of onset in varieties of phobia. *Amer. J. Psychiat.* **123**, 218-221.

MENDEL, J. G. C. and KLEIN, D. F. (1969). Anxiety attacks with subsequent agoraphobia. *Comprehens. Psychiat.* **10**, 190-195.

ROBERTS, A. H. (1964). Housebound housewives—a follow up study of a phobic anxiety state. *Brit. J. Psychiat.* **110**, 191-197.

ROTH, M. (1959). The phobic anxiety-depersonalization syndrome. *Proc. roy. Soc. Med.* 52, 587-595.

ROTH, M. (1969). Anxiety neuroses and phobic states. I Clinical features. *Brit. med. J.* 1, 489-492.

SNAITH, R. P. (1968). A clinical investigation of phobias. *Brit. J. Psychiat.* **114**, 673-697.

TAYLOR, F. K. (1966). *Psychopathology: its Causes and Symptoms.* London.

BEHAVIOUR THERAPY OF PHOBIC DISORDERS

The term Behaviour Therapy refers to a number of different types of treatment, which have in common the aim of relieving symptoms directly, and which have been developed by behaviourists from knowledge of the psychological mechanisms involved in learning, and in particular from Pavlov's work on conditioning. Useful reviews of the wide variety of treatments used by behaviour therapists have been published by Rachman (1963) and Gelder (1967).

Phobias are regarded by behaviourists as conditioned fear responses associated with avoidance behaviour analogous to those observed in experimental animals after repeated presentation of a neutral (conditioned) stimulus followed by a noxious (unconditioned) stimulus. Conditioned avoidance and apparent fear of the previously neutral stimulus tend to persist even if there is no further presentation of the noxious stimulus, for two reasons. First, because avoidance is rewarding in that it reduces the fear and secondly, because the fear cannot be extinguished unless the avoidance response is prevented (Baum, 1966).

In spite, however, of the obvious similarity between clinical and experimentally derived phobias, Gelder (1967) points out that there are discrepancies between knowledge derived from the psychological laboratory and clinical experience of behaviour therapy and he advises a pragmatic approach to the latter.

Two main techniques of behaviour therapy have been used in the treatment of phobias, namely systematic desensitization (also known as treatment by reciprocal inhibition, counterconditioning or deconditioning) and implosion (or "flooding"). Since the latter is used infrequently at present it will be considered separately later.

REFERENCES

BAUM, M. (1966). Rapid extinction of an avoidance response following a period of response prevention in the avoidance apparatus. *Psychol. Rep.* **18**, 59-64.
GELDER, M. G. (1967). Behaviour therapy. *Hosp. Med.* **1**, 306-313.
RACHMAN, S. (1963). Introduction to behaviour therapy. *Behav. Res. Ther.* **1**, 3-15.

Technique of Systematic Desensitization

There are two procedures preparatory to treatment; first, some measure is undertaken to reduce or counteract anxiety—usually training the patient to relax—and secondly a list or hierarchy of the feared stimuli is constructed and graded according to the amount of anxiety each produces. The treatment itself consists of exposing the anxiety-free patient to the stimuli, starting with the one that produces the least fear. The stimuli may be real situations (*in vivo* desensitization, desensitization in practice, graded retraining) or visually imagined scenes (imaginal desensitization, desensitization in imagination). Each stimulus is repeated until it no longer evokes any emotional disturbance and then the next stimulus in the hierarchy is dealt with in a similar way. The two preparatory procedures and the treatment itself are now considered in more detail.

Anxiety Reduction

Many methods to reduce anxiety have been used, but the most common is relaxation by verbal instruction, an abbreviation of the method of Progressive Relaxation described by Jacobson (1938). The patient is instructed to make himself comfortable in a chair or on a couch and then to note the sensations arising from his muscles when they are deliberately tensed and relaxed in turn; this is continued until he can fully relax the muscles voluntarily. The therapist may start by asking the patient to clench and unclench a fist and note the sensations from his forearm and hand. When he has learnt to relax those muscles, other groups are dealt with both individually and together so that eventually he has complete control over muscle tension and can become deeply relaxed at will. Detailed instructions of the procedure are given by Wolpe and Lazarus (1966), Rachman (1968) and Beech (1969). Usually about six 30-minute sessions are devoted to training and in addition the patient is asked to practise daily at home. When relaxation is poor it may be enhanced by the use of meprobamate or chlorpromazine given one hour before inter-view (Wolpe, 1961).

Use of Methohexitone

Intravenously administered methohexitone sodium (methohexital sodium, U.S.; "Brietal", "Brevital") has been used by Friedman (1966a, 1968), by Brady (1966) and by Bloomfield (1969) as an alternative to relaxation training. Methohexitone is an ultra-short acting barbiturate with effects which usually last for a few minutes only. The technique advocated by Friedman (1968) involves the initial injection of 0·5 ml of a 2·5 per cent solution (i.e. 12·25 mg). Further injections are given during the desensitization procedure should the patient become anxious. Since the needle is left in the vein, in vivo desensitization is usually not possible, although Friedman (1966b) reported the treatment of a deaf mute with a dog phobia who was exposed, while sedated with methohexitone, to pictures of dogs in ascending order of size and ferocity. The total dose given during a treatment session is on average 25 to 50 mg and is about one-quarter of that required to produce anaesthesia. Friedman (1968) advised giving a preliminary test dose of 0·1 ml at the beginning of the first treatment to detect possible allergy to the drug.

The suggested advantages of methohexitone over verbal instructions are first, that it is effective in patients unable to relax; secondly, that all anxiety disappears with the drug, whereas with verbal instruction some anxiety may persist even where there is good evidence of muscle relaxation; and thirdly, that it is more economical in time both as regards number and duration of treatment sessions (Friedman and Silverstone, 1967; Friedman, 1968). Using methohexitone, Friedman and Silverstone (1967) have reported a series of 20 phobic patients, all of whom were much improved after a mean of 13 treatment sessions, each of 15 to 20 minutes' duration, and they suggest that systematic desensitization using methohexitone is the treatment of choice for phobic symptoms.

No adverse effects of methohexitone were noted by Friedman (1968) in a series of 100 cases and he states that all patients are able to leave unac-companied and to drive within 10 minutes of the treatment ending. Using larger doses of methohexitone (100-200 mg) during each one-hour session, Sergeant and Yorkston (1968) have however noted a number of untoward effects. Six of their 18 patients failed to relax, and 10 showed slowing of their thinking and speech with consequent hindrance of the desensitization pro-cedure. Following the treatment, 12 patients complained of memory im-pairment, usually mild and short lived, but sometimes more severe and lasting for days or weeks. Fourteen patients complained of drowsiness and one, at the end of a long course, showed evidence of barbiturate dependence and withdrawal symptoms. It would seem prudent therefore to administer the drug in short courses where possible, to combine its use with verbal instruc-tion to relax, and to advise out-patients not to leave unaccompanied or to drive home.

Construction of Hierarchies

A hierarchy is a list of anxiety-provoking situations ranked in order according to the amount of anxiety each produces.

During treatment, the items of the hierarchy are presented to the patient in turn starting with those which are least feared, and if they are ranked properly the elimination of anxiety in any one situation should indicate that all less feared situations are also well tolerated. With single well-circumscribed phobias it is usually relatively easy to construct a hierarchy which has this ideal characteristic. Situations which the patient has not actually encountered but which he imagines would cause anxiety may be included, and in addition the therapist may use the principle of primary stimulus generalization to contrive further situations for inclusion in the hierarchy (Meyer and Gelder, 1963). This principle implies that exposure to situations similar to but not identical with the feared one will elicit less anxiety, and the greater the dissimilarity the less the anxiety provoked. Thus a hierarchy for a patient with a fear of heights may be constructed on the basis of the less the height the less the fear, while that for a patient with a fear of large black hairy spiders might include spiders of varying size, colour and hairiness, and at various distances from the patient. The principles of hierarchy construction have been propounded by Wolpe (1961, 1969), Wolpe and Lazarus (1966) and Beech (1969).

An example of a fairly simple hierarchy constructed by Wolpe and Lazarus (1966) for a young woman with a fear of examinations is as follows: (the situations are ranked in decreasing order of anxiety provocation).

1. On the way to the university on the day of an examination.
2. In the process of answering an examination paper.
3. Before the unopened doors of the examination room.
4. Awaiting the distribution of the examination papers.
5. The examination paper lying face down in front of her.
6. The night before an examination.
7. On the day before an examination.
8. Two days before an examination.
9. Three days before an examination.
10. Four days before an examination.
11. Five days before an examination.
12. A week before an examination.
13. Two weeks before an examination.
14. A month before an examination.

An example of a somewhat more complex hierarchy has been given by Wolpe (1961), constructed for a woman whose fears included fear of death:

1. Being at a burial (the most feared situation).
2. Being at a house of mourning.
3. The word *death*.
4. Seeing a funeral procession (the nearer, the more disturbing).

5. The sight of a dead animal.

6. Driving past a cemetery (the nearer, the more disturbing).

This patient's other fears included those relating to enclosed spaces, and to illness and for each of these a similar hierarchy had to be constructed.

Sometimes, careful interrogation is required to discover the actual source of the anxiety in a particular situation since merely ranking the situations may not lead to successful treatment. For example, a patient complaining of anxiety in certain social situations may say that he experiences most anxiety at weddings, least anxiety attending musical evenings and that parties are intermediate. Further examination of these situations may however reveal that it is the number of people present in the situation rather than the situation itself which determines the degree of anxiety, and the hierarchy should be constructed with this in mind (Wolpe, 1961).

Hierarchical construction is best spread over several sessions, most conveniently on the same occasions that the patient attends for relaxation training. At any time during treatment however the hierarchy can be modified, particularly when the gradation does not appear to be fine enough and new intermediate items need to be inserted.

Desensitization in Imagination

With the patient relaxed, he is asked to imagine as clearly as possible the least disturbing item on the hierarchy for about 5 to 15 seconds, the actual time depending on the degree of anxiety expected. Following this the patient is instructed to concentrate on relaxing for a further 15 to 30 seconds. If the patient has indicated that he has felt anxious during the presentation of the scene (by making a prearranged signal, say by raising his right index finger), it is presented again and the sequence (presentation of scene—pause—relaxation—pause) is repeated until the scene no longer causes anxiety. Whenever a clearly visualized scene evokes no disturbance the next scene on the hierarchy may be dealt with. The number of presentations before all anxiety is extinguished varies; in a study by Agras (1965) it ranged from 2 to 14 with a mean of 6·0. If a scene elicits a great deal of anxiety, the visualization should be stopped immediately, and after a period of relaxation a less anxiety-provoking item substituted. It is also important to ensure before each presentation that the patient has recovered from the effects of the previous one. During the course of a one-hour treatment session it is usually possible to deal with four or five items on a hierarchy. In between treatments the patients should attempt to enter those situations to which he has been desensitized.

Various investigators have studied skin conductance during desensitization Clark, 1963; (Agras, 1965; Hoenig and Reed, 1966); Seager and Brown, 1967. As might be expected exposure to a scene which evokes anxiety is associated with a psychogalvanic reflex and, in general, as desensitization occurs so the size of the reflex decreases. Hoenig and Reed (1966) however noted that two of their patients who showed clinical improvement with desensitization showed no concomitant diminution in the size of the PGR when exposed to the feared situation.

Desensitization In Vivo

Although there is some evidence that exposure to real-life situations is more effective than desensitization in imagination (Barlow, Leitenberg, Agras and Wincze, 1969), *in vivo* desensitization has been largely supplanted for a variety of reasons (Meyer and Crisp, 1966). First, it is a tedious and time-consuming procedure—it is hardly possible for example to deal with four or five elements in an agoraphobic's hierarchy in the course of one hour. Secondly, it may be impossible to devise the situations precisely as represented in the hierarchy, as for example when a fear of thunder or fear of vomiting is being treated. Lastly, in certain situations such as crowded streets, it may be difficult to remove the patient when anxiety occurs and both the fear and the avoidance behaviour may become intensified as a result. Nevertheless, for patients who find difficulty in visualization, or who do not feel anxious when they do imagine the scenes or who fail to relax, desensitization *in vivo* may be the only feasible method.

REFERENCES

AGRAS, W. S. (1965). An investigation of the decrement of anxiety responses during systematic desensitization therapy. *Behav. Res. Ther.* **2**, 267-270.

BARLOW, D. H., LEITENBERG, H., AGRAS, W. S. and WINCZE, J. P. (1969). The transfer gap in systematic desensitization: an analogue study. *Behav. Res. Ther.* **7**, 191-196.

BEECH, H. R. (1969). *Changing Man's Behaviour*. Harmondsworth.

BLOOMFIELD, E. (1969). The treatment of examination phobia by desensitization with methohexitone. A report of a case. *Practitioner*, **202**, 668-671.

BRADY, J. P. (1966). Brevital-relaxation treatment of frigidity. *Behav. Res. Ther.* **4**, 71-77.

CLARK, D. F. (1963). The treatment of monosymptomatic phobia by systematic desensitization. *Behav. Res. Ther.* **1**, 63-68.

FRIEDMAN, D. (1966a). A new technique for the systematic desensitization of phobic symptoms. *Behav. Res. Ther.* **4**, 139-140.

FRIEDMAN, D. (1966b). Treatment of a case of dog phobia in a deaf mute by behaviour therapy. *Behav. Res. Ther.* **4**, 141.

FRIEDMAN, D. (1968). A new technique for desensitization. In *Progress in Behaviour Therapy* (Editor Freeman, H.). Bristol.

FRIEDMAN, D. E. I. and SILVERSTONE, J. T. (1967). Treatment of phobic patients by systematic desensitization. *Lancet*, **1**, 470-472.

HOENIG, J. and REED, G. F. (1966). The objective assessment of desensitization. *Brit. J. Psychiat.* **112**, 1279-1283.

JACOBSON, E. (1938). *Progressive Relaxation* (2nd edition). Chicago.

MEYER, V. and CRISP, A. H. (1966). Some problems in behaviour therapy. *Brit. J. Psychiat.* **112**, 367-381.

MEYER, V. and GELDER, M. G. (1963). Behaviour therapy and phobic disorders. *Brit. J. Psychiat.* **109**, 19-28.

RACHMAN, S. (1968). *Phobias. Their Nature and Control.* Springfield, Ill.

SEAGER, C. P. and BROWN, B. H. (1967). An indicator of tension during reciprocal inhibition. *Brit. J. Psychiat.* **113**, 1129-1132.

SERGEANT, H. G. S. and YORKSTON, N. J. (1968). Some complications of using methohexitone to relax anxious patients. *Lancet,* **2**, 653-655.

WOLPE, J. (1961). The systematic desensitization treatment of neuroses. *J. nerv. ment. Dis.* **132**, 189-203.

WOLPE, J. (1969). *The Practice of Behavior Therapy.* New York.

WOLPE, J. and LAZARUS, A. A. (1966). *Behavior Therapy Techniques. A Guide to the Treatment of Neuroses.* Oxford.

Efficacy of Desensitization in Phobic Disorders

There are now a large number of published reports of uncontrolled studies of the treatment of phobic patients by desensitization. Typical is that described by Hain, Butcher and Stevenson (1966) who treated 27 patients with various types of phobia by desensitization in imagination. After a mean of 19 treatment sessions, 78 per cent showed improvement in their phobic symptoms and 70 per cent showed marked improvement in their general condition. In this type of investigation however, where no control patients are included, it is not possible to deduce whether the improvement was spontaneous, due to the desensitization itself, or due to other aspects of the treatment.

Controlled Retrospective Studies

Cooper (1963), Marks and Gelder (1965) and Cooper, Gelder and Marks (1965) have reported a retrospective controlled study of 41 phobic patients treated by desensitization at the Maudsley Hospital. The control patients, treated by methods other than desensitization, were similar as regards type and severity of phobia, duration of symptoms, age and sex. The severity of the symptoms, as reported in the case notes of each patient, was rated before treatment and at various later times up to and including one year after the end of treatment. In the group which had received desensitization, there were 29 cases of agoraphobia and 12 cases of other (specific) phobias (e.g. of animals, insects, thunder) and all of these except one were matched by similar cases in the control group. The exception was a patient with a specific phobia for whom a control could not be found. Desensitization consisted of graded retraining in all patients and 12 received desensitization in imagination as well. The controls had been treated by various other methods including sedative and other drugs, group or individual psychotherapy, occupational therapy etc. The improvements noted at the end of treatment and at one month and one year later are shown in Table 5.5. Agoraphobics fared slightly better (though to a statistically insignificant degree) when treated by desensitization. Patients with other phobias showed a very much better immediate response with desensitization than with other treatments, but one year later this difference was no longer significant.

Controlled Prospective Studies

Lazarus (1961) studied 35 subjects with various phobias such as fear of heights, claustrophobia and sexual phobias. He treated 18 by desensitization in imagination and 17 by group psychotherapy. Desensitization led to recovery in 13 subjects (72 per cent) while with psychotherapy only two subjects (12 per cent) recovered—statistically, a highly significant difference.

At the Maudsley Hospital, Gelder and his colleagues have reported a series of controlled prospective studies. Their first investigation (Gelder and Marks, 1966) compared the effects of desensitization in imagination combined with graded retraining with those of individual psychotherapy. There were

Table 5.5

OUTCOME OF TREATMENT OF PHOBIC PATIENTS
(Cooper *et al.*, 1965)

Type of phobia	*No. of cases*	*Mean no. of sessions*	*Mean duration of treatment (months)*	*Percentage improved at:*		
				End of treatment	*One month's follow up*	*One year's follow up*
Results of Desensitization						
Agoraphobia	29	56	6	69	59	72
Other phobias	12	27	4	100	91	67
Results of Control Treatments						
Agoraphobia	29	30	5	55	58	60
Other phobias	11	27	9	27	-	45

10 severely agoraphobic hospitalized patients in each group and treatment was carried out three times weekly for five to six months. The severity of the symptoms was rated by the patients, by the therapists and by independent assessors, using rating scales shown to be reliable, before and during treatment and at various times up to one year after treatment had been completed. Although desensitization produced slightly better initial results than psychotherapy, at the end of one year there was no difference in the effects of treatment. Both desensitization and psychotherapy gave better results in patients with fewer symptoms and with better work records prior to treatment.

In a second study, Gelder, Marks and Wolff (1967) randomly allocated 42 less severely phobic outpatients to three types of treatment:

(*a*) desensitization in imagination (16 patients)
(*b*) analytically orientated individual psychotherapy (10 patients)
(*c*) analytically orientated group psychotherapy (16 patients).

The groups matched one another as regards severity of phobia, presence of other symptoms, age and sex, and each contained both agoraphobics and patients with other phobias. Improvement with desensitization was much more rapid than with psychotherapy, although the intervals between treatments were the same in all groups. At the end of the follow-up period (an average of seven months after the completion of treatment) desensitization was still the most effective, but not to a statistically significant degree, and there were no significant long term differences in outcome between the three treatments.

In an extension of this investigation, Gelder and Marks (1968) desensitized seven of the patients who had not responded to group psychotherapy. They noted a more rapid response among these patients than among patients who had had no previous psychotherapy and they concluded that psychotherapy may facilitate desensitization. Lazarus (1961) also observed that the response to desensitization was more rapid if preceded by group psychotherapy and he came to the same conclusion.

Variables Related to Outcome

The response to desensitization appears to be related to a number of clinical features (Gelder et al., 1967). Agoraphobic patients, particularly those severely affected, fare less well than patients with other phobias. This finding is demonstrated in Table 5.6. Patients with many symptoms other than their phobias also respond less well, particularly if there is severe

Table 5.6

EFFICACY OF DESENSITIZATION IN PHOBIAS

	Percentage much improved at end of treatment	
	Desensitization	*Control*
Specific phobias (Retrospective study Cooper et al., 1965)	58	18
Mixed phobias (Prospective study Gelder et al., 1967)	56	19
Severe agoraphobia (Retrospective study Cooper et al., 1965)	41	21
Severe agoraphobia (Prospective study Gelder et al., 1967)	40	20

generalized anxiety or difficulties in interpersonal relationships, but obsessions, depression and hypochondriasis also tend to be associated with a poorer result. Gelder (1967, 1968) has pointed out the necessity for treating these other disturbances by sedative drugs, counselling, social work and possibly psychotherapy. These measures are probably better undertaken before desensitization but Brady (1968) has reported a case where psychotherapy after desensitization was effective. Modified leucotomy, to be considered only in the most severe and protracted cases resistant to other treatments, tends to benefit agoraphobia, particularly when there is severe general anxiety, and it may facilitate desensitization, probably because it reduces the level of anxiety (Marks, Birley and Gelder, 1966). Patients with anxious or shy premorbid personalities or who have prominent depressive symptoms appear to respond less well to operation.

That general anxiety tends to be associated with a poor response to desensitization has been demonstrated by Lader, Gelder and Marks (1967) who studied the palmar skin conductance of 36 phobic patients before treatment and related their findings to a number of clinical and psychological variables and to response. Patients who benefited most from desensitization tended to have low levels of arousal as evidenced by a rapid rate of habituation of the PGR, few spontaneous fluctuations in skin conductance and little in the way of anxiety outside feared situations. Patients with specific phobias tended to have low levels of arousal and treatment was more effective in this group. Lader *et al.* (1967) suggest that generalized anxiety interferes with desensitization in two ways. First, anxiety may inhibit desensitization itself, possibly by slowing habituation; this hypothesis is further discussed below. Secondly, anxiety predisposes to panic attacks during which new phobias are formed, and old phobias, previously treated successfully by desensitization, regenerated. Hence in anxious patients not only must desensitization be more prolonged and intense to be effective, but relapse is more likely.

Martin, Marks and Gelder (1969) have shown that the response to desensitization is better in patients who demonstrate rapid acquisition of conditioned eyelid responses. Patients with specific phobias tend both to condition rapidly and to respond to desensitization but even among agoraphobics, where response to treatment is generally less good, outcome is also related to the rate of conditioning.

REFERENCES

BRADY, J. P. (1968). Psychotherapy by a combined behavioural and dynamic approach. *Comprehens. Psychiat.* **9**, 536-543.

COOPER, J. E. (1963). A study of behaviour therapy in thirty psychiatric patients. *Lancet*, **1**, 411-415.

COOPER, J. E., GELDER, M. G. and MARKS, I. M. (1965). Results of behaviour therapy in 77 psychiatric patients. *Brit. med. J.* **1**, 1222-1225.

GELDER, M. G. (1967). Behaviour therapy. *Hosp. Med.* **1**, 306-313.

GELDER, M. G. (1968). Indications for behaviour therapy. In *Progress in Behaviour Therapy* (Editor, Freeman, H.). Bristol.

GELDER, M. G. and MARKS, I. M. (1966). Severe agoraphobia: a controlled prospective trial of behaviour therapy. *Brit. J. Psychiat.* **112**, 309-319.

GELDER, M. G. and MARKS, I. M. (1968). Desensitization and phobias: a cross-over study. *Brit. J. Psychiat.* **114**, 323-328.

GELDER, M. G., MARKS, I. M. and WOLFF, H. H. (1967). Desensitization and psychotherapy in the treatment of phobic states: a controlled enquiry. *Brit. J. Psychiat.* **113**, 53-73.

HAIN, J. D., BUTCHER, R. H. G. and STEVENSON, I. (1966). Systematic desensitization therapy: an analysis of results in twenty-seven patients. *Brit. J. Psychiat.* **112**, 295-307.

LADER, M. H., GELDER, M. G. and MARKS, I. M. (1967). Palmar skin conductance measures as predictors of response to desensitization. *J. psychosom. Res.* **11**, 283-290.

LAZARUS, A. A. (1961). Group therapy of phobic disorders by systematic desensitization. *J. abnorm. soc. Psychol.* **63**, 504-510.
MARKS, I. M., BIRLEY, J. L. T. and GELDER, M. G. (1966). Modified leucotomy in severe agoraphobia: a controlled serial enquiry. *Brit. J. Psychiat.* **112**, 757-769.
MARKS, I. M. and GELDER, M. G. (1965). A controlled retrospective study of behaviour therapy in phobic patients. *Brit. J. Psychiat.* **111**, 561-573.
MARTIN, I., MARKS, I. M. and GELDER, M. (1969). Conditioned eyelid responses in phobic patients. *Behav. Res. Ther.* **7**, 115-124.

Mechanism of Action of Systematic Desensitization

There is now clear evidence that both relaxation and repeated exposure to graded phobic stimuli are essential for systematic desensitization to be effective. Lang and Lazovik (1963) treated 11 students with an intense fear of snakes, by relaxation combined with repeated exposure and noted a significant reduction of the fear compared to that obtained by treating 13 similar subjects by relaxation alone. Relaxation combined with repeated exposure has been noted to be more effective than relaxation alone in other similar studies on subjects with snake phobias (Davison, 1968) on spider phobics (Rachman, 1965) on students with examination anxiety (Johnson and Sechrest, 1968) and on rat phobics (Cooke, 1968). Moore (1965) has reported significantly greater improvement in ventilatory function among patients with bronchial asthma treated with relaxation and repeated exposure than with relaxation alone.

In similar studies, repeated exposure to graded phobic stimuli combined with relaxation has been shown to be more effective than repeated exposure alone (Rachman, 1965; Lomont and Edwards, 1967; Davison, 1968), but Cooke (1968) who studied normal subjects with an intense fear of rats found that repeated exposure was equally beneficial whether combined with relaxation or not. It is important to note that none of these studies were on patients referred for treatment, and that conclusions drawn from them may not be applicable to neurotic subjects. Mathews and Gelder (1969) however, have noted no effect of relaxation training on the symptoms of anxious or phobic patients.

Originally, Wolpe (1958) introduced relaxation on the basis of assertions made by Jacobson (1938), that the subjective experience of emotion is largely derived from intensive proprioceptive stimulation, and that complete *muscular* relaxation is incompatible with anxiety. Davison (1966), however, has pointed out that muscular paralysis produced by curare does not interfere with the experience of anxiety. Reluctant to abandon the idea that muscular relaxation inhibits anxiety he suggests two possible explanations, alternative to Jacobson's hypothesis. First, that muscular relaxation may produce a pleasant affective state, and secondly that emotional experience may be determined by activity of the efferent (rather than afferent) nerves to the muscles. There is however some doubt whether the muscles are in any way important in relaxation and Rachman (1968) argues that muscular relaxation may not be essential for desensitization to be effective. He cites evidence supporting this view, notably that treatment may be successful even if the patient has had little or no training in muscle relaxation, and that the electromyographic activity of the muscles may not change during relaxation. He suggests that what may be essential is a feeling of calmness or *mental* relaxation and that this can be achieved even if the muscles are active.

While both relaxation and repeated exposure to graded phobic stimuli seem to be important in systematic desensitization there is some evidence that other effects, such as those of sympathetic support, of the relationship of the patient to the therapist, and of suggestion, may also play a part. Paul (1966) compared the effects of various treatments on normal subjects who experienced anxiety while speaking in public. Though systematic desensitization was much superior to brief insight-oriented psychotherapy, the latter was significantly more effective than no treatment. Gelder, Marks and Wolff (1967) and Gelder and Marks (1968) have also shown that psychotherapy is beneficial in phobic states. That a psychotherapeutic relationship between the patient and therapist may be important has been emphasized by Meyer and Gelder (1963) who noted that the results of behaviour therapy of phobic patients were better where the patient-therapist relationship was particularly good. Moreover, Agras and Leitenberg (1969) have shown that encouragement and praise by the therapist may benefit the treatment.

Suggestion may also play a part in systematic desensitization. Paul (1966) observed that treatment by suggestion and placebo, though not as beneficial as systematic desensitization, had a significantly better effect than no treatment. Marks, Gelder and Edwards (1968) allocated at random 28 phobic patients to two treatment groups. One group received systematic desensitization; the other was treated by hypnosis with forceful suggestion that the phobias would gradually disappear. Patients who did not improve with one treatment were then given the other. Both treatments led to significant reduction in the intensity of the phobias, but although there was a tendency for greater improvement with systematic desensitization, this was not statistically significantly different from that obtained by suggestion.

Theories of Systematic Desensitization

Two broad theories, neither of which has yet been confirmed or refuted, have been proposed to explain the efficacy of systematic desensitization. The first, by Wolpe (1958) is dependent on the supposition that phobias are conditioned responses, the result of a repeated previous association between an object or situation (the conditioned stimulus) and unconditioned stimuli producing a fear reaction. Wolpe (1958) suggests that relaxation inhibits anxiety and that the repeated presentation of a phobic stimulus to a relaxed patient will, by "reciprocal inhibition", weaken the bond between that stimulus and anxiety. Thus Wolpe's theory suggests that systematic desensitization is effective because it teaches the patient to relax rather than to become anxious in the feared situation; i.e. that it is a counter-conditioning process, or alternatively that it leads to extinction of the conditioned response.

The second theory, by Lader and Mathews (1968) suggests that relaxation reduces the level of arousal and that if the level of arousal is sufficiently low, repeated presentation of the phobic stimulus will be associated with habituation of the response such that eventually the stimulus will cease to produce anxiety. Certainly relaxation does appear to reduce the level of arousal as evidenced by a decrease in the number of spontaneous fluctuations in the electrical resistance of the skin (Mathews and Gelder, 1969); also the rate of habituation is increased as the level of arousal is reduced (Lader, 1969). This is an attractive theory because it is consistent with various clinical observations e.g. that the response to systematic desensitization is better in patients (a) with low anxiety, (b) with high habituation rates of the PGR to auditory stimuli, and (c) whose arousal level has been reduced by sedative drugs (Lader and Mathews, 1968).

REFERENCES

AGRAS, S. and LEITENBERG, H. (1969). The role of selective positive reinforcement in the modification of phobic behaviour. *Canad. psychiat. Ass. J.* **14**, 69-70.

COOKE, G. (1968). Evaluation of the efficacy of the components of reciprocal inhibition psychotherapy. *J. abnorm. Psychol.* **73**, 464-467.

DAVISON, G. C. (1966). Anxiety under total curarization: implications for the role of muscular relaxation in the desensitization of neurotic fears. *J. nerv. ment. Dis.* **143**, 443-448.

DAVISON, G. C. (1968). Systematic desensitization as a counter-conditioning process. *J. abnorm. Psychol.* **73**, 91-99.

GELDER, M. G. and MARKS, I. M. (1968). Desensitization and phobias: a cross-over study. *Brit. J. Psychiat.* **114**, 323-328.

GELDER, M. G., MARKS, I. M. and WOLFF, H. H. (1967). Desensitization and psychotherapy in the treatment of phobic states: a controlled enquiry. *Brit. J. Psychiat.* **113**, 53-73.

JACOBSON, E. (1938). *Progressive Relaxation* (2nd edition). Chicago.

JOHNSON, S. M. and SECHREST, L. (1968). Comparison of desensitization and progressive relaxation in treating test anxiety. *J. cons. clin. Psychol.* **32**, 280-286.

LADER, M. H. (1969). Psychophysiological aspects of anxiety. In *Studies of Anxiety* (Editor, Lader, M. H.). British Journal of Psychiatry Special Publication No. 3. Ashford.

LADER, M. H. and MATHEWS, A. M. (1968). A physiological model of phobic anxiety and desensitization. *Behav. Res. Ther.* **6**, 411-421.

LANG, P. J. and LAZOVIK, A. D. (1963). Experimental desensitization of a phobia. *J. abnorm. soc. Psychol.* **66**, 519-525.

LOMONT, J. F. and EDWARDS, J. E. (1967). The role of relaxation in systematic desensitization. *Behav. Res. Ther.* **5**, 11-25.

MARKS, I. M., GELDER, M. G. and EDWARDS, G. (1968). Hypnosis and desensitization for phobias: a controlled prospective trial. *Brit. J. Psychiat.* **114**, 1263-1274.

MATHEWS, A. M. and GELDER, M. G. (1969). Psycho-physiological investigations of brief relaxation training. *J. psychosom. Res.* **13**, 1-12.

MEYER, V. and GELDER, M. G. (1963). Behaviour therapy and phobic disorders. *Brit. J. Psychiat.* **109**, 19-28.

MOORE, N. (1965). Behaviour therapy in bronchial asthma. A controlled study. *J. psychosom. Res.* **9**, 257-276.

PAUL, G. L. (1966). *Insight vs. Desensitization in Psychotherapy*. Stanford.
RACHMAN, S. (1965). Studies in desensitization. I The separate effects of relaxation and desensitization. *Behav. Res. Ther.* **3**, 245-251.
RACHMAN, S. (1968). The role of muscular relaxation in desensitization therapy. *Behav. Res. Ther.* **6**, 159-166.
WOLPE, J. (1958). *Psychotherapy by Reciprocal Inhibition*. Stanford.

Implosive Therapy

Implosion or flooding is a form of behaviour therapy which has been developed in recent years and which shows indications of being faster and more effective than desensitization in the treatment of phobic disorders. The essence of the treatment is that the patient is repeatedly exposed, either in imagination or in real life, to the most intensely phobic situations for up to one hour at a time. The patient initially experiences severe anxiety, as evidenced by his reports and behaviour and by psychophysiological measures; after some minutes the anxiety tends to subside but can be revived by introducing variation into the stimulus. Hogan (1968) and Boulougouris and Marks (1969) give detailed examples of how the method may be applied.

Although the theoretical basis is uncertain, implosive therapy may be analogous to the extinction of conditioned fear responses in experimental animals by the repeated presentation of the unconditioned stimulus, while at the same time the avoidance response is prevented by physical restraint. Some therapists however emphasize the psychodynamic determination of the symptoms and present to the patient anxiety-producing material that seems to have been repressed. Thus in treating fear of snakes the therapist may attempt to arouse anxiety by instructing the patient to imagine scenes in which the snake behaves as a phallus (Hogan, 1968). The introduction of other repressed anxiety-provoking situations is advocated by Stampfl and Levis (1967); these include the presentation of scenes in which aggressive or sexual impulses are expressed towards the parents and other members of the family, and instructing the patient to experience in imagination events involving castration, fellatio and homosexuality. In the present state of knowledge it is not certain what relevance these dynamic elements have to the effectiveness of the treatment.

Most reports on the use of implosive therapy have been concerned with the treatment of well-circumscribed fears, such as of snakes, rats or spiders, in normal volunteers. Hogan and Kirchner (1967) reported a series of 43 students who were fearful of rats, of whom 21 were treated by one hour's implosive therapy. Fourteen of these subjects showed marked improvement whereas none of 22 untreated controls showed any change in their symptoms. In a further study of 30 female students with snake phobias, Hogan and Kirchner (1968) obtained better results using implosive therapy than two other psychological treatments. To be effective, exposure to the feared situation must be prolonged. Indeed Rachman (1966) showed that fear of spiders might be aggravated if the subject was asked to imagine a maximally feared situation for only two minutes at a time.

There have been very few reports on the treatment of patients with phobic disorders by implosion. Malleson (1959) described a student with an intense fear of examinations who presented in acute panic 48 hours before he was due to sit an important examination. He was instructed to imagine all the terrible consequences if he failed—the humiliation, the disappointment of his family, the financial loss etc.—and within half-an-hour he was calm. Over the next 48 hours the patient assiduously practised experiencing the fear every half hour or so and before the examination (which he passed without difficulty) he was almost unable to be frightened by the situation. Boulougouris and Marks (1969) have treated four phobic patients—two agoraphobic, one with a spider phobia and one with a fear of vomiting—by implosive therapy. Initially treatment consisted of exposure in imagination to the feared situations and the patients were asked to try and experience these fantasies at home in between the treatment sessions. With time the patients could imagine the scenes without experiencing anxiety and they were then exposed to the feared situation in real life. Three of the four patients became almost free of symptoms after a mean of 14 treatment sessions. This was much better and faster than could have been expected with conventional treatment. The patient who feared vomiting did not respond, but she had much free-floating anxiety and the authors suggest that this may have been responsible for the poor outcome.

Wolpe (1969) has reported two patients who responded to implosive therapy. One, a dentist who was unable to give injections because of a fear that his patients might die as a result, was treated successfully by getting him to imagine the most feared situation as vividly as possible, while the second patient, an agoraphobic, improved with *in vivo* implosive therapy. He points out however that some of his patients have been made worse by the treatment.

Clearly, before more definite conclusions can be drawn concerning the usefulness of implosive therapy, further investigation is necessary.

REFERENCES

BOULOUGOURIS, J. C. and MARKS, I. M. (1969). Implosion (flooding)—a new treatment for phobias. *Brit. med. J.* 2, 721-723.

HOGAN, R. A. (1968). The implosive technique. *Behav. Res. Ther.* 6, 423-431.

HOGAN, R. A. and KIRCHNER, J. H. (1967). Preliminary report on the extinction of learned fears via short-term implosive therapy. *J. abnorm. Psychol.* 72, 106-109.

HOGAN, R. A. and KIRCHNER, J. H. (1968). Implosive, eclectic verbal and bibliotherapy in the treatment of fears of snakes. *Behav. Res. Ther.* 6, 167-171.

MALLESON, N. (1959). Panic and phobia. A possible method of treatment. *Lancet*, 1, 225-227.

RACHMAN, S. (1966). Studies in desensitization—II: flooding. *Behav. Res. Ther.* 4, 1-6.

STAMPFL, T. G. and LEVIS, D. J. (1967). Essentials of implosive therapy: a learning-theory-based psychodynamic behavioural therapy. *J. abnorm. Psychol.* 72, 496-503.

WOLPE, J. (1969). *The Practice of Behavior Therapy.* New York.

Drug Therapy of Phobias

Behaviour therapy is a time-consuming procedure and before embarking on it, it is often worth trying the effect of drugs. *Anxiety relieving drugs* are of particular value when taken half to one hour before entering the feared situation and many patients have observed that alcohol has a similar effect. For patients who enter the phobic situation frequently, more regular medication—three or more times daily—may be desirable. Of the sedatives available barbiturates (e.g. sodium amylobarbitone, 60 mg) are the most effective in preventing panic but their use may lead to addiction, particularly in agoraphobics who may require several doses a day and whose illnesses tend to persist for years. Indeed Sim and Houghton (1966) noted a 20·9 per cent incidence of dependence on sedative drugs or alcohol in their series of 191 patients with phobic anxiety. Other effective anxiety-relieving drugs are meprobamate ("Equanil", "Miltown") 400 mg, chlordiazepoxide ("Librium") 10 mg, diazepam ("Valium") 5 mg and oxazepam ("Serenid D") 10 mg—all of which may be taken up to six doses per day, although in large amounts they tend to cause drowsiness. Nitrazepam ("Mogadon") 5 mg, usually prescribed as an hypnotic, may be useful where other anxiety relieving drugs have failed.

Antidepressant drugs may be effective in phobic states—particularly in the agoraphobic syndrome, even in the absence of any overt depression. King (1962) described a series of 28 patients with phobic anxiety and depersonalization who had been ill for an average of five years (range five months to 30 years); most had had previous psychiatric treatment without benefit. Within one month of starting treatment with phenelzine 15 mg three times daily, the phobic symptoms were relieved in 75 per cent of cases, and within three months in 84 per cent. Complete relief of depersonalization was noted in almost 90 per cent of patients. Sargant (1969*a*, *b*) has given a preliminary report on over 200 patients with phobic anxiety treated by monoamine oxidase inhibitors and followed up for one year or more; in 80 per cent improvement was noted. He advocates the administration of the monoamine oxidase inhibitor in divided doses during the day, with the addition of a single dose of a tricyclic antidepressant (amitriptyline or trimipramine, 50 to 150 mg) at night, if there is early morning wakening. During the first few weeks of treatment it is preferable to prescribe chlordiazepoxide or diazepam as well. Frommer (1967) in a controlled trial noted that phenelzine 15 mg with chlordiazepoxide 10 mg (both twice daily) was more effective in treating phobic children than phenobarbitone 30 mg twice daily. Similarly beneficial results have been reported using imipramine. Klein (1964) treated 22 patients with the agoraphobic syndrome by imipramine 75 to 150 mg daily. He noted that the panic attacks ceased within 3 to 14 days of starting treatment and that 6 out of 10 patients relapsed within one month of stopping the drug.

Other drugs. Intravenous injections (two or three times weekly) of acetylcholine (Sim and Houghton, 1966) or thiopentone (King and Little, 1959) have also been advocated in the treatment of agoraphobia, but they have not been widely used.

REFERENCES

FROMMER, E. A. (1967). Treatment of childhood depression with antidepressant drugs. *Brit. med. J.* **1**, 729-732.

KING, A. (1962). Phenelzine treatment of Roth's calamity syndrome. *Med. J. Aust.* **1**, 879-883.

KING, A. and LITTLE, J. C. (1959). Thiopentone treatment of the phobic anxiety-depersonalization syndrome. *Proc. roy. Soc. Med.* **52**, 595-596.

KLEIN, D. F. (1964). Delineation of two drug-responsive anxiety syndromes. *Psychopharmacologia (Berl.)*, **5**, 397-408.

SARGANT, W. (1969*a*). Physical treatments of anxiety. In *Studies of Anxiety* (Editor Lader, M. H.). British Journal of Psychiatry Special Publication No. 3. Ashford.

SARGANT, W. (1969*b*). Treatment of the phobic anxiety state. *Brit. med. J.* **2**, 49.

SIM, M. and HOUGHTON, H. (1966). Phobic anxiety and its treatment. *J. nerv. ment. Dis.* **143**, 484-491.

CHAPTER 6

GRIEF

Typical (Uncomplicated) Grief

GRIEF is the normal response to the loss of a love object such as a close relative or friend or sometimes an animal pet, material valuables or even a non-material possession such as reputation (Averill, 1968). It usually comes to the attention of psychiatrists only when it is anomalous in some way and for this reason the common reaction to bereavement ("typical" or "uncomplicated" grief) has been defined only recently. Marris (1958) interviewed 72 women living in the East End of London, aged 25 to 56 years, whose husbands had died on average two years and two months previously; Gorer (1965) has reported a study on 359 British men and women who had lost a first-degree relative during the previous five years, and 80 of these he investigated in detail; Clayton, Desmarais and Winokur (1968) traced the relatives of a number of hospital patients who had died, and interviewed them within a few days of the loss and again two to four months later, while Parkes (1969) has reported a study of 22 unselected widows whom he interviewed at set intervals during the first year of bereavement. The health of unselected widows has been studied by Parkes (1964b) and by Maddison and Viola (1968), while descriptions of typical grief have also been given by Lindemann (1944), Parkes, (1965a), Hinton (1967) and Averill (1968).

From these accounts can be derived a description of the usual reaction to the death of a close relative. Following the loss there may be a period of apparent failure to realize fully that the death has occurred. When this happens it lasts usually for only a few hours or days but sometimes for as much as two weeks, and during this time the bereaved person may experience no distress and indeed by his behaviour give strength to the rest of the family. An example has been reported by Marris (1958) who describes how a young woman went home after learning of the death of her husband and there read the newspapers as if nothing had happened. Alternatively, during the latent period the bereaved may experience a sense of numbness and inability to appreciate any emotional reaction. This numbness is perhaps akin to the phenomena of depersonalization and derealization which were reported by six per cent of the subjects in the series studied by Clayton *et al.* (1968).

With the realization of the extent of the loss, the full reaction appears characterized by various mental and physical changes which are discussed in detail below. The usual duration of these disturbances has been estimated variously. Lindemann (1944) found that most of the subjects he studied were distressed for only four to six weeks; Clayton *et al.* (1968) noted that improvement usually occurred after six to ten weeks; Gorer (1965) has asserted that grief usually remains severe for six to twelve weeks, while Parkes (1965a) states that the intensity of the symptoms declines after one to six weeks and is minimal by six months. Nevertheless, it appears that a proportion of mourners continue to grieve for long periods of time. Only 14 of the 72 widows studied by Marris (1958) considered themselves to be recovered at the time they were interviewed some two years after bereavement, while 19 per cent of Gorer's subjects reported that their grief had been unlimited in duration and that they would never completely recover.

The characteristics of grief include preoccupation with memories of the deceased, perceptual disturbances, mental distress, physical symptoms, behavioural changes and hostility, and these are now considered in turn.

Preoccupation with Memories of the Deceased

The thoughts of the bereaved are concentrated on the person who has died, particularly during the early months of the loss. Parkes (1969) noted that 19 of the 22 widows he studied experienced an overwhelming preoccupation during the first month and that one year later 12 spent much of their time thinking of their husband. He also found that most of the widows retained a very clear visual mental picture of the deceased and that this correlated significantly with the amount of preoccupation. Marris (1958) observed that widows welcomed the opportunity to talk at length about their loss and that 5 of the 72 he interviewed seemed to be obsessed with memories of their husband or of the circumstances in which he died. Marris also noted that in their preoccupation the bereaved tended to idealize the lost person and to overlook his faults. Vivid dreams of the deceased were reported to Gorer (1965) by 31 of the 80 mourners he interviewed, particularly by women who had lost their husbands. The majority found that the dreams were comforting and only six informants were distressed by them.

Perceptual Disturbances

A proportion of bereaved persons report unusual sensory experiences which are understandable in the light of their preoccupation. Most commonly they take the form of illusions, where for example the mourner hears ill-defined sounds in the house and misinterprets them as the dead person's footsteps, or where strangers in the street are fleetingly misidentified as the deceased; nine of Parkes' (1969) 22 widows reported such experiences. Sometimes hallucinatory phenomena, usually auditory or visual, are described. Five of the 80 bereaved subjects interviewed by Gorer (1965) reported visual hallucinations of the dead and one described auditory hallucinations, while Marris (1958) gives some examples, including one of a woman who would hear her dead husband turn his key in the door and the swish of his coat along the balcony. Of the 40 bereaved persons studied by Clayton et al. (1968) three per cent reported hallucinatory experiences. Phenomenologically they are pseudohallucinations since the subject realizes that they have no basis in reality. They are more often comforting than frightening, but even so may lead the person who experiences them to fear that he is becoming mentally deranged.

Another strange experience is a feeling of the presence of the dead person which was reported by 50 per cent of the women in Marris' (1958) series and by 68 per cent of the widows studied by Parkes (1969). The latter found that this phenomenon was associated, in a statistically significant way, with clear visual memories of the deceased and with preoccupation with thoughts relating to him, and that it tended to be a comforting experience in that it was often associated with a lessening of the yearning and of the mental distress. Difficulty in accepting the loss which was reported by 24 per cent of Marris' widows is perhaps a related phenomenon.

Mental Distress

Depression, with or without associated symptoms such as crying, insomnia, lack of interest in work or leisure pursuits, anorexia, tiredness, self neglect, attacks of panic, apathy, a sense of futility, guilt feelings and suicidal ideas, is a more or less constant feature of the grief and is aggravated by reminders of the loss. Parkes (1964b) studied the family doctors' medical records of 44 unselected widows and calculated that during the six-month period following the bereavement the consultation rate for psychiatric symptoms such as anxiety, depression, insomnia and tiredness was about three times that during the period before the loss. The increase was particularly notable among the younger and middle-aged widows (i.e. those under the age of 65 years) where there was a 240 per cent increase in number of consultations for mental symptoms; among older widows, the increase was only 25 per cent. More severe mental disorder is usually referred to psychiatric attention and will be discussed later, but 9 of the 80 unselected mourners interviewed by Gorer (1965) were very seriously depressed when he saw them at least twelve months after the bereavement.

Maddison and Viola (1968) have reported data on the health of 375 widows during the year following the death of their husbands and of 199 matched married-women controls. Table 6.1 sets out those symptoms which were significantly more common among the widows. Increased difficulty in sleeping was reported by 40·8 per cent of the bereaved compared with 12·6 per cent of controls. In other series insomnia has also been a prominent symptom; it was complained of by 85 per cent of the subjects studied by Clayton *et al.* (1968), by 80 per cent of Gorer's (1965) widows and widowers and by 79 per cent of Marris' (1958) subjects. Twenty-one of the 44 unselected widows whose medical records were examined by Parkes (1964b) received a sedative drug from their family doctor at some time during the 18 months following bereavement; in this series increased use of sedatives was particularly common among the younger widows.

The more severely distressed mourners tend to have suicidal ideas which can often be understood as arising from guilt feelings and self-recriminations, that they were responsible in some way for the death or that they did not do enough for the deceased when he was alive. Such guilt was expressed by 11 per cent of the widows studied by Marris (1958) and by 13 per cent of those in the series reported by Clayton *et al.* (1968). Some feel suicidal because they believe (often with some justification) that life holds nothing for them or because they wish to join the dead person in an after-life.

Physical Symptoms

Lindemann (1944) emphasized the physical distress suffered by mourners. The somatic symptoms include feelings of tightness in the throat, choking sensations with shortness of breath, sighing and an empty feeling in the abdomen; they tend to occur in bouts lasting 20 minutes to one hour at a

Table 6.1

PREVALENCE OF VARIOUS SYMPTOMS AMONG WIDOWS DURING YEAR FOLLOWING
BEREAVEMENT AND AMONG CONTROLS.

(Only those symptoms which are significantly more common (p < 0·01)
among the widows are included)

(Maddison and Viola, 1968)

	Widows *N=375*	*Controls* *N=199*
	%	%
General nervousness	41·3	16·1
Depression	22·7	5·5
Feelings of panic	12·0	2·5
Persistent fears	12·0	3·0
Nightmares	8·8	1·0
Insomnia	40·8	12·6
Trembling	10·4	2·0
Repeated peculiar thoughts	8·5	2·0
Fear of nervous breakdown	13·1	2·0
Reduced work capacity	46·7	26·1
Gross fatigue	29·6	11·6
Increased drug intake	37·3	11·1
Increased alcohol intake	6·7	2·0
Increased smoking	11·7	1·5
Headache	17·6	9·0
Indigestion	9·9	4·5
Vomiting	2·7	0
Excessive appetite	5·4	0·5
Anorexia	13·1	1·0
Weight loss	13·6	2·0
Palpitations	12·5	4·0
Chest pain	10·1	4·5
Dyspnoea	12·0	4·5
Frequent infections	2·1	0
General aching	8·4	4·0

time and are associated with aggravation of the mental distress. The physical complaints of the widows studied by Maddison and Viola (1968) are set out in Table 6.1. Other investigators have also described the somatic aspects of grief. Lasting deterioration in health was reported by 43 per cent of the widows studied by Marris (1958); the physical symptoms of these women included loss of weight, rheumatism and fibrositis, indigestion and recurrence of peptic ulceration, rashes and headache. Nineteen per cent of the mourners interviewed by Clayton *et al.* (1968) complained of multiple somatic symptoms, such as headache, blurred vision and dyspnoea. In Gorer's (1965) series, loss of weight was reported by 36 per cent of all the subjects and by 71 per cent of widows and widowers. Parkes (1964*b*) found that there was a significant increase of physical complaints after loss of a husband, especially of symptoms referable to the muscles and joints. Hinton (1967) has pointed out that occasionally mourners complain of symptoms similar to those which the dead person experienced during his illness, presumably due to unconscious identification with the deceased, but this phenomenon may be more character-istic of "atypical" than of "typical" grief. While many of the physical com-plaints of the bereaved undoubtedly have no organic basis, grief is associated with an increased mortality risk and this is discussed further below.

Behavioural Changes

These include restlessness, withdrawal from social contact and conduct aimed at keeping alive the memories of the deceased. Parkes (1969) noted that 20 of the 22 widows he studied showed motor hyperactivity during the first month of bereavement, confirming an observation by Lindemann (1944) that grief is associated with restlessness and continuous aimless movement. Consistent with these findings is Marris' report (1958) that 18 per cent of the widows he interviewed had impulses to wander away from home to escape the distressing memories and that some had moved away permanently. With-drawal from social contact and rejection of consolation was found in 37·5 per cent of Marris' widows, sometimes due to preoccupation with thoughts of the deceased, and sometimes because meeting people, particularly married couples, reminded them of their loss.

Although revival of memories tends to increase the grief, many mourners feel drawn towards the environment associated with the deceased. Six of the widows studied by Parkes (1969) felt the need to visit places which they and their husbands had frequented, several felt attracted to the cemetery where he was buried or to the hospital where he had died, and 19 treasured posses-sions belonging to him. Similar impulses to keep alive memories by clinging to the belongings of the deceased, by frequently gazing at his photographs or by returning to old haunts have been described also by Marris (1958) and by Gorer (1965). Indeed, of the 80 mourners interviewed by Gorer, six (four widowers and two widows) had preserved their houses and the possessions of the dead (clothes, pipes, tobacco etc.) exactly as if the dead person were still alive; Gorer uses the term "mummification" to describe this phenomenon.

Some mourners cultivate the feeling that the dead person is present by talking to him or by otherwise behaving as if he were present (Marris, 1958; Gorer, 1965; Parkes, 1969). In addition, it is not uncommon for bereaved persons to forget their loss unwittingly, and for example to prepare a cup of tea for a husband who has been dead for some time; 15 of Marris' widows reported such behaviour.

Since recovery from grief might be hastened by the development of new interests and by the establishment of new relationships, much of the behaviour of mourners, such as the withdrawal from social contact, the rejection of consolation and the cultivation of memories, seems to be maladaptive. Averill (1968) attempts to explain these paradoxical aspects by suggesting that they have a biological purpose, namely that the cohesiveness of society may depend to some extent on the existence of mechanisms which cause intensely painful and long-lasting reactions to the dissolution of strong interpersonal relationships. Another theory, not inconsistent with this, has been proposed by Parkes (1969) who suggests that the behaviour of bereavement is analogous to that associated with separation anxiety in children or young animals and is the expression of a search for the lost object. Thus Parkes argues that the motor hyperactivity, the preoccupation with memories of the deceased, the illusions and misidentifications and the focusing of attention on those parts of the environment which have been associated with the dead person are all manifestations of the urge to recover that which is lost. Since the bereaved realize that searching for a dead person is irrational, few will admit that this is what motivates their behaviour, but four of Parkes' widows did in fact do so.

Hostility

Anger and resentment may be expressed by the grief-stricken, who may accuse the doctor of incompetence or even assault or take legal action against him. Some feel hostile towards God or the clergy and may change or denounce their religion, while occasionally members of the family are accused of contributing to the death (Lindemann, 1944; Marris, 1958; Hinton, 1967). Other aspects of this animosity are feelings of irritability, resentment and bitterness associated with a loss of normal compassion for the sufferings of others and a pervasive feeling of the injustice of their loss. Of the widows studied by Marris (1958), 18 per cent expressed such general resentment and 15 per cent blamed specific people.

Variation in Symptomatology

The intensity of these disturbances varies. First it depends on the closeness of the relationship between the bereaved and the deceased. Gorer (1965) found that the most distressing and long-lasting grief is that of a parent for a full-grown child, that reactions to the death of infants or of young children are usually much less severe and that loss of a spouse is commonly much more painful than death of a sib or parent. But grief may be experienced even when there existed a hostile relationship; of the 72 widows interviewed by Marris (1958), five admitted that their marriages had been unhappy and yet they showed typical reactions to the loss. Secondly, the age of the mourner appears to influence the intensity; it tends to be greatest among young adults and less severe in childhood and old age (Parkes 1965b). Thirdly, the severity may depend on how the bereaved perceives the environment. In studies on widows, Maddison and his colleagues found that deterioration in physical or mental health was associated with reports of failure by others to be helpful during the first few months after their husbands' deaths (Maddison and Walker, 1967; Maddison, Viola and Walker, 1969).

Atypical (Complicated) Grief

Typical grief, as described above is a normal phenomenon; the disturbance generally lasts for less than six months and is not so severe that the mourner stays away from work for more than two weeks, attempts suicide, isolates himself so as to be inaccessible to relatives or friends, or is referred to a psychiatrist (Parkes, 1965a). But occasionally the reaction is distorted, or exaggerated and therefore does come to psychiatric attention. Wretmark (1959) has described 28 patients with such "atypical" or "complicated" grief and Parkes (1965a) has studied 21 similar patients whose mental illness had begun within six months of the death of a close relative. The characteristics and symptoms of these patients differ in some ways from those of typical grief-stricken subjects. First, there is a preponderance of women (93 per cent of Wretmark's and 81 per cent of Parkes' patients were female). Secondly, delayed reactions appear to be more common: there was an interval of more than two weeks between the bereavement and the onset of symptoms in 43 per cent of Wretmark's patients and in 38 per cent in Parkes' series. Thirdly, the duration of the disturbance tends to be longer than normal: 52 per cent of Parkes' patients had reactions lasting more than one year (including 28 per cent where they lasted for two years or more, and one patient whose symptoms persisted for six years) while the illness of one of the patients reported by Wretmark lasted for 19 years. Fourthly, the intensity of the reaction tends to be more severe among patients than among typical grief-stricken persons, and tends to lead to social isolation and a well-marked impairment of the capacity to work.

Parkes (1965a) showed that certain symptoms, particularly difficulty in accepting the loss and feelings of guilt, were more common in atypical than typical reactions. Persisting difficulty in accepting the loss, sometimes to the point of refusing to believe that the death had occurred was noted in two-thirds of his patients, and a similar proportion expressed ideas of guilt and self-blame. Marked hostility to individuals connected with the death (doctors, nurses, clergy etc.) also appeared to be more common; it was expressed by 38 per cent of Parkes' patients including one who was preoccupied with the idea of killing her sister's murderer. From this study, Parkes (1965a) also concludes that the presence of hypochondriacal symptoms similar to those suffered by the deceased during his last illness, and attacks of acute anxiety precipitated by reminders of the loss are characteristic of atypical grief. Suicidal ideas too tend to be more pronounced: 28 per cent of Wretmark's

(1959) patients expressed suicidal ideas and 11 per cent had attempted suicide, compared with an incidence of suicidal thoughts of only 13 per cent in the series of unselected mourners studied by Clayton *et al.* (1968). The increased risk of suicide after bereavement is discussed below.

Although grief (either typical or atypical) is the usual response to bereavement, Parkes (1965*b*) points out other psychiatric reactions may occur. These latter illnesses are however non-specific in that they are also seen in the absence of bereavement. They include psychosomatic disorders, psychoneuroses (such as agoraphobia—see Chapter 5), affective disorders (usually depressive psychosis but very rarely mania) and alcoholism.

The extent to which recent bereavement may be a cause of mental disturbance leading to admission to psychiatric hospital has been investigated by Parkes (1964*a*). He examined the case records of 3245 patients admitted to Bethlem Royal and Maudsley Hospitals during the years 1949-51 and noted that 94 (2·9 per cent) developed their illnesses within six months of the death of a parent, spouse, sib or child. Comparison of these patients with the other (non-bereaved) admissions showed a preponderance of women among the bereaved and a significant association between bereavement and a diagnosis of affective disorder. On the basis of the Registrar-General's statistics for England and Wales, Parkes calculated how many of the total number of patients would be expected to have lost a parent or spouse during the six months before admission. Table 6.2 compares the expected numbers with those observed, and shows that actual loss of a spouse was some six times greater than expected, suggesting that the bereavement was a causative factor

Table 6.2

COMPARISON OF OBSERVED AND EXPECTED NUMBERS OF BEREAVED PATIENTS
ADMITTED TO BETHLEM ROYAL AND MAUDSLEY HOSPITALS 1949-51
(Parkes, 1964*a*)

| | Male patients | | Female patients | | All patients | |
	Observed	Expected	Observed	Expected	Observed	Expected
Losing a father	10	8·1	13	7·0	23	15·1
Losing a mother	10	10·6	11	13·2	21	23·8
Losing a spouse	6	1·5	24	3·4	30	4·9
Total	26	20·2	48	23·6	74	43·8

in the aetiology of these patients' illnesses. These data also indicate that loss of a husband is more likely to lead to hospital admission than loss of a wife. Although the numbers admitted following death of a parent did not differ very much from those expected, a possible cause and effect relationship here is suggested by Parkes' observation that over half of these patients had been living with the parent who died for more than one year before the death. Further evidence that recent parental death may be a cause of mental illness, particularly of severe depression, has been adduced by Birtchnell (1970*a*, *b*).

Stein and Susser (1969) have also investigated the relationship between bereavement and subsequent mental disorder. They examined the records of all adults in Salford (Lancs.) who came into contact with agencies providing psychiatric care during 1959-63. They found that mental disorders were much commoner among widows and widowers than among married persons of the same age and sex, particularly depressive illnesses in women, addiction (mainly alcoholism) in men and organic and senile dementias in both men and women. Comparison of the time elapsed since bereavement with data relating to a random sample of households in the community showed a significantly increased rate of referral to psychiatric care during the first year after the death. These authors also reported that mental illness consequent on the loss of a spouse had a better prognosis and was less likely to lead to chronic disability than illness not associated with bereavement.

The Mortality of Bereavement

Grief is associated with an increased mortality risk. This is partly due to the higher prevalence of suicide among mourners than in the general population. MacMahon and Pugh (1965) showed that loss of a spouse predisposes to suicide in the period immediately following the bereavement, particularly in males. They estimated that the suicide risk is maximal in the year following the loss, when it is about 2·5 times higher than that four or more years later. But death from other causes is also more common in the bereaved. A follow-up study of 4486 men over the age of 54 years whose wives had died in 1957 has been reported by Young, Benjamin and Wallis (1963) and by Parkes, Benjamin and Fitzgerald (1969). During the first four years following bereavement more of these widowers died than would be expected on the basis of data relating to married men of the same age, but thereafter the risk of dying was a little lower than expected. Figure 6.1 shows that the increase was particularly

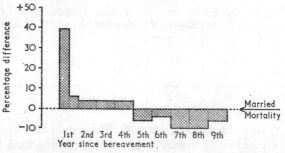

Figure 6.1 Percentage difference between morality rate of widowers aged over 54 years and that of married men of the same age, by years since bereavement. (Parkes *et al.* 1969)

notable during the first six months following bereavement when it amounted to more than 40 per cent (213 actual deaths compared with 148 expected). Parkes *et al.* (1969) analysed the causes of death during the first six months and found that coronary thrombosis and other arteriosclerotic and degenerative heart disease was especially common. Seventy-seven of the 213 deaths were attributed to these diseases whereas only 46 would be expected among married men of the same age, a statistically significant difference. Deaths due to other diseases of the cardiovascular system, to respiratory infections and to cancer were also more common than expected but not to a statistically significant extent.

The mortality risk of bereavement has also been studied by Cox and Ford (1964) and by Rees and Lutkins (1967). The former investigated the Government Actuary's records of 60,000 women who had been awarded widows' pensions during 1927 and found that during the second and third years after bereavement there was a slightly higher death rate than expected. Rees and Lutkins (1967) studied the first-order kin of 371 men and women who had died in a small Welsh semi-rural community during the six-year period 1960-65, and a control group consisting of the relatives of persons who had not died but who matched the deceased as regards age, sex and marital status. During the first year after the loss, 4·76 per cent of bereaved relatives died compared with 0·86 per cent of the controls. In subsequent years also deaths among the bereaved were commoner than among the controls, but the differences were less well marked. The death rate of the bereaved varied with their sex and with their relationship to the deceased. It was higher among males than females and greater among those who had lost a spouse than among other relatives of the dead. It was also higher in the families of those who had died away from home. The greatest mortality risk was observed among widowers, of whom 19·6 per cent died in the first year, compared with 3·9 per cent of control husbands.

REFERENCES

AVERILL, J. R. (1968). Grief: its nature and significance. *Psychol. Bull.* **70**, 721-748.

BIRTCHNELL, J. (1970*a*). Recent parent death and mental illness. *Brit. J. Psychiat.* **116**, 289-297.

BIRTCHNELL, J. (1970*b*). Depression in relation to early and recent parent death. *Brit. J. Psychiat.* **116**, 299-306.

CLAYTON, P., DESMARAIS, L. and WINOKUR, G. (1968). A study of normal bereavement. *Amer. J. Psychiat.* **125**, 168-178.

COX, P. R. and FORD, J. R. (1964). The mortality of widows shortly after widowhood. *Lancet*, **1**, 163-164.

GORER, G. (1965). *Death, Grief and Mourning in Contemporary Britain.* London.

HINTON, J. (1967). *Dying.* Harmondsworth.

LINDEMANN, E. (1944). Symptomatology and management of acute grief. *Amer. J. Psychiat.* **101**, 141-148.

MACMAHON, B. and PUGH, T. F. (1965) Suicide in the widowed. *Amer. J. Epidem.* **81**, 23-31.

MADDISON, D. and VIOLA, A. (1968). The health of widows in the year following bereavement. *J. psychosom. Res.* **12**, 297-306.

MADDISON, D., VIOLA, A. and WALKER, W. L. (1969). Further studies in conjugal bereavement. *Aust. N.Z. J. Psychiat.* **3**, 63-66.

MADDISON, D. and WALKER, W. L. (1967). Factors affecting the outcome of conjugal bereavement. *Brit. J. Psychiat.* **113**, 1057-1067.

MARRIS, P. (1958). *Widows and their Families.* London.

PARKES, C. M. (1964a). Recent bereavement as a cause of mental illness. *Brit. J. Psychiat.* **110**, 198-204.

PARKES, C. M. (1964b). Effects of bereavement on physical and mental health—a study of the medical records of widows. *Brit. med. J.* **2**, 274-279.

PARKES, C. M. (1965a). Bereavement and mental illness. Part 1. A clinical study of the grief of bereaved psychiatric patients. *Brit. J. med. Psychol.* **38**, 1-12.

PARKES, C. M. (1965b). Bereavement and mental illness. Part 2. A classification of bereavement reactions. *Brit. J. med. Psychol.* **38**, 13-26.

PARKES, C. M. (1969). Separation anxiety: an aspect of the search for a lost object. In *Studies of Anxiety* (Editor, Lader, M. H.). British Journal of Psychiatry Special Publication No. 3. Ashford.

PARKES, C. M., BENJAMIN, B. and FITZGERALD, R. G. (1969). Broken heart; a statistical study of increased mortality among widowers. *Brit. med. J.* **1**, 740-743.

REES, W. D. and LUTKINS, S. G. (1967). Mortality of bereavement. *Brit. med. J.* **4**, 13-16.

STEIN, Z. and SUSSER, M. (1969). Widowhood and mental illness. *Brit. J. prev. soc. Med.* **23**, 106-110.

WRETMARK, G. (1959). A study in grief reactions. *Acta psychiat. scand.* Supplement 136, pp. 292-299.

YOUNG, M., BENJAMIN, B. and WALLIS, C. (1963). The mortality of widowers. *Lancet,* **2**, 454-456.

CHAPTER 7

SYMPTOMATIC MENTAL DISORDERS

Anti-cholinergic Drugs. Drugs used in the Treatment of Tuberculosis.
Hypotensive Drugs. Bromides. Cushing's Syndrome and Cortisone
Psychosis. Thyroid Disorders. Parathyroid Disorders. Systemic Lupus
Erythematosus. Acute Intermittent Porphyria.

MENTAL disturbances arising during the course of physical disease very commonly represent an emotional reaction to the illness. Sometimes, however, they are symptomatic and are caused directly by the altered physical state, or they may be side-effects of treatment. In this chapter are discussed a few of the very numerous physical illnesses with mental symptoms and some of the adverse mental effects of drugs. Organic brain disease associated with mental disorder is considered in Chapter 8, while puerperal psychoses and psychiatric conditions arising from the use of oral contraceptive preparations are described in Chapter 9.

ANTI-CHOLINERGIC DRUGS

Atropine and Related Compounds

Intoxication with atropine, hyoscine (scopolamine, U.S.) and related anti-cholinergic drugs is characterized by delirium associated with symptoms due to parasympathetic receptor blockade. Intoxication can arise in various ways:

(a) by the accidental ingestion of plants containing atropine-like alkaloids such as *Atropa belladonna* ("deadly nightshade"), *Hyoscyamus niger* ("henbane") and *Datura stramonium* ("thorn apple"; "Jimson weed"; "stinkblaar"; etc.): examples have been reported by Dewberry (1959), Rosen and Lechner (1962) and by Meiring (1966).

(b) following the use of atropine or homatropine eye drops (Hoefnagel, 1961; Shah, 1966): Baker and Farley (1958) have described a patient who developed a toxic psychosis after repeated ocular instillation of 1 per cent atropine sulphate, necessitating her admission to a psychiatric hospital: cyclopentolate, an atropine-like substance used as a mydriatic may also cause severe mental disturbance when applied locally to the eye (Simcoe, 1962; Mark, 1963; Binkhorst, Weinstein, Baretz and Clahane, 1963).

(c) after deliberate self-overdose with proprietary sedative preparations containing hyoscine (Beach, Fitzgerald, Holmes *et al.*, 1964; Whitlock and Fama, 1966; Bernstein and Leff, 1967; Leff and Bernstein, 1968; Ullman, Groh and Wolff, 1970).

(d) when atropine is used to increase the heart rate of patients with severe bradycardia due to myocardial infarction, delirious states have occasionally been reported as a complication (Thomas and Woodgate, 1966; Kimball and Killip, 1968; Erikssen, 1969).

(e) following deliberate ingestion of large amounts of stramonium preparations by young people for their hallucinogenic effect: several reports from the United States have been published (Dean, 1963; Muller, 1967; Keller and Kane, 1967; Goldsmith, Frank and Ungerleider, 1968; Di Giacomo, 1968; Teitelbaum, 1968; Graff, 1969).

A uniform clinical picture is found, independent of the type of poisoning, and identical to that observed by Forrer and Miller (1958) who used large doses of atropine to treat psychiatric patients and by Crowell and Ketchum (1967) who produced hyoscine intoxication in healthy volunteers. The effects are noted within half-an-hour of the administration of the drug. Initially, these are the peripheral anti-cholinergic actions producing a dry flushed appearance of the skin, dryness of the mouth, tachycardia and widely dilated unreactive pupils. Somewhat later, the mental disturbances dominate the condition: disorientation, confusion, clouding of consciousness, vivid visual hallucinations (particularly of animals) and bizarre non-purposive behaviour such as plucking at the bed-clothes. Illusions, auditory hallucinations and abnormal conduct such as the smoking of imaginary cigarettes have also been reported, but anxiety does not appear to be a feature of the delirium. Neurological changes include ataxia, slurring of speech and extensor plantar responses.

The mental effects reach their maximum about 90 minutes after the drug has been taken and as a rule persist for only a few hours. Complete recovery, apart from amnesia for the delirious period, is usually noted within 24 hours, but in the cases reported by Baker and Farley (1958) and by Korolenko, Yevseyeva and Volkov (1969) the mental disturbance persisted for some days.

A possibly useful diagnostic test for anti-cholinergic poisoning, described by Dameshek and Feinsilver (1937) is based on the observation that atropine-like drugs block the parasympathomimetic actions of methacholine; 10 to 20 mg methacholine is injected subcutaneously and if there is then no sign of sweating, lacrimation, salivation, rhinorrhoea or increased peristalsis, the diagnosis of anticholinergic intoxication is proved.

Anti-cholinesterase drugs antagonize the effects of anticholinergic drugs, and physostigmine which crosses the blood-brain barrier and therefore has central as well as peripheral effects has been used with success to treat patients with atropine intoxication. Duvoisin and Katz (1968) and Ullman et al. (1970) found that one or two injections of 1 mg physostigmine given at an interval of 15 mins. restored the mental state to normal within a few minutes, but Forrer and Miller (1958) and Crowell and Ketchum (1967) observed that larger doses (up to 4 mg) were required and that further injections might be needed at intervals of one to two hours if the confusion returned. Hypnotic drugs such as chloral hydrate and paraldehyde may be administered if the patient is markedly overactive; chlorpromazine has a theoretical disadvantage in that it has intrinsic anticholinergic activity. Atropine is excreted in the urine and this may be hastened by the administration of diuretics (Groden and Williams, 1964).

Antiparkinson Agents

Drugs used in the treatment of Parkinsonism are anti-cholinergic and may give rise to mental disturbances similar to those observed in atropine poisoning. Most reports of such disturbances have been due to intoxication with benzhexol (trihexyphenidyl, U.S.P.: "Artane"; "Pipanol") and these have been reviewed by Stephens (1967). Similar mental disorder has been reported also in association with the administration of benztropine ("Cogentin"), procyclidine ("Kemadrin") and biperidin ("Akineton") (Medina, Kramer and Kurland, 1962; Warnes, 1967; Dunlap and Miller, 1969).

The clinical features of the intoxication have been summarized by Stephens (1967). Physically, they include peripheral anticholinergic effects and the total abolition of all pre-existing symptoms of Parkinsonism; there is also a tendency to urinary and faecal incontinence. Mentally, the patient is pathologically excited, anxious and disorientated, and has delusions of persecution and vivid visual hallucinations. These disturbances commonly last for 24 to 48 hours after withdrawal of the drug and the patient is usually amnesic for the whole episode.

Intoxication may arise during treatment, either of Parkinsonism or of the extra-pyramidal side-effects of phenothiazine or butyrophenone drug therapy in psychiatric patients. Porteous and Ross (1956) reported 52 Parkinsonian patients treated with benzhexol, of whom 10 developed severe mental disturbance attributable to the drug; in three instances, the disorder was so great that transfer to a psychiatric hospital was necessary. Stephens (1967) has observed that such adverse mental effects are most likely in patients (a) who are over the age of 60 years, (b) who are arteriosclerotic, (c) who are receiving 7·5 mg/day or more of the drug and (d) who have a previous history of confusion induced by sedatives. Warnes (1967) reported nine psychiatric patients who developed toxic psychoses while receiving major tranquillizers and antiparkinson drugs. When this happens there is a risk that the toxic effects of the latter may be wrongly attributed to the underlying psychiatric disorder (Stephens, 1967).

Intoxication may also arise following deliberate self-overdosage, by persons with suicidal intent (Singh, 1961; Morgenstern, 1962; Stephens, 1967), by irresponsible patients (Bolin, 1960; Stephens, 1967) and perhaps by young persons dependent on drugs who take benzhexol for its hallucinogenic effect (Bachrich, 1964; Stephens, 1967).

Treatment of poisoning by antiparkinson agents is similar to that of atropine intoxication, and Duvoisin and Katz (1968) have found that the parenteral administration of 1 mg physostigmine salicylate leads to immediate improvement in the mental state.

REFERENCES

BACHRICH, P. B. (1964). New drugs of addiction. *Brit. med. J.* **1**, 834.

BAKER, J. P. and FARLEY, J. D. (1958). Toxic psychosis following atropine eye drops. *Brit. med. J.* **2**, 1390-1392.

BEACH, G. O., FITZGERALD, R. P., HOLMES, R., PHIBBS, B. and STUCKENHOFF, H. (1964). Scopolamine poisoning. *New Engl. J. Med.* **270**, 1354-1355.

BERNSTEIN, S. and LEFF, R. (1967). Toxic psychosis from sleeping medicines containing scopolamine. *New Engl. J. Med.* **277**, 638-639.

BINKHORST, R. D., WEINSTEIN, G. W., BARETZ, R. M. and CLAHANE, A. C. (1963). Psychotic reaction induced by cyclopentolate (Cyclogyl). *Amer. J. Ophthal.* **55**, 1243-1245.

BOLIN, R. R. (1960). Psychiatric manifestations of artane toxicity. Case report illustrating the effect of trihexyphenidyl on affective state and personality functioning. *J. nerv. ment. Dis.* **131**, 256-259.

CROWELL, E. B. and KETCHUM, J. S. (1967). The treatment of scopolamine-induced delirium with physostigmine. *Clin. Pharmacol. Ther.* **8**, 409-414.

DAMESHEK, W. and FEINSILVER, O. (1937). Human autonomic pharmacology XIV. The use of acetyl-beta-methyl choline chloride (mecholyl) as a diagnostic test for poisoning by the atropine series of drugs. *J. Amer. med. Ass.* **109**, 561-564.

DEAN, E. S. (1963). Self-induced stramonium intoxication. *J. Amer. med. Ass.* **185**, 882.

DEWBERRY, E. B. (1959). *Food Poisoning.* London.

DI GIACOMO, J. N. (1968). Toxic effect of stramonium simulating LSD trip. *J. Amer. med. Ass.* **204**, 265-267.

DUNLAP, J. C. and MILLER, W. C. (1969). Toxic psychosis following the use of benztropine methanesulphonate (Cogentin). *J. S.C. med. Ass.* **65**, 203-204.

DUVOISIN, R. C. and KATZ, R. (1968). Reversal of central anticholinergic syndrome in man by physostigmine. *J. Amer. med. Ass.* **206**, 1963-1965.

ERIKSSEN, J. (1969). Atropine psychosis. *Lancet*, **1**, 53.

FORRER, G. R. and MILLER, J. J. (1958). Atropine coma: a somatic therapy in psychiatry. *Amer. J. Psychiat.* **115**, 455-458.

GOLDSMITH, S. R., FRANK, I. and UNGERLEIDER, J. T. (1968). Poisoning from stramonium-belladonna mixture. Flower power gone sour. *J. Amer. med. Ass.* **204**, 169-170.

GRAFF, H. (1969). Marihuana and scopolamine "high". *Amer. J. Psychiat.* **125**, 1258-1259.

GRODEN, B. M. and WILLIAMS, W. D. (1964). Atropine poisoning treated by forced diuresis. *Postgrad. med. J.* **40**, 28-29.

HOEFNAGEL, D. (1961). Toxic effects of atropine and homatropine eye drops in children. *New Engl. J. Med.* **264**, 168-171.

KEELER, M. H. and KANE, F. J. (1967). The use of hyoscyamine as a hallucinogen and intoxicant. *Amer. J. Psychiat.* **124**, 852-854.

KIMBALL, J. T. and KILLIP, T. (1968). Aggressive treatment of arrhythmias in acute myocardial infarction: procedures and results. *Progr. cardiovasc. Dis.* **10**, 483-504.

KOROLENKO, C. P., YEVSEYEVA, T. A. and VOLKOV, P. P. (1969). Data for a comparative account of toxic psychoses of various aetiologies. *Brit. J. Psychiat.* **115**, 273-279.

LEFF, R. and BERNSTEIN, S. (1968). Proprietary hallucinogens. *Dis. nerv. Syst.* **29**, 621-626.

MARK, H. H. (1963). Psychotogenic properties of cyclopentolate. *J. Amer. med. Ass.* **186**, 430-431.

MEDINA, C., KRAMER, M. D. and KURLAND, A. A. (1962). Biperiden in the treatment of phenothiazine-induced extrapyramidal reactions. *J. Amer. med. Ass.* **182**, 1127-1129.

MEIRING, P. de V. (1966). Poisoning by Datura stramonium. *S. Afr. med. J.* **40**, 311-312.

MORGENSTERN, G. F. (1962). Trihexyphenidyl (Artane) intoxication due to overdose with suicidal intent. *Canad. med. Ass. J.* **87**, 79-80.

MULLER, D. J. (1967). Unpublicized hallucinogens. The dangerous belladonna alkaloids. *J. Amer. med. Ass.* **202**, 650-651.

PORTEOUS, H. B. and ROSS, D. N. (1956). Mental symptoms in parkinsonism following benzhexol hydrochloride therapy. *Brit. med. J.* **2**, 138-140.

ROSEN, C. S. and LECHNER, M. (1962). Jimson weed intoxication. *New Engl. J. Med.* **267**, 448-450.

SHAH, P. M. (1966). Toxic effects of atropine eye drops. *Indian J. Pediat.* **33**, 13-17.

SIMCOE, C. W. (1962). Cyclopentolate (Cyclogyl) toxicity. *Arch. Ophthal.* **67**, 406-408.

SINGH, S. P. (1961). Benzhexol hydrochloride poisoning. *Brit. med. J.* **1**, 130.

STEPHENS, D. A. (1967). Psychotoxic effects of benzhexol hydrochloride (Artane). *Brit. J. Psychiat.* **113**, 213-218.

TEITELBAUM, D. T. (1968). Stramonium poisoning in "teenyboppers". *Ann. intern. Med.* **68**, 174-175.

THOMAS, M. and WOODGATE, D. (1966). Effect of atropine on bradycardia and hypotension in acute myocardial infarction. *Brit. Heart J.* **28**, 409-413.

ULLMAN, K. C., GROH, R. H. and WOLFF, F. W. (1970). Treatment of scopolamine induced delirium. *Lancet*, **1**, 252.

WARNES, H. (1967). Toxic psychosis due to antiparkinsonian drugs. *Canad. psychiat. Ass. J.* **12**, 323-326.

WHITLOCK, F. A. and FAMA, P. G. (1966). Hyoscine poisoning in psychiatric practice. *Med. J. Aust.* **2**, 763-764.

DRUGS USED IN THE TREATMENT OF TUBERCULOSIS

Isoniazid

Isoniazid, the most effective anti-tuberculosis agent, is used frequently as a primary treatment, usually in combination with streptomycin or para-aminosalicylic acid. Toxic effects are rare but when they occur they most commonly involve the nervous system and produce peripheral neuropathy, toxic psychoses, encephalopathy or myelopathy. The peripheral neuropathy is due to pyridoxine deficiency and can be prevented by the concurrent administration of pyridoxine 50 to 100 mg daily (Biehl and Vilter, 1954), but this however does not seem to prevent the toxic effects of isoniazid on the central nervous system.

Toxic Psychosis

Duncan and Kerr (1962) have described three examples of toxic psychosis due to isoniazid and have analysed published reports of 35 other cases arising in patients with no history of previous mental disorder. The psychosis may occur at any time during treatment; in the cases they reviewed the duration of therapy before the onset of symptoms varied from 2 days to 10 months. Although more common in patients receiving relatively high doses of the drug (more than 5 mg/kg body weight per day) it sometimes arises when the dose is much less. Occasionally the psychosis begins suddenly but in most cases there is a prodromal period of some days or weeks during which symptoms of anxiety, irritability and involuntary muscular twitching may be noted. The mental disturbance itself is characterized by agitation and anxiety, confusion, paranoid delusions and auditory and visual hallucinations, and, if the drug is withdrawn, recovery is the rule although this may take many months. Although Duncan and Kerr (1962) point out that pyridoxine does not appear to prevent this complication, they advocate giving multi-vitamin preparations for two weeks after withdrawal of isoniazid. Certainly, vitamin therapy does sometimes seem to have a dramatic effect, as in a patient reported by Aspinall (1964) who developed a depressive illness with periods of confusion and deterioration of memory, 11 months after starting treatment with isoniazid. Physical examination revealed glossitis and angular stomatitis, patchy pigmentation of the skin and peripheral neuropathy, suggestive of vitamin B deficiency. Withdrawal of the anti-tuberculosis drugs and administration of nicotinic acid 100 mg thrice daily and of intravenous vitamin-B complex led to notable improvement in the mental state within three days and in the physical condition within two weeks. Cases of typical pellagra have also been described as a complication of isoniazid therapy (McConnell and Cheetham, 1952; Jones and Jones, 1953) and this provides further good reason for the routine treatment of isoniazid psychosis with vitamin B.

Encephalopathy and Myelopathy

Occasionally, the administration of isoniazid is associated with severe damage to the central nervous system. Hunter (1952) reported such a case which presented as a toxic confusional psychosis, which improved when the isoniazid was withdrawn, but which left the patient with a severe Korsakoff-like state. Adams and Davies (1961) have described two patients, both of whom developed serious lesions of the nervous system during treatment with isoniazid; in one case there were signs of a left parietal lobe lesion and in the other there was a spastic paraplegia, and both had been severely depressed. Adams and White (1965) have reported a similar case of a patient who became delirious and paraplegic while taking the drug; the mental state improved when the isoniazid was withdrawn and vitamin B administered, but the paraplegia persisted. When encephalopathy or myelopathy occurs, quite clearly the isoniazid must be discontinued; in addition, high dosage vitamin B therapy should probably be given, although the usefulness of this measure is doubtful.

Memory Impairment

An investigation by Olsen and Tørning (1968) indicates that isoniazid may cause some impairment of memory and difficulty in concentration which persists for as long as the drug is taken. Of 38 patients studied before and during treatment with isoniazid, 13 complained of impairment of memory and psychological testing gave objective evidence of this in 12 of these. A further 15 patients showed a deterioration in their ability to perform the tests while on the drug, but had no relevant symptoms.

REFERENCES

ADAMS, B. G. and DAVIES, B. M. (1961). Neurological changes associated with P.A.S. and I.N.A.H. therapy. *J. ment. Sci.* **107**, 943-947.

ADAMS, P. and WHITE, C. (1965). Isoniazid-induced encephalopathy. *Lancet*, **1**, 680-682.

ASPINALL, D. L. (1964). Multiple deficiency state associated with isoniazid therapy. *Brit. med. J.* **2**, 1177-1178.

BIEHL, J. P. and VILTER, R. W. (1954). Effects of isoniazid on pyridoxine metabolism. *J. Amer. med. Ass.* **156**, 1549-1552.

DUNCAN, H. and KERR, D. (1962). Toxic psychosis due to isoniazid. *Brit. J. Dis. Chest* **56**, 131-138.

HUNTER, R. A. (1952). Confusional psychosis with residual organic cerebral impairment following isoniazid therapy. *Lancet*, **2**, 960-962.

JONES, W. A. and JONES, G. P. (1953). Peripheral neuropathy due to isoniazid. Report of two cases. *Lancet*, **1**, 1073-1074.

McCONNELL, R. B. and CHEETHAM, H. D. (1952). Acute pellagra during isoniazid therapy. *Lancet*, **2**, 959-960.

OLSEN, P. V. and TØRNING, K. (1968). Isoniazid and loss of memory. *Scand. J. resp. Dis.* **49**, 1-8.

Cycloserine

Cycloserine, an antibiotic product of *Streptomyces orchidaceus*, is a powerful anti-tuberculosis agent which is effective when given by mouth, but toxic effects are common in therapeutic doses and it is therefore usually used only when the tubercle bacillus is resistant to streptomycin, isoniazid and para-aminosalicylic acid. The toxic actions involve the central nervous system particularly, causing epileptic seizures and, less commonly, mental disturbances such as depression and confusion. Of 13 tuberculous patients treated with cycloserine by Walker and Murdoch (1957), five developed psychiatric disorders—mainly confusional states—within a few days of starting to take the drug, and all became mentally normal within a few days of stopping it. Lewis, Calden, Thurston and Gilson (1957) reported that 15 of their 30 patients showed mental changes ranging from mild depression and irritability to acute toxic psychosis within one month of starting cycloserine therapy. In both these series the dose was much higher than now recommended; four of Walker and Murdoch's five cases were receiving 1·5 G daily while Lewis *et al.* gave 1 G daily to their patients. Of 116 patients treated by only 0·5 G/day by Ruiz (1964), the incidence of mental disturbance was much lower; five patients had symptoms of depression which disappeared within 24 to 48 hours of withdrawal of the drug, three became confused and there was one instance of hysteria. But one patient committed suicide, possibly the result of drug-induced depression and Ruiz recommends immediate withdrawal of cycloserine if depression is evident. Cycloserine, in a dose of 0·5 G daily, was used by Landes, Lyon, Burch and Dávila (1960) to treat 111 patients with acute urinary infections, and they noted two cases of depression and one of hypomania with recovery within 24 hours of stopping medication.

The mental disturbance may develop suddenly and lead to emergency admission to a psychiatric hospital, as in a case reported by Bankier (1965). This patient had been treated for six months by cycloserine (0·5 G daily) and para-aminosalicylic acid (12 G daily) and developed an acute paranoid psychosis with grandiose and persecutory delusions, disorientation and homicidal behaviour. The anti-tuberculous drugs were stopped and treatment with chlorpromazine led to complete recovery of the mental disorder within four days. While para-aminosalicylic acid does rarely cause a psychotic reaction (Chandra, 1963) cycloserine was very probably responsible in this case and examples of manic-depressive, schizophreniform and paranoid psychoses attributable to cycloserine have been reported by Tani and Poppius (1963).

Although cycloserine may produce serious mental disorder, it is not absolutely contra-indicated in mentally ill patients. Burnett and Brodie (1961) gave cycloserine to 27 psychotic patients with tuberculosis and noted only one instance where the drug appeared to increase the mental disturbance.

REFERENCES

BANKIER, R. G. (1965). Psychosis associated with cycloserine. *Canad. med. Ass. J.* **93**, 35-37.
BURNETT, P. C. and BRODIE, D. (1961). Report on the use of cycloserine and isoniazid in twenty-seven cases of pulmonary tuberculosis in psychotic patients. *Dis. Chest*, **39**, 403-406.
CHANDRA, S. (1963). Psychotic reaction to para-aminosalicylic acid. *J. Indian med. Ass.* **40**, 229-230.
LANDES, R. L., LYON, E. W., BURCH, J. F. and DÁVILA, J. M. (1960). Cycloserine in the treatment of acute urinary infections. *J. Urol. (Baltimore)* **83**, 490-492.
LEWIS, W. C., CALDEN, G., THURSTON, J. R. and GILSON, W. E. (1957). Psychiatric and neurological reactions to cycloserine in the treatment of tuberculosis. *Dis. Chest* **32**, 172-182.
RUIZ, R. C. (1964). D-cycloserine in the treatment of pulmonary tuberculosis resistant to the standard drugs. A study of 116 patients. *Dis. Chest* **45**, 181-186.
TANI, P. and POPPIUS, H. (1963). Side-effects of an anti-tuberculous five-drug regimen: ethionamide, cycloserine, pyrizanamide, viomycin and isoniazid. *Acta tuberc. scand.* **43**, 256-264.
WALKER, W. C. and MURDOCH, J. McC. (1957). Cycloserine in the treatment of pulmonary tuberculosis. *Tubercle (Lond.)* **38**, 297-302.

Ethionamide and Prothionamide

Ethionamide and its *n*-propyl derivative prothionamide are, like isoniazid, derivatives of isonicotinic acid, and are used mainly to treat tuberculosis where the organisms are resistant to the primary drugs. Mental side-effects, mainly depression, occur frequently: Weinstein, Hallett and Sarauw (1962) treated 11 patients with ethionamide and noted the development of severe depression in six of them; of 52 patients taking ethionamide 1 G daily and isoniazid 400 mg/day reported by Lees (1965a), there were seven instances of depression, the onset varying from 3 weeks to 18 months after starting treatment, while of 112 patients treated by Schwartz (1966) with ethionamide, two developed psychoses attributable to the drug. In a series of 80 similar patients receiving only 750 mg ethionamide daily (Lees, 1965b) there were four cases of depression, one of a toxic psychosis resembling schizophrenia and one patient who became tremulous and anxious. Withdrawal of the drug is usually followed within a few days by complete recovery of the mental disturbance.

The British Tuberculosis Association (1968) have shown that the mental side-effects of prothionamide are similar to those of ethionamide. Of 53 patients receiving prothionamide 750 mg daily, three became depressed and one developed an acute psychosis during the second week of treatment which resolved when the drug was withdrawn; there were two instances of depression among the 48 patients receiving ethionamide, 750 mg/day.

REFERENCES

BRITISH TUBERCULOSIS ASSOCIATION (1968). A comparison of prothionamide and ethionamide. *Tubercle (Lond.)*, **49**, 125-135.
LEES, A. W. (1965a). Ethionamide 1000 mg and isoniazid 400 mg in previously untreated cases of pulmonary tuberculosis. *Brit. J. Dis. Chest*, **59**, 228-232.
LEES, A. W. (1965b). Ethionamide 750 mg daily, plus isoniazid 450 mg daily in previously untreated cases of pulmonary tuberculosis. *Amer. Rev. resp. Dis.* **92**, 966-969.
SCHWARTZ, W. S. (1966). Comparison of ethionamide with isoniazid in original treatment cases of pulmonary tuberculosis. *Amer. Rev. resp. Dis.* **93**, 685-692.
WEINSTEIN, H. J., HALLETT, W. Y. and SARAUW, A. S. (1962). The absorption and toxicity of ethionamide. *Amer. Rev. resp. Dis.* **86**, 576-578.

HYPOTENSIVE DRUGS

Four types of drugs used in the treatment of hypertension are of interest to the psychiatrist viz. the rauwolfia alkaloids, adrenergic neuronal blocking agents, alpha-methyldopa and the ganglion-blocking drugs.

Rauwolfia Alkaloids

The main features of reserpine-induced depression have been known for some years and they have been reviewed by Bunney and Davis (1965). The incidence of this side effect among patients receiving rauwolfia or reserpine has been estimated variously from about one in ten to about one in four. Lemieux, Davignon and Genest (1956) found that depression occurred in 15 per cent of their series of 195 patients; Platt and Sears (1956) reported 10 cases (18 per cent) including one suicide, among their 54 patients, while in the series of 202 patients described by Quetch, Achor, Litin and Faucett (1959) the incidence of depression was 26 per cent; Smith, Thurm and Bromer (1969) noted that

11·3 per cent of their hypertensive patients receiving rauwolfia whole root or reserpine became depressed. Depression is particularly likely when the dose is high, and because of this few physicians now prescribe more than 0·5 mg daily of reserpine (or the equivalent dose of other preparations) but depression may occur on less than this as in one patient (reported by Freis, 1954) who was taking only 0·25 mg daily. A previous history of depression definitely seems to indicate a predisposition: Quetch *et al.* (1959) observed that of their patients who became depressed on rauwolfia, 21 per cent gave a past history of depression, whereas of those who did not become depressed on rauwolfia, there was a previous history of depression in only 5 per cent (Table 7.1).

Table 7.1

DEPRESSION DURING RAUWOLFIA THERAPY AND PAST PSYCHIATRIC HISTORY
(Quetch *et al.*, 1959)

Previous history of depression

		Yes	No	Total
Depression with rauwolfia	Yes	11	42	53
	No	8	141	149
Total		19	183	202

There is a delay from the start of treatment to the onset of the depression, usually of several months but varying in duration from a few days to two years or more. The intensity of the depression also shows considerable variation; it may be relatively mild or extremely severe and suicide has been reported. In the majority of patients, withdrawal of the reserpine leads to immediate improvement and in the milder cases reducing the dose may have the same effect. Rarely, electroconvulsive treatment is required but its administration to patients taking reserpine may be dangerous (Gonzalez and Imahara, 1964) and the drug should be withdrawn first.

All the rauwolfia alkaloids can produce depression. Early reports that methoserpidine ("Decaserpyl") was free of this tendency have now been refuted and Layland, Leishman, Matthews and Smith (1962) noted the development of depression in 18·5 per cent of 119 patients taking this drug.

The administration of reserpine causes a profound fall in the concentration in the brain of 5-hydroxytryptamine and of noradrenaline (Shore, 1962) and it is this that is probably responsible for the depression (see Chapter 1). The exact mechanism by which monoamine depletion occurs is not known with certainty, although there is some evidence that reserpine releases into the cytoplasm part of the intraneuronal store of monoamines allowing their deamination by monoamine oxidase (see Figure 1.4, Chapter 1).

REFERENCES

BUNNEY, W. E. and DAVIS, J. M. (1965). Norepinephrine in depressive reactions. *Arch. gen. Psychiat.* 13, 483-494.

FREIS, E. D. (1954). Mental depression in hypertensive patients treated for long periods with large doses of reserpine. *New Engl. J. Med.* 251, 1006-1008.

GONZALEZ, J. R. and IMAHARA, J. K. (1964). Electroshock therapy with the pheno-thiazines and reserpine: a survey and report. *Amer. J. Psychiat.* **121**, 253-256.

LAYLAND, W. R., LEISHMAN, A. W. D., MATTHEWS, H. L. and SMITH, A. J. (1962). Methoserpidine ("Decaserpyl") and depression. *Brit. med. J.* **1**, 639.

LEMIEUX, G., DAVIGNON, A. and GENEST, J. (1956). Depressive states during rauwolfia therapy for arterial hypertension. A report of 30 cases. *Canad. med. Ass. J.* **74**, 522-526.

PLATT, R. and SEARS, H. T. N. (1956). Reserpine in severe hypertension. *Lancet*, **1**, 401-403.

QUETCH, R. M., ACHOR, R. W. P., LITIN, E. M. and FAUCETT, R. L. (1959). Depressive reactions in hypertensive patients. A comparison of those treated with rauwolfia and those receiving no specific antihypertensive treatment. *Circulation*, **19**, 366-375.

SHORE, P. A. (1962). Release of serotonin and catecholamines by drugs. *Pharmacol. Rev.* **14**, 531-550.

SMITH, W. M., THURM, R. H. and BROMER, L. (1969). Comparative evaluation of rauwolfia whole root and reserpine. *Clin. Pharmacol. Ther.* **10**, 338-343.

Adrenergic Neuronal Blocking Agents

These drugs, which include guanethidine sulphate ("Ismelin"), bethanidine sulphate ("Esbatal") and debrisoquine ("Declinax") are effective in the treatment of hypertension because they interfere with postganglionic sympathetic neurotransmission. In addition, guanethidine has a reserpine-like action in that it depletes the intraneuronal stores of catecholamines, and it is this action that is probably responsible for the occasional development of depression in patients on the drug. Bethanidine and debrisoquine, however, have little or no effect on monoamine stores, except possibly after long continued administration, and they cause depression much less commonly.

Of 28 hypertensive patients treated with guanethidine by Bauer, Croll, Goldrick *et al.* (1961), four became depressed; one of these patients committed suicide and another was admitted to psychiatric hospital, while a third recovered within 24 hours of withdrawal of the drug. Dollery, Emslie-Smith and Milne (1960) observed severe depression and suicidal tendencies in two of the 80 patients they treated with guanethidine, but the condition of both improved when administration of the drug was stopped. Evanson and Sears (1960) have reported a patient who developed a paranoid psychosis 10 days after starting treatment with guanethidine 25 mg/day and who recovered when the drug was withdrawn but relapsed when it was reintroduced, and Prichard, Johnston, Hill and Rosenheim (1968) noted that one-fifth of their patients on guanethidine admitted to mild depression. There were, however, no instances of mental disturbance among the 100 patients taking guanethidine in the two series reported by Leishman, Matthews and Smith (1959) and by Lowther and Turner (1963).

The incidence of depressive side-effects is much less with bethanidine. Johnston, Prichard and Rosenheim (1964) treated 31 hypertensive patients with this drug and noted no evidence of mental disturbance, while in the series of 30 patients reported by Prichard *et al.* (1968), there were no spontaneous complaints of depression, although on direct questioning, two patients admitted to having mild depressive symptoms. Gifford (1965) reported two cases of depression among 23 patients on bethanidine, and one of these committed suicide, but there was no convincing evidence that bethanidine was responsible in any way for the second patient's mental disturbance.

The effects of debrisoquine on the mental state have been noted by Rosendorff, Marsden and Cranston (1968); of 63 patients who had taken the drug for at least six months, only one patient complained of slight depression necessitating a dose reduction.

REFERENCES

BAUER, G. E., CROLL, F. J. T., GOLDRICK, R. B., JEREMY, D., RAFTOS, J., WHYTE, H. M. and YOUNG, A. A. (1961). Guanethidine in the treatment of hypertension. *Brit. med. J.* 2, 410-415.

DOLLERY, C. T., EMSLIE-SMITH, D. and MILNE, M. D. (1960). Clinical and pharmacological studies with guanethidine in the treatment of hypertension. *Lancet*, 2, 381-387.

EVANSON, J. M. and SEARS, H. T. N. (1960). Comparison of bretylium tosylate with guanethidine in the treatment of severe hypertension. *Lancet*, 2, 387-389.

GIFFORD, R. W. (1965). Bethanidine sulfate—a new anti-hypertensive drug. *J. Amer. med. Ass.* 193, 901-905.

JOHNSTON, A. W., PRICHARD, B. N. C. and ROSENHEIM, M. L. (1964). The use of bethanidine in the treatment of hypertension. *Lancet*, 2, 659-661.

LEISHMAN, A. W. D., MATTHEWS, H. L. and SMITH, A. J. (1959). Guanethidine. Hypotensive drug with prolonged action. *Lancet*, 2, 1044-1048.

LOWTHER, C. P. and TURNER, R. W. D. (1963). Guanethidine in the treatment of hypertension. *Brit. med. J.* 2, 776-781.

PRICHARD, B. N. C., JOHNSTON, A. W., HILL, I. D. and ROSENHEIM, M. L. (1968). Bethanidine, guanethidine and methyldopa in treatment of hypertension: a within-patient comparison. *Brit. med. J.* 1, 135-144.

ROSENDORFF, C., MARSDEN, D. and CRANSTON, W. I. (1968). Clinical evaluation of debrisoquin in the treatment of hypertension. *Arch. intern. Med.* 122, 487-490.

Alpha-Methyldopa

The hypotensive effect of this drug is due to its interference with the synthesis of noradrenaline at sympathetic nerve endings. It competes with dopa so that α-methylnoradrenaline, which has relatively little pressor activity, is synthesized instead of noradrenaline (Day and Rand, 1963). Similar actions within the brain probably account for the fall in cerebral concentrations of noradrenaline and 5-hydroxytryptamine associated with its administration (Sourkes, 1965) and may explain, on the monoamine theory of depression, the development of depression in some patients receiving the drug (see Chapter 1).

Table 7.2 lists a number of studies in which mental depression has been reported during treatment with α-methyldopa; it also includes some series where specific mention is made that there were no cases of depression. Two recent studies by Johnson, Kitchin, Lowther and Turner (1966) and by Prichard, Johnston, Hill and Rosenheim (1968) merit further description. Johnson *et al.* reported a series of 114 patients of whom one attempted suicide, while in another case the drug had to be withdrawn because of severe depression; including these two more serious developments, six

Table 7.2

INCIDENCE OF DEPRESSION WITH ALPHA-METHYLDOPA

Authors	Number of patients treated	Number of cases of depression
Gillespie *et al.* (1962)	52	3
Baumgarten (1962)	19	3
Dollery and Harington (1962)	59	2
Daley and Evans (1962)	20	0
Irvine *et al.* (1962)	15	0
Doyle and Trevaks (1962)	40	0
Hamilton and Kopelman (1963)	69	3
Smirk (1963)	53	5
Lauwers *et al.* (1963)	28	2
Colwill *et al.* (1964)	29	1
Johnson *et al.* (1966)	114	6
Prichard *et al.* (1968)	30	5
Total	528	30 (5·7%)

patients in all became depressed while on the drug. Prichard *et al.* treated 30 patients with α-methyldopa and withdrew it in two cases because of the development of well-marked depression; a further three patients admitted to mild depression on direct questioning.

Bunney and Davis (1965) have reviewed 15 published reports of patients becoming depressed during treatment with α-methyldopa. In only 10 instances was there any information concerning the previous psychiatric history, but nine of these had in fact been clinically depressed in the past. Bunney and Davis observed that the depression, often severe, could arise within 72 hours of the initial dose of α-methyldopa, and that it frequently remitted within one week of stopping the drug. Sometimes, however, convulsive therapy was needed to improve the mental condition. The remarkable way in which the depression may suddenly develop and remit is exemplified by three cases reported by Gillespie, Oates, Crout and Sjoerdsma (1962). Two of their patients became agitated and depressed, associated with insomnia and the expression of suicidal ideas, within 48 hours of starting treatment, and all these disturbances rapidly subsided within 24 hours of discontinuing the drug; their third patient became depressed more slowly but showed the same dramatic improvement when α-methyldopa was withdrawn. McKinney and Kane (1967) have described a patient who became severely depressed after some months' treatment and who improved when the drug was withdrawn but relapsed within one week of re-institution of therapy; of interest in this man's history was a previous episode of reserpine-induced depression necessitating treatment in hospital.

Mental disturbances other than depression have been reported during treatment with α-methyldopa. Nightmares have been noted by Irvine, O'Brien and North (1962), by Smirk (1963) and by Johnson *et al.* (1966). Dubach (1963) has reported a patient with carcinoid syndrome who became confused with auditory illusions and hallucinations while on the drug, and Fullerton and Morton-Jenkins (1963) have described a puerperal patient who developed similar symptoms. A patient of Paykel (1966) who was receiving pargyline, a monoamine oxidase inhibitor, became hallucinated when α-methyldopa was added.

REFERENCES

BAUMGARTEN, A. (1962). Clinical trial of a new hypotensive drug, methyl dopa ("Aldomet"). *Med. J. Aust.* 2, 52-55.

BUNNEY, W. E. and DAVIS, J. M. (1965). Norepinephrine in depressive reactions. *Arch. gen. Psychiat.* 13, 483-494.

COLWILL, J. M., DUTTON, A. M., MORRISSEY, J. and YU, P. N. (1964). Alpha methyldopa and hydrochlorothiazide. A controlled study of their comparative effectiveness as antihypertensive agents. *New Engl. J. Med.* 271, 696-703.

DALEY, D. and EVANS, B. (1962). Another hypotensive agent—methyldopa. *Brit. med. J.* 2, 156-158.

DAY, M. D. and RAND, M. J. (1963). A hypothesis for the mode of action of α methyldopa in relieving hypertension. *J. Pharm. Pharmacol.* 15, 221-224.

DOLLERY, C. T. and HARINGTON, M. (1962). Methyldopa in hypertension. Clinical and pharmacological studies. *Lancet*, 1, 759-763.

DOYLE, A. and TREVAKS, G. (1962). Alpha methyl dopa in the treatment of hypertension. *Med. J. Aust.* 2, 55-56.

DUBACH, U. C. (1963). Methyldopa and depression. *Brit. med. J.* 1, 261-262.

FULLERTON, A. G. and MORTON-JENKINS, D. (1963). Methyldopa and depression. *Brit. med. J.* 1, 538-539.

GILLESPIE, L., OATES, J. A., CROUT, J. R. and SJOERDSMA, A. (1962). Clinical and chemical studies with α-methyl dopa in patients with hypertension. *Circulation*, 25, 281-291.

HAMILTON, M. and KOPELMAN, H. (1963). Treatment of severe hypertension with methyldopa. *Brit. med. J.* 1, 151-155.

IRVINE, R. O. H., O'BRIEN, K. P. and NORTH, J. D. K. (1962). Alpha methyl dopa in treatment of hypertension. *Lancet*, 1, 300-303.

JOHNSON, P., KITCHIN, A. H., LOWTHER, C. P. and TURNER, R. W. D. (1966). Treatment of hypertension with methyldopa. *Brit. med. J.* 1, 133-137.

LAUWERS, P., VERSTRAETE, M. and JOOSSENS, J. V. (1963). Methyldopa in the treatment of hypertension. *Brit. med. J.* 1, 295-300.

McKINNEY, W. T. and KANE, F. J. (1967). Depression with the use of alpha-methyldopa. *Amer. J. Psychiat.* 124, 80-81.

PAYKEL, E. S. (1966). Hallucinosis on combined methyldopa and pargyline. *Brit. med. J.* 1, 803.

PRICHARD, B. N. C., JOHNSTON, A. W., HILL, I. D. and ROSENHEIM, M. L. (1968). Bethanidine, guanethidine and methyldopa in treatment of hypertension: a within-patient comparison. *Brit. med. J.* 1, 135-144.

SMIRK, H. (1963). Hypotensive action of methyldopa. *Brit. med. J.* 1, 146-150.

SOURKES, T. L. (1965). The action of α-methyldopa in the brain. *Brit. med. Bull.* 21, 66-69.

Ganglion Blocking Drugs

Ganglion blocking agents such as hexamethonium tartrate, ("Vegolysen T"), pempidine tartrate ("Perolysen"), pentolinium tartrate ("Ansolysen") and mecamylamine hydrochloride ("Inversine") are effective in the treatment of hypertension, but nowadays are rarely used since newer drugs generally control the blood pressure more smoothly. Because they block neurotransmission at the autonomic ganglia and do not affect catecholamine metabolism they have some advantage over the more recently introduced drugs in that they do not cause depression. Treatment with mecamylamine in high dosage is, however, sometimes associated with a neuro-psychiatric disturbance similar to that seen in delirium tremens. The symptoms include tremor of the limbs, confusion and hallucinations (Harington and Kincaid-Smith, 1958; Munster, 1961). Other ganglion blocking agents do not cause mental disturbance and their use may be indicated where other hypotensive therapy has been discontinued because of severe depression.

REFERENCES

HARINGTON, M. and KINCAID-SMITH, P. (1958). Psychosis and tremor due to mecamylamine. *Lancet*, **1**, 499-501.
MUNSTER, A. M. (1961). The side effects of mecamylamine hydrochloride. A review of 50 cases. *Med. J. Aust.* **1**, 247-249.

BROMIDES

After continued ingestion, bromide tends to accumulate in the body and to reach toxic levels with the development of prominent mental disturbances, usually typical of an organic reaction. When the intoxication is mild these consist of impairment of memory, irritability and emotional lability and when more severe there is clouding of consciousness and disorientation and sometimes a full-blown delirious state with hallucinations, delusions and intense restlessness (Martin, 1967). An unexplained and not uncommon finding is that the delirium starts one or two days after the drug has been stopped. In some cases of bromide psychosis, there is little or no impairment of consciousness or disorientation and the clinical picture may closely resemble that of paranoid schizophrenia or more rarely that of a non-schizophrenic hallucinosis (Levin, 1960). Neurological disturbances, mainly ataxia, dysarthria and nystagmus commonly occur and if bromism is not diagnosed, brain disease may be suspected (Morgan and Weaver, 1969) especially since diffuse electroencephalographic abnormalities and increased amounts of protein in the CSF—sometimes as much as 100 mg per 100 ml—are not uncommon (Green, 1961).

Descriptions of chronic bromism usually include reference to acneiform or proliferative nodular skin lesions. These are attributable to allergic hypersensitivity and their occurrence seems independent of the intensity of the intoxication (Rook and Rowell, 1968). While occasionally the skin mani-festations give a clue to the diagnosis, they are in fact somewhat uncommon; only three of 28 patients with bromism reported by Trethowan and Pawloff (1962) and only 2 of 24 cases described by Green (1961) had rashes.

The diagnosis of bromism is made by demonstrating a high serum bromide concentration. Bromide estimation is a fairly simple procedure: bromide solutions form a brown colour with gold chloride, the intensity of which is proportional to the concentration. Normally the serum contains little or no bromide; levels above 10 mEq/1 (80 mg/100 ml) may be associated with symptoms but evidence of severe intoxication is usually found only when the concentration is above 20 mEq/1 (160 mg/100 ml). A rapid screening test for bromism has recently been described by Gaff, Rand and Diamond (1969), based on the fact that bromide is secreted in the saliva. Drops of saliva are placed on prepared paper which changes colour in the presence of bromide and this test is positive even when the serum bromide concentration is below the toxic level.

Carbromal ("Adalin", "Dormupax" etc.) and bromvaletone (bromi-sovalum, "Bromural" etc.) are monoureide sedatives which contain bromine and which are hydrolysed in the body to release bromide ions. Trethowan and Pawloff (1962) studied volunteers who had taken either potassium bromide or doses of bromureide containing equivalent amounts of bromine and noted that the rate of increase in serum bromide concentration was indepen-dent of the type of preparation given. Hence the ingestion of bromureides over prolonged periods of time tends to cause chronic bromism, but Harenko (1967a) has noted some differences in the toxic effects of the two types of drug. First, neurological symptoms are almost constantly present with bromureide poisoning, whereas with bromide they occur in about 60 per cent of cases only, and secondly the serum bromide level in chronic bromureide poisoning is about half that found among patients with bromide intoxication with symptoms of comparable severity. These differences suggested to Harenko that bromide ion is not entirely responsible for the features of bromureide intoxication, a point also made previously by Copas, Kay and Longman (1959).

While in the past, bromism was mainly iatrogenic, this is no longer so, although cases are still being reported of long term treatment with bromides (e.g. for epilepsy) and resulting intoxication (Pozuelo-Utanda, Crawford and Anderson, 1966), and of cases where preparations such as "Carbrital" (containing carbromal and pentobarbitone) have been prescribed for long periods of time (Boyles and Martin, 1967; Fisher and Akhtar, 1970). Some-times intoxication occurs when the patient presents the same prescription repeatedly over many years (Segal, 1964; Mackay, 1969) while Drysdale and Theriault (1964) have reported a case of bromism arising when, by mistake, a patient with familial periodic paralysis was given potassium bromide instead of potassium chloride. Nowadays most cases of bromism occur as the result of self-medication with preparations which can be obtained without prescription, and for this reason prohibition of the direct sale of bromides and bromureides to the public has been advocated in recent years in the United States (Ewing and Grant, 1965; Muller, 1968; Morgan and Weaver, 1969) in Canada (Emery and Richards, 1963; Mackay, 1969) and in Australia (Martin, 1967). In the United Kingdom, carbromal and bromvaletone have been included for some years in Schedule 4 of the Poisons Rules, but bromides continue to be available without prescription and to be a hazard (Nugi, Richardson, Goggin and Bayliss, 1966).

Treatment of Bromism

Bromide is dealt with in the body almost in the same way as chloride. It is distributed throughout the extracellular fluid where it displaces chloride so that the total halide concentration remains constant. Blumberg and Nelp (1967) have reported a patient whose serum bromide was 44·6 mEq/1 and, using radioisotope dilution techniques, they showed that about 45 per cent of the total body chloride had been replaced by bromide. Since bromide is excreted slowly in the urine—more slowly than choride since it is reabsorbed more readily from the renal tubules—the serum concentration, in untreated cases of bromism, often takes some weeks to fall to non-toxic levels; Söremark (1960) has estimated that the blood level falls by half in about 12 days. The administration of chloride, either as the sodium or ammonium salt, may increase urinary excretion (Harenko, 1967b), but diuretics seem to be much more effective. Blumberg and Nelp (1967) treated a patient by intravenous infusions of isotonic saline (3 litres daily) and by mercaptomerin sodium (280 mg daily) and in four days the body was rid of 60 per cent of its bromide content. Nugi et al. (1966) also report favourably on the effect of mercurial diuretics while thiazides have been advocated by Wooster, Dunlop and Joske (1967).

Chloruretic agents such as ethacrynic acid ("Edecrin") and frusemide ("Lasix") have a theoretical advantage over other diuretics in that they promote chloride excretion. Adamson, Flanigan and Ackerman (1966) have described a confused patient whose serum bromide level was 45 mEq/1 and who was treated by intravenous injection of ethacrynic acid and by mannitol infusions. A dramatic fall in serum bromide was observed, followed more slowly by improvement in the mental state, and after four days the patient was symptom-free. A slightly slower response—recovery in six days—has been observed in a similar case treated with ethacrynic acid 50 mg daily by Seliskar, Shipman and Kennison (1966). Haemodialysis has also been used with good effect, but this is not advocated except when the intoxication is very severe or where there is poisoning by other drugs as well (Jørgensen and Wieth, 1963; Wieth and Funder, 1963).

Bromide delirium sometimes responds dramatically and inexplicably to convulsive therapy. Arneson and Ourso (1965) have reported two such patients who showed progressive and striking improvement following three applications, but treatment along these lines is probably unnecessary if diuretics are used.

REFERENCES

ADAMSON, J. S., FLANIGAN, W. J. and ACKERMAN, G. L. (1966). Treatment of bromide intoxication with ethacrynic acid and mannitol diuresis. *Ann. intern. Med.* **65**, 749-752.

ARNESON, G. A. and OURSO, R. (1965). Bromide intoxication and electroshock therapy. *Amer. J. Psychiat.* **121**, 1115-1116.

BLUMBERG, A. and NELP, W. B. (1967). Total body bromide excretion in a case of prolonged bromide intoxication. *Helv. med. Acta.* **33**, 330-333.

BOYLES, A. F. and MARTIN, D. J. (1967). Bromism. *Brit. med. J.* **4**, 806.

COPAS, D. E., KAY, W. W. and LONGMAN, V. H. (1959). Carbromal intoxication. *Lancet*, **1**, 703-705.

DRYSDALE, R. D. and THERIAULT, J. C. (1964). Familial periodic paralysis and bromide intoxication. *Canad. med. Ass. J.* **90**, 789-791.

EMERY, A. W. and RICHARDS, A. G. (1963). Bromide poisoning over the counter. *Canad. med. Ass. J.* **89**, 354-355.

EWING, J. A. and GRANT, W. J. (1965). The bromide hazard. *Sth. med. J. (Bgham, Ala).* **58**, 148-152.

FISHER, W. J. and AKHTAR, S. N. (1970). A case of bromism. *Canad. psychiat. Ass. J.* **15**, 87-93.

GAFF, G., RAND, M. J. and DIAMOND, J. (1969). Rapid screening test for bromism. *Med. J. Aust.* **1**, 967-969.

GREEN, D. (1961). Bromide intoxication. A survey of 15 years' experience at S.U.I. hospitals. *J. Iowa St. med. Soc.* **51**, 189-194.

HARENKO, A. (1967a). On the differences between chronic bromide and bromisovalum intoxications. *Acta neurol. scand.* Supplement 31, pp 150-151.

HARENKO, A. (1967b). Serum bromide level and its reduction in chronic bromisovalum poisoning. *Ann. Med. intern. Fenn.* **56**, 177-180.

JØRGENSEN, H. E. and WIETH, J. O. (1963). Dialysable poisons. Haemodialysis in the treatment of acute poisoning. *Lancet*, **1**, 81-84.

LEVIN, M. (1960). Bromide hallucinosis. *Arch. gen. Psychiat.* **2**, 429-433.

MACKAY, J. (1969). A case of bromism. *Canad. med. Ass. J.* **100**, 730-731.

MARTIN, I. (1967). Bromism induced by "safe" medications, old and new: some psychological considerations. *Med. J. Aust.* **1**, 95-98.

MORGAN, J. E. and WEAVER, E. N. (1969). Chronic bromism simulating neurological diseases. *Virginia med. Mth.* **96**, 262-264.

MULLER, D. J. (1968). Bromide intoxication continues to occur. *Tex. Med.* **64**, No. 4. 72-73.

NUGI, G., RICHARDSON, P., GOGGIN, M. J. and BAYLISS, R. I. S. (1966). Four cases of bromism. *Brit. med. J.* **2**, 390-391.

POZUELO-UTANDA, J., CRAWFORD, D. C. and ANDERSON, J. C. (1966). Bromism and epilepsy. *Int. J. Neuropsychiat.* **2**, 90-97.

ROOK, A. and ROWELL, N. R. (1968). Drug reactions. In *Textbook of Dermatology* (Editors, Rook, A., Wilkinson, D. S. and Ebling, F. J. G.). Volume 1, Chapter 16. London.

SEGAL, M. (1964). Excessive consumption of drugs. *Brit. med. J.* **2**, 942-943.

SELISKAR, J. E., SHIPMAN, K. H. and KENNISON, H. B. (1966). Bromide intoxication treated with ethacrynic acid. *Ann. intern. Med.* **65**, 1341-1342.

SÖREMARK, R. (1960). The biological half-life of bromide ions in human blood. *Acta physiol. scand.* **50**, 119-123.

TRETHOWAN, W. H. and PAWLOFF, T. (1962). A clinical and experimental study of bromide intoxication with special reference to bromureides. *Med. J. Aust.* **1**, 229-232.

WIETH, J. O. and FUNDER, J. (1963). Treatment of bromide poisoning. Comparison of forced halogen turnover and haemodialysis. *Lancet*, **2**, 327-329.

WOOSTER, A. G., DUNLOP, M. and JOSKE, R. A. (1967). Use of an oral diuretic (Doburil) in treatment of bromide intoxication. *Amer. J. med. Sci.* **253**, 23-26.

CUSHING'S SYNDROME AND CORTISONE PSYCHOSIS

Cushing's Syndrome

Excessive production of glucocorticoids by the adrenal cortex is the cause of this clinical syndrome. Bilateral adrenocortical hyperplasia is the commonest pathological finding, and sometimes this is associated with a tumour of the pituitary—particularly a basophil adenoma. Less common than hyperplasia are functional tumours of the adrenal cortex which may be benign or malignant.

Mental disturbances, usually not severe, are frequently observed. Of 50 cases studied by Ross, Marshall-Jones and Friedman (1966), 20 showed psychiatric abnormalities; six patients complained of depression when first seen and others admitted to it on direct questioning, while one patient complained of inability to concentrate and failure of memory. Apart from one patient whose paranoid schizophrenia was probably independent of the endocrine disorder, treatment by adrenalectomy or irradiation of the pituitary led to complete remission of all mental symptoms, although sometimes transient post-operative emotional lability was observed; after operation one patient attempted suicide and another required psychiatric treatment because of severe anxiety.

About one-third to one-half of all patients with Cushing's syndrome show some psychiatric disturbance. Ross *et al.* (1966) reviewed 601 cases in 11 published series (including their own) and noted a 42 per cent incidence of "psychological difficulty". Of 123 patients reported by O'Neal (1964), 21·1 per cent had mental symptoms, while depression was evident in 39 per cent of a personal series of 36 patients studied by Mattingly (1968), and in 66 per cent of the series of 35 cases reported by Lauler and Thorn (1966) there were "personality changes" ranging from "irritability or emotional lability to severe depression, confusion or even frank psychosis".

The more severe mental manifestations of Cushing's syndrome have been reviewed by Woodbury (1958) and by Michael and Gibbons (1963). Severe depression, often associated with hallucinations and paranoid delusions, is the commonest psychosis, but typical schizophrenia is not seen. Treatment of the endocrine disorder usually leads to improvement in the mental state and grossly disturbed patients may become quite normal mentally within a few days or weeks of operation. Occasionally, the patient may present with a purely psychiatric disorder and the other manifestations of the condition may be delayed for many months.

Non-pituitary neoplasms, particularly oat-cell carcinoma of the bronchus, sometimes produce a corticotrophin-like substance leading to bilateral hyperplasia of the adrenal cortex (O'Riordan, Blanchard, Moxham and Nabarro, 1966; Friedman, Marshall-Jones and Ross, 1966). Patients with these conditions rarely show the florid physical features of Cushing's syndrome (i.e. hirsutes, purple striae and bruising of the skin, a plethoric appearance etc.), but mental disturbances occur commonly and of 33 cases reviewed by O'Neal (1964), 11 had psychiatric manifestations. Sometimes the condition presents as a mental disorder; Friedman *et al.* (1966) described such a patient who had been admitted to a psychiatric unit with a history of depression and recent mental confusion. Investigation showed evidence of hyperfunction of the adrenal cortex and at autopsy an oat-cell carcinoma of the bronchus was demonstrated. Another case presenting as a psychiatric condition has been reported by Strott, Nugent and Tyler (1968): this patient's symptoms included emotional lability and impotence and the initial diagnosis was acute paranoid schizophrenia, but there was biochemical evidence of excessive corticosteroid secretion and X-ray examination revealed a tumour in the left lung. Surgical removal of the tumour—a bronchial adenoma containing corticotrophin—relieved the patient's symptoms completely.

Non-pituitary corticotrophin secreting tumours commonly cause hypokalaemic alkalosis, a disturbance not seen in classical Cushing's syndrome. The hypokalaemia may be responsible for mental aberration, as in a case reported by Landon, James and Peart (1967) of a man with a bronchial neoplasm whose presenting symptoms included mental confusion. The plasma potassium concentration was only 1·7 mEq/1, and when this was corrected the mental state improved.

Cortisone Psychosis

The continued administration of corticotrophin or of natural or synthetic glucocorticosteroids is associated with mental side-effects in a high proportion of cases (Woodbury, 1958; Michael and Gibbons, 1963). Most commonly these consist of mild disturbances of mood only, more often euphoria than depression, but in about 5 per cent of patients there are more severe mental changes, similar to those seen in Cushing's syndrome, and these are particularly likely to occur where high doses have been given for long periods of time. Severe affective disorders, either depression or mania, are most frequent, but sometimes the patient develops a confusional state with severe disorientation and non-specific psychotic features; withdrawal of the drug leads to recovery. Cass, Alexander and Enders (1966) have described five such instances of steroid psychosis occurring in patients with multiple sclerosis, three to six weeks after starting treatment with corticotrophin. Various mental abnormalities were noted, including confusion, memory disturbance, agitation, insomnia, disorientation, hostility, depression with suicidal ideas, and, in one case, delusions of grandeur. The mental state reverted to normal in all patients within five days to three weeks of reducing the dose or of withdrawal of the drug; while awaiting recovery, phenothiazines were administered. The mechanism by which cortisone and allied compounds produce mental disturbances is not known, but there is some evidence that they interfere with normal tryptophan metabolism and with the synthesis of 5-hydroxytryptamine in the brain and that this might be the basis for the psychiatric symptomatology (see Chapter 1).

The reported incidence of mental disturbances during steroid therapy varies widely (Table 7.3), but this is, at least in part, due to lack of uniform criteria. Thus Nielsen, Drivsholm, Fischer *et al.* (1963) reported an incidence of 24 per cent, but in only 10 per cent did the severity of the mental disturbance necessitate withdrawal of the drug, while Smyllie and Connolly (1968), who noted an incidence of only 1·8 per cent, excluded from this figure all mental conditions which were not severe enough to warrant advice and treatment from a psychiatrist. A further study, not included in Table 7.3, has been reported by Marx and Barker (1967). These authors compared the

Table 7.3

INCIDENCE OF MENTAL DISORDER DURING TREATMENT WITH
CORTICOTROPHIN OR CORTICOSTEROIDS

Authors	*Condition treated*	No. of cases	% Incidence mental disorder
Bernsten and Freyberg (1961)	Rheumatoid arthritis	183	13·1
Medical Research Council (1961)	Systemic lupus erythematosus	107	8·4
Rees and Williams (1962)	Bronchial asthma	317	0
Nielsen *et al.* (1963)	Rheumatoid arthritis	50	24·0
Treadwell *et al.* (1964)	Rheumatoid arthritis	110	15·4
Cass *et al.* (1966)	Multiple sclerosis	47	10·6
Vincent and de Gruchy (1967)	Aplastic anaemia	40	7·5
Joseph (1968)	Bronchial asthma	135	0
Smyllie and Connolly (1968)	Respiratory disease	550	1·8

course of 50 patients with ulcerative colitis who had received steroid therapy with that of 81 similar patients who had not received the drug, and noted that the incidence of post-operative psychoses in the two groups was 12 per cent and 2·5 per cent respectively.

REFERENCES

BERNSTEN, C. A. and FREYBERG, R. H. (1961). Rheumatoid patients after five or more years of corticosteroid treatment: a comparative analysis of 183 cases. *Ann. intern. Med.* **54**, 938-953.

CASS, L. J., ALEXANDER, L. and ENDERS, M. (1966). Complication of corticotropin therapy in multiple sclerosis. *J. Amer. med. Ass.* **197**, 173-178.

FRIEDMAN, M., MARSHALL-JONES, P. and ROSS, E. J. (1966). Cushing's syndrome: adrenocortical hyperactivity secondary to neoplasms arising outside pituitary-adrenal system. *Quart. J. Med.* **35**, 193-214.

JOSEPH, M. (1968). Corticosteroids in the treatment of chronic asthma. *Med. J. Aust.* **1**, 166-170.

LANDON, J., JAMES, V. H. T. and PEART, W. S. (1967). Cushing's syndrome associated with a "corticotrophin" producing bronchial neoplasm. *Acta endocr. (Kbh.)* **56**, 321-332.

LAULER, D. P. and THORN, G. W. (1966). Diseases of the adrenal cortex. In *Principles of Internal Medicine*. 5th edition. (Editors Harrison, T. R. *et al.*), pp. 449-484. New York.

MATTINGLY, D. (1968). Disorders of the adrenal cortex and pituitary gland. In *Recent Advances in Medicine*. 15th edition. (Editors Baron, D. N., Compston, N. and Dawson, A. M.), pp. 125-169. London.

MARX, F. W. and BARKER, W. F. (1967). Surgical results in patients with ulcerative colitis treated with and without corticosteroids. *Amer. J. Surg.* **113**, 157-163.

MEDICAL RESEARCH COUNCIL (1961). Treatment of systemic lupus erythematosus with steroids. *Brit. med. J.* **2**, 915-920.

MICHAEL, R. P. and GIBBONS, J. L. (1963). Interrelationships between the endocrine system and neuropsychiatry. *Int. Rev. Neurobiol.* **5**, 243-302.

NIELSEN, J. B., DRIVSHOLM, A., FISCHER, F. and BRØCHNER-MORTENSEN, K. (1963). Long term treatment with corticosteroids in rheumatoid arthritis (over a period of 9-12 years). *Acta med. scand.* **173**, 177-183.

O'NEAL, L. W. (1964). Pathologic anatomy in Cushing's syndrome. *Ann. Surg.* **160**, 860-869.

O'RIORDAN, J. L. H., BLANCHARD, G. P., MOXHAM, A. and NABARRO, J. D. N. (1966). Corticotrophin-secreting carcinomas. *Quart. J. Med.* **35**, 137-147.

REES, H. A. and WILLIAMS, D. A. (1962). Long term steroid therapy in chronic intractable asthma. *Brit. med. J.* **1**, 1575-1579.

ROSS, E. J., MARSHALL-JONES, P. and FRIEDMAN, M. (1966). Cushing's syndrome: diagnostic criteria. *Quart. J. Med.* **35**, 149-192.

SMYLLIE, H. C. and CONNOLLY, C. K. (1968). Incidence of serious complications of corticosteroid therapy in respiratory disease. A retrospective survey of patients in the Brompton Hospital. *Thorax.* **23**, 571-581.

STROTT, C. A., NUGENT, C. A. and TYLER, F. H. (1968). Cushing's syndrome caused by bronchial adenomas. *Amer. J. Med.* **44**, 97-104.

TREADWELL, B. L. J., SEVER, E. D., SAVAGE, O. and COPEMAN, W. S. C. (1964). Side-effects of long-term treatment with corticosteroids and corticotrophin. *Lancet*, **1**, 1121-1123.

VINCENT, P. C. and DE GRUCHY, G. C. (1967). Complications and treatment of acquired aplastic anaemia. *Brit. J. Haemat.* **13**, 977-999.

WOODBURY, D. M. (1958). Relation between the adrenal cortex and the central nervous system. *Pharmacol. Rev.* **10**, 275-357.

THYROID DISORDERS

Hyperthyroidism

Neurotic Symptoms in Hyperthyroidism

Minor mental disturbances, particularly anxiety, irritability and emotional lability are extremely common in thyrotoxicosis, and many of the manifestations resemble those seen in psychoneurotic patients. Of 247 hyperthyroid subjects studied by Williams (1964), 99 per cent complained of nervousness, 91 per cent of increased sweating, more than 80 per cent of palpitations, loss of weight and fatigue and more than 70 per cent of dyspnoea and weakness, while diarrhoea was a symptom in 23 per cent of cases. Wayne (1954) compared the symptoms of 90 patients with proven hyperthyroidism with those of 72 other patients, most of whom were suffering from anxiety states but who were initially suspected of having overactive thyroids. He found a similar incidence in the two groups of complaints of nervousness, dyspnoea on exertion, palpitation, tiredness and excessive sweating.

Differentiation of thyrotoxicosis from other conditions, particularly psychiatric disturbances with similar symptoms, can, however, often be made on purely clinical grounds. Crookes, Murray and Wayne (1959) have constructed a Clinical Diagnostic Index of symptoms and signs which they and Crown, Crisp and Ellis (1966) have shown can make the discrimination in the majority of cases. They demonstrated that the symptoms most strongly indicative of thyrotoxicosis are preference for cold weather, excessive sweating, loss of weight and increased appetite, and that if all these are absent the diagnosis is unlikely. The response of the pulse rate to sedation can also be useful in distinguishing thyrotoxicosis from other conditions, but Crown *et al.* (1966) showed that the sleeping heart rate of thyrotoxic patients is significantly higher than that of other patients only after the administration of a barbiturate and they found that a sleeping pulse rate of more than 80/min after 400 mg pentobarbitone sodium suggested toxicity. In an attempt to differentiate thyrotoxicosis from anxiety, Turner, Granville-Grossman and Smart (1965) observed the effects of intravenously administered adrenergic-receptor-blocking agents (propranolol and phentolamine) and of amylobarbitone sodium on the sinus tachycardia of eight patients with anxiety and eight patients with hyperthyroidism. Both groups of patients showed a sustained fall in heart rate after the administration of 5 mg propranolol and a transient rise after 5 mg phentolamine; intravenous amylobarbitone sodium (62·5 mg) had no significant effect on the tachycardia in either condition and it was not possible to make a diagnosis on the basis of the responses to the drugs given (Figure 7.1).

Adrenergic Activity in Hyperthyroidism

The resemblance of many of the symptoms of thyrotoxicosis to those of anxiety has provoked considerable discussion. A most extreme view has been expressed by Moschcowitz and Bernstein (1944) who suggested that neuro-circulatory asthenia—regarded nowadays as a form of anxiety in which diminished exercise tolerance is a prominent symptom—is very closely related to primary hyperthyroidism and they cite a number of case histories in which there appeared to be a transition from one condition to the other. More modern work (reviewed by Harrison, 1964, and by Waldstein, 1966) emphasizes the similarity between the pharmacological actions of thyroid hormone and of the catecholamines, and Waldstein (1966) points out that the symptoms of phaeochromocytoma and hyperthyroidism may resemble each other very closely. There is, however, no evidence of increased production of catecholamines in hyperthyroidism (Wiswell, Hurwitz, Coronho

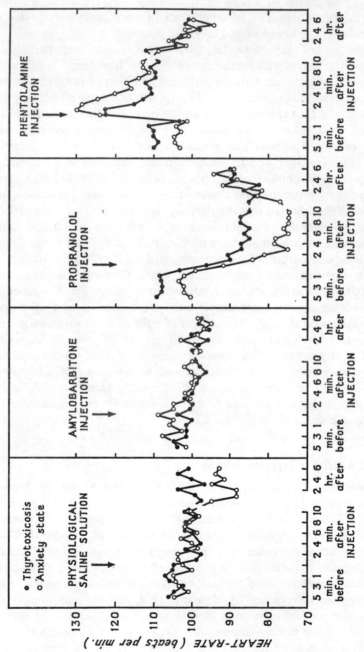

Figure 7.1 Effect on heart-rate of propranolol 5 mg, phentolamine 5 mg, amylobarbitone sodium 62·5 mg and physiological saline solution 5 ml in patients with thyrotoxicosis and anxiety states. Each point represents the mean of observations in eight patients. (Turner, Granville-Grossman and Smart, 1965)

et al., 1963; Harrison, 1964) and both Harrison (1964) and Waldstein (1966) have concluded that thyroid hormone increases the sensitivity of the tissues to the effects of normal catecholamine activity and sympathetic stimulation. There is, however, some doubt concerning this assertion. Aoki, Wilson, Theilen *et al.* (1967) induced hyperthyroidism in normal volunteers by administering tri-iodothyronine, and noted no increased effect of adrenaline on the cardiovascular system. McDevitt, Shanks, Hadden *et al.* (1968) and Frick, Heikkilä and Kahanpää, (1967) isolated the heart from nervous and hormonal influences by administering atropine and propranolol, using a technique described by Jose (1966); the heart rate in these circumstances (the intrinsic heart rate) is higher than normal in thyrotoxic subjects and subnormal in hypothyroidism, indicating that thyroid hormone has a direct action on the heart independent of autonomic nervous activity. Cairoli and Crout (1967) made similar observations on thyroxine-treated rats and reached the same conclusion. In contrast, in anxiety the intrinsic heart rate is quite normal (Frick *et al.*, 1967) indicating that the cardiovascular changes in this condition are mediated entirely through the autonomic nervous system.

Although the precise extent of involvement of sympathetic activity in hyperthyroidism is at present uncertain, there is good evidence that adrenergic blocking drugs affect many of the manifestations of the condition and that they are useful in treatment. Adrenergic neuronal-blocking agents such as guanethidine and reserpine, abolish many of the symptoms of thyrotoxicosis, including anxiety and nervousness (Canary, Schaaf, Duffy and Kyle, 1957; Lee, Bronsky and Waldstein, 1962). Eye-lid retraction and lid lag associated with primary hyperthyroidism are abolished after instillation of guanethidine eye drops in 10% concentration (Sneddon and Turner, 1966) while orally administered guanethidine corrects the impairment of glucose tolerance associated with this condition (Woeber, Arky and Braverman, 1966).

Propranolol and other β-adrenergic receptor blocking drugs resemble guanethidine and reserpine in that they do not affect thyroid function, yet abolish many of the peripheral manifestations of thyrotoxicosis. The heart rate is slowed and the cardiac output is reduced (Turner *et al.*, 1965; Howitt and Rowlands, 1966; Marsden, Gimlette, McAllister *et al.*, 1968; Turner and Hill, 1968) the amplitude of finger tremor is reduced and the abnormal briskness of the tendon reflexes is corrected (Marsden *et al.*, 1968).

Propranolol has been shown to be effective in the symptomatic treatment of hyperthyroidism. Its administration by mouth in a dose of 10 to 40 mg four times daily relieves the agitation, nervousness, tremor, palpitations and sweating (Vinik, Pimstone and Hoffenberg, 1968; Pimstone, 1969; Pimstone, Joffe, Pimstone *et al.*, 1969; Shanks, Hadden, Lowe *et al.*, 1969), and since these effects are immediate the drug is of particular value when given before thyroidectomy or while waiting for specific anti-thyroid therapy to control the condition. Stout, Weiner and Cox (1969) have obtained similar results using a combination of alpha- and beta-receptor blocking agents. Pimstone *et al.* (1969) have used propranolol as the only treatment in 27 thyrotoxic

H

patients, some of whom became completely symptom-free while on the drug, and in a few cases thyroid function became normal, and remained so when propranolol treatment was discontinued. The muscular power of thyrotoxic patients with proximal myopathy may also improve with propranolol therapy (Pimstone, Marine and Pimstone, 1968).

Thyroid Crisis

Thyroid crisis or storm, a sudden exacerbation of all the symptoms and signs of thyrotoxicosis, is characterized by fever, tachycardia and other cardiac arrhythmias, diarrhoea, tremor, pronounced restlessness, emotional lability, confusion and occasional frank psychosis (Ingbar, 1966). The condition is usually precipitated by infection, trauma or operation (including, sometimes, thyroidectomy). Waldstein, Slodki, Kaganiec and Bronsky (1960) described 21 examples, 19 of which were associated with profound mental and emotional disturbances; there were six episodes associated with psychosis (including one which presented the clinical picture of catatonic schizophrenia) and six examples of confusional states with severe disorientation. More recently, Parsons and Jewitt (1967), Greer and Parsons (1968), Buckle (1968) and Nelson and Becker (1969) have described patients with hyperthyroid crisis with similar severe mental symptoms, while Schottstaedt and Smoller (1966) have reported a patient without thyroid disease who was admitted to a psychiatric unit in a state of thyroid crisis due to the deliberate ingestion, over a period of three or four days, of 800 grains (52 grammes) of thyroid extract. All the 21 patients with thyroid crisis in Nelson and Becker's (1969) series were mentally agitated, 11 were delirious and four showed disorientation without delirium.

Many of the symptoms of hyperthyroid crisis are similar to those of intense adrenergic stimulation, and measures which inhibit sympathetic nerve activity or its effects often lead to very notable symptomatic improvement. Thus spinal anaesthesia, producing a functional interruption of autonomic pathways may have a dramatic effect on the clinical state, particularly on the tachycardia and hyperthermia (Harrison, 1964). Waldstein et al. (1960) have found that reserpine is an effective treatment, and guanethidine has also been noted to improve the condition (Waldstein, West, Lee and Bronsky, 1964; Mazzaferri and Skillman, 1969), but the effect of these adrenergic neuronal blocking agents appears to be less certain than that of β-receptor blockade. Buckle (1968) and Das and Krieger (1969) have described patients whose condition responded remarkably well to propranolol after having failed to show any improvement when treated by reserpine or guanethidine.

The mental disturbance of most patients with thyroid crisis is that of an organic reaction, but Greer and Parsons (1968) have described the case of a man admitted to hospital in thyroid crisis yet who showed no disorientation or impairment of memory. He was however anxious, suspicious and perplexed, was experiencing feelings of derealization and visual and auditory hallucinations, and he showed evidence of a paranoid delusional system with ideas of reference. This schizophrenia-like state responded dramatically to propranolol 60 mg/day and chlorpromazine 400 mg/day and within 48 hours all psychotic manifestations had gone, the fever had subsided and the pulse rate notably slowed. It was at this stage that antithyroid treatment (methylthiouracil) was introduced. Greer and Parsons discussed the possible mechanisms by which propranolol and chlorpromazine may have been effective, but were unable to decide which of the two drugs was responsible for the improvement.

Psychosis in Hyperthyroidism

Apart from thyroid crisis where psychotic disturbance is common, major mental disorders sometimes occur in less severe forms of hyperthyroidism, and this complication has been reviewed by Bursten (1961), Gibson (1962), Michael and Gibbons (1963), Greer and Parsons (1968), Whybrow, Prange and Treadway (1969) and by Clower, Young and Kepas (1969). There is considerable variation in the form that the psychosis takes, but affective psychoses and confusional states appear to be most common, while schizophrenia-like disorders are rare, although paranoid symptoms are often extremely prominent. Martin (1963) has described four examples of thyrotoxic confusional state where disorientation, restlessness and overactivity were important features, but paranoid delusions and violent behaviour were also observed.

REFERENCES

AOKI, V. S., WILSON, W. R., THEILEN, E. O., LUKENSMEYER, W. W. and LEAVERTON, P. E. (1967). The effects of triiodothyronine on haemodynamic responses to epinephrine and norepinephrine in man. *J. Pharmacol. exp. Ther.* **157**, 62-68.

BUCKLE, R. M. (1968). Treatment of thyroid crisis by beta-adrenergic blockade. *Acta endocr. (Kbh.)* **57**, 168-176.

BURSTEN, B. (1961). Psychoses associated with thyrotoxicosis. *Arch. gen. Psychiat.* **4**, 267-273.

CAIROLI, V. J. and CROUT, J. R. (1967). Role of the autonomic nervous system in the resting tachycardia of experimental hyperthyroidism. *J. Pharmacol. exp. Ther.* **158**, 55-65.

CANARY, J. J., SCHAAF, M., DUFFY, B. J. and KYLE, L. H. (1957). Effects of oral and intramuscular administration of reserpine in thyrotoxicosis. *New Engl. J. Med.* **257**, 435-442.

CLOWER, C. G., YOUNG, A. J. and KEPAS, D. (1969). Psychotic states resulting from disorders of thyroid function. *Johns Hopk. med. J.* **124**, 305-310.

CROOKS, J., MURRAY, I. P. C. and WAYNE, E. J. (1959). Statistical methods applied to the clinical diagnosis of thyrotoxicosis. *Quart. J. Med.* **28**, 211-234.

CROWN, S., CRISP, A. H. and ELLIS, J. P. (1966). Some aspects of the diagnosis of thyrotoxicosis. *J. psychosom. Res.* **10**, 209-214.

DAS, G. and KRIEGER, M. (1969). Treatment of thyrotoxic storm with intravenous administration of propranolol. *Ann. intern. Med.* **70**, 985-988.

FRICK, M. H., HEIKKILÄ, J. and KAHANPÄÄ, A. (1967). Combined parasympathetic and beta-receptor blockade as a clinical test. *Acta med. scand.* **182**, 621-628.

GIBSON, J. G. (1962). Emotions and the thyroid gland: a critical appraisal. *J. psychosom. Res.* **6**, 93-116.

GREER, S. and PARSONS, V. (1968). Schizophrenia-like psychosis in thyroid crisis. *Brit. J. Psychiat.* **114**, 1357-1362.

HARRISON, T. S. (1964). Adrenal medullary and thyroid relationships. *Physiol. Rev.* **44**, 161-185.

HOWITT, G. and ROWLANDS, D. J. (1966). Beta-sympathetic blockade in hyperthyroidism. *Lancet*, **1**, 628-631.

INGBAR, S. H. (1966). Thyrotoxic storm. *New Engl. J. Med.* **274**, 1252-1254.

JOSE, A. D. (1966). Effect of combined sympathetic and parasympathetic blockade on heart rate and cardiac function in man. *Amer. J. Cardiol.* **18**, 476-478.

LEE, W. L., BRONSKY, D. and WALDSTEIN, S. S. (1962). Studies of thyroid and sympathetic nervous system interrelationships. II. Effects of guanethidine on manifestations of hyperthyroidism. *J. clin. Endocr.* **22**, 879-885.

MARSDEN, C. D., GIMLETTE, T. M. D., McALLISTER, R. G., OWEN, D. A. L. and MILLER, T. N. (1968). Effect of β adrenergic blockade on finger tremor and achilles reflex time in anxious and thyrotoxic patients. *Acta endocr.* (*Kbh.*) **57**, 353-362.

MARTIN, E. A. (1963). Thyrotoxic confusional state: a report of four cases. *Irish J. med. Sci.* **448**, 187-196.

MAZZAFERRI, E. K. and SKILLMAN, T. G. (1969). Thyroid storm. A review of 22 episodes with special emphasis on the use of guanethidine. *Arch. intern. Med.* **124**, 684-690.

McDEVITT, D. G., SHANKS, R. G., HADDEN, D. R., MONTGOMERY, D. A. D. and WEAVER, J. A. (1968). The role of the thyroid in the control of the heart rate. *Lancet*, **1**, 998-1000.

MICHAEL, R. P. and GIBBONS, J. L. (1963). Interrelationships between the endocrine system and neuropsychiatry. *Int. Rev. Neurobiol.* **5**, 243-302.

MOSCHCOWITZ, E. and BERNSTEIN, S. S. (1944). The relationship of neurocirculatory asthenia to Grave's disease. *Amer. Heart J.* **28**, 177-198.

NELSON, N. C. and BECKER, W. F. (1969). Thyroid crisis: diagnosis and treatment. *Ann. Surg.* **170**, 263-273.

PARSONS, V. and JEWITT, D. (1967). Beta-adrenergic blockade in the management of acute thyrotoxic crisis, tachycardia and arrhythmias. *Postgrad. med. J.* **43**, 756-762.

PIMSTONE, B. L. (1969). Beta-adrenergic blockade in thyrotoxicosis. *S. Afr. med. J.* Supplement, December 6th, pp. 27-29.

PIMSTONE, B., JOFFE, B., PIMSTONE, N., BONNICI, F. and JACKSON, W. P. U. (1969). Clinical response to long-term propranolol therapy in hyperthyroidism. *S. Afr. med. J.* **43**, 1203-1205.

PIMSTONE, N., MARINE, N. and PIMSTONE, B. (1968). Beta-adrenergic blockade in thyrotoxic myopathy. *Lancet*, **2**, 1219-1220.

SCHOTTSTAEDT, E. S. and SMOLLER, M. (1966). "Thyroid storm" produced by acute thyroid hormone poisoning. *Ann. intern. Med.* **64**, 847-849.

SHANKS, R. G., HADDEN, D. R., LOWE, D. C., McDEVITT, D. G. and MONTGOMERY, D. A. D. (1969). Controlled trial of propranolol in thyrotoxicosis. *Lancet*, **1**, 993-994.

SNEDDON, J. M. and TURNER, P. (1966). Adrenergic blockade and the eye signs of thyrotoxicosis. *Lancet*, **2**, 525-527.

STOUT, B. D., WIENER, L. and COX, J. W. (1969). Combined alpha and beta sympathetic blockade in hyperthyroidism. *Ann. intern. Med.* **70**, 963-970.

TURNER, P., GRANVILLE-GROSSMAN, K. L. and SMART, J. V. (1965). Effect of adrenergic receptor blockade on the tachycardia of thyrotoxicosis and anxiety state. *Lancet*, **2**, 1316-1318.

TURNER, P. and HILL, R. C. (1968). A comparison of three beta-adrenergic receptor-blocking drugs in thyrotoxic tachycardia. *J. clin. Pharmacol.* **8**, 268-271.

VINIK, A. I., PIMSTONE, B. L. and HOFFENBERG, R. (1968). Sympathetic nervous system blocking in hyperthyroidism. *J. clin. Endocr.* **28**, 725-727.

WALDSTEIN, S. S. (1966). Thyroid-catecholamine interrelations. *Ann. Rev. Med.* **17**, 123-132.

WALDSTEIN, S. S., SLODKI, S. J., KAGANIEC, G. I. and BRONSKY, D. (1960). A clinical study of thyroid storm. *Ann. intern. Med.* **52**, 626-642.

WALDSTEIN, S. S., WEST, G. H., LEE, W. Y. and BRONSKY, D. (1964). Guanethidine in hyperthyroidism. *J. Amer. med. Ass.* **189**, 609-612.

WAYNE, E. J. (1954). The diagnosis of thyrotoxicosis. *Brit. med. J.* **1**, 411-419.

WHYBROW, P. C., PRANGE, A. J. and TREADWAY, C. R. (1969). Mental changes accompanying thyroid gland dysfunction. *Arch. gen. Psychiat.* **20**, 48-63.

WILLIAMS, R. H. (1946). Thiouracil treatment of thyrotoxicosis. 1. The results of prolonged treatment. *J. clin. Endocr.* **6**, 1-22.

WISWELL, J. G., HURWITZ, G. E., CORONHO, V., BING, O. H. L. and CHILD, D. L. (1963). Urinary catechol amines and their metabolites in hyperthyroidism and hypothyroidism. *J. clin. Endocr.* **23**, 1102-1106.

WOEBER, K. A., ARKY, R. and BRAVERMAN, L. E. (1966). Reversal by guanethidine of abnormal oral glucose tolerance in thyrotoxicosis. *Lancet*, **1**, 895-898.

Hypothyroidism

Minor mental disturbances, particularly loss of interest and initiative, impairment of memory and psychomotor retardation occur commonly in hypothyroidism. Of 100 proven cases studied by Wayne (1960), 85 complained of mental lethargy and 40 of decreased appetite, while evidence of slow cerebration was observed in 48. These symptoms are however not specific to hypothyroidism, and a comparison of the clinical features of patients with proven hypothyroidism with those of euthyroid controls showed that they are of little diagnostic value (Billewicz, Chapman, Crooks *et al.*, 1969). These authors noted that the manifestations most suggestive of the condition were diminished sweating, hoarseness of the voice, paraesthesiae, intolerance of cold, slowing of the ankle jerk, slowing of voluntary movements and coarseness of the skin. Other minor mental disturbances, such as irritability, nervousness, emotional lability and decreased libido, similar to those seen in neurotic patients have also been reported as a common occurrence (Schon, 1964).

More serious mental disorders, though relatively infrequent, have been described in association with hypothyroidism and the more recent reviews include those by Browning, Atkins and Weiner (1954), Michael and Gibbons (1963), Logothetis (1963), Whybrow, Prange and Treadway (1969) and Clower, Young and Kepas (1969). Logothetis (1963) in summarizing some 100 previously published cases, points out that the psychosis usually begins several months or years after the appearance of the physical manifestations, although, sometimes, it is the presenting symptom as in four patients of his own and in one case described by Bernstein (1965). Identical psychiatric disturbances however sometimes arise when thyrotoxicosis has been over-treated with anti-thyroid medication and in these circumstances the psychosis may develop within a few weeks of starting therapy (Brewer, 1969; Herridge and Abey-Wickrama, 1969.) Logothetis (1963) has further observed that the clinical manifestations usually suggest an organic type of mental reaction with prominent confusion, memory impairment, visual and auditory hallucinations and paranoid delusions, and that even in those not uncommon cases where the main disturbance is an affective change, there is usually some evidence of a confusional state. Jellinek (1962) has reported five patients with short-lived confusional episodes whose symptoms were reminiscent of those seen in parietal-lobe disturbances, while more persistent confusional states have been noted by Browning et al. (1954) and by Logethetis (1963).

Hypothyroidism is associated with a decreased rate of blood flow through the cerebral cortex (O'Brien and Harris, 1968) and with slowing of the EEG alpha rhythm (Hermann and Quarton, 1964). These abnormalities disappear with thyroid treatment suggesting that they are due to thyroid deficiency and this supports the view that the impairment of intellectual function and other mental abnormalities of hypothyroidism are directly due to the effects of hormonal lack on the brain. A further contributing factor to the mental disturbance may be hypothermia, to which hypothyroid subjects are particularly prone (Ward and Rastall, 1967).

There is some evidence of a closer causal relationship of hypothyroidism to organic mental reactions than to functional type of disturbances, in that where there are both organic and functional features, thyroid medication may affect the former much more obviously and much more rapidly than the latter (Browning et al., 1954; Pitts and Guze, 1961; Logothetis, 1963). While thyroid medication improves the mental disturbances associated with hypothyroidism within a few weeks in about 75 per cent of cases (Logothetis, 1963), Tonks (1964) has reported 18 patients, of whom only six showed a good response as regards their mental symptoms when the hypothyroid state was corrected, but he noted that a favourable response did appear to be significantly associated with evidence of disturbed consciousness, confusion and disorientation. Hypothyroidism may present with mental symptoms strongly suggestive of progressive presenile or senile dementia and Bentley and Brown (1969) and Olivarius and Röder (1970) have described examples where the intellectual deterioration and other mental abnormalities improved with replacement therapy. An exception to the general contention that organic symptoms respond better to thyroid treatment than do functional ones is the experience of Easson (1966) who found no evidence that disturbance of consciousness tended to correlate with clinical recovery. Moreover, long continued hypothyroidism can lead to irreversible dementia; Jellinek (1962) reported six such cases, whose mean age was 58 years, who had had untreated myxoedema for some years and who showed no improvement with thyroid medication. Tonks (1964) has also noted that in long-standing myxoedema, improvement in the mental symptoms with treatment is less likely.

Mental symptoms similar to those seen in functional disorders occur commonly, usually in association with disorientation, confusion or memory impairment. Paranoid disturbances are particularly frequent and were prominent in all the 19 patients in Easson's (1966) series. Jellinek (1962), in his report of 56 hypothyroid patients with neurological manifestations noted functional-type mental disturbances—paranoia, depression, agitation or hypomania—in 18 cases; some of these disturbances occurred only after thyroid treatment was started, in which case they were usually transient. Sometimes the "functional" disturbances dominate the clinical picture as in the case of a patient described by Libow and Durell (1965) whose myxoedema was associated with agitation and depression but no evidence of any organic mental reaction; both the mental and physical state responded to treatment with triiodothyronine, and when this drug was withdrawn there was a return of the mental symptoms. Pitts and Guze (1961) and Clower et al. (1969) have also reported examples of hypothyroidism presenting as a purely depressive illness (with no obvious cognitive dysfunction) which responded to treatment of the endocrine disorder, but sometimes improvement may not be noted until antidepressant medication, tranquillizing drugs or ECT are given (Pitts and Guze, 1961; Glucksman and Stokes, 1967). Although the mental state in hypothyroidism may be so disturbed as to warrant the administration of major tranquillizing agents such as chlorpromazine and other phenothiazine derivatives, these are best avoided as on occasion they have been known to precipitate hypothermic coma (Mitchell, Surridge and Willison, 1959; Harper and Earnshaw, 1970).

REFERENCES

BENTLEY, R. J. and BROWNE, R. J. S. (1969). Paralytic ileus and dementia in a case of myxoedema. *Postgrad. med. J.* **45**, 779-781.

BERNSTEIN, I. C. (1965). A case of hypothyroidism presenting as a psychiatric illness. *Psychosomatics*, **6**, 215-216.

BILLEWICZ, W. Z., CHAPMAN, R. S., CROOKS, J., DAY, M. E., GOSSAGE, J., WAYNE, E. and YOUNG, J. A. (1969). Statistical methods applied to the diagnosis of hypothyroidism. *Quart. J. Med.* **38**, 255-266.

BREWER, C. (1969). Psychosis due to acute hypothyroidism during the administration of carbimazole. *Brit. J. Psychiat.* **115**, 1181-1183.

BROWNING, T. B., ATKINS, R. W. and WEINER, H. (1954). Cerebral metabolic disturbances in hypothyroidism. *Arch. intern. Med.* **93**, 938-950.

CLOWER, C. G., YOUNG, A. J. and KEPAS, D. (1969). Psychotic states resulting from disorders of thyroid function. *Johns Hopk. med. J.* **124**, 305-310.

EASSON, W. M. (1966). Myxedema with psychosis. *Arch. gen. Psychiat.* **14**, 277-283.

GLUCKSMAN, M. L. and STOKES, P. E. (1967). Psychopathologic and metabolic changes in a patient with myxedema psychosis treated with *l*-tri-iodothyronine. *Amer. J. Psychiat.* **123**, 1291-1294.

HARPER, M. A. and EARNSHAW, B. A. (1970). Combined adrenal and thyroid deficiency (Schmidt's syndrome) presenting as an acute psychosis. *Med. J. Aust.* **1**, 546-548.

HERMANN, H. T. and QUARTON, G. C. (1964). Changes in alpha frequency with change in thyroid hormone level. *Electroenceph. clin. Neurophysiol.* **16**, 515-518.

HERRIDGE, C. F. and ABEY-WICKRAMA, I. (1969). Acute iatrogenic hypothyroid crisis. *Brit. med. J.* **3**, 154.

JELLINEK, E. H. (1962). Fits, faints, coma and dementia in myxoedema. *Lancet*, **2**, 1010-1012.

LIBOW, L. S. and DURELL, J. (1965). Clinical studies on the relationship between psychosis and the regulation of thyroid activity. II Psychotic symptoms and thyroid regulation in a case of post-thyroidectomy depressive psychosis. *Psychosom. Med.* **27**, 377-382.

LOGOTHETIS, J. (1963). Psychotic behavior as the initial indicator of adult myxedema. *J. nerv. ment. Dis.* **136**, 561-568.

MICHAEL, R. P. and GIBBONS, J. L. (1963). Interrelationships between the endocrine system and neuropsychiatry. *Int. Rev. Neurobiol.* **5**, 243-302.

MITCHELL, J. R. A., SURRIDGE, D. H. C. and WILLISON, R. G. (1959). Hypothermia after chlorpromazine in myxoedematous psychosis. *Brit. med. J.* **2**, 932-933.

O'BRIEN, M. D. and HARRIS, P. W. R. (1968). Cerebral-cortex perfusion rates in myxoedema. *Lancet*, **1**, 1170-1172.

OLIVARIUS, B. de F. and RÖDER, E. (1970). Reversible psychosis and dementia in myxedema. *Acta psychiat. scand.* **46**, 1-13.

PITTS, F. N. and GUZE, S. B. (1961). Psychiatric disorders and myxedema. *Amer. J. Psychiat.* **118**, 142-147.

SCHON, M. (1964). Hypothyroidism. A psychoendocrinological evaluation. *Psychosomatics*, **5**, 203-212.

TONKS, C. M. (1964). Mental illness in hypothyroid patients. *Brit. J. Psychiat.* **110**, 706-710.

WARD, D. J. and RASTALL, M. L. (1967). Prognosis in "myxoedematous madness". *Brit. J. Psychiat.* **113**, 149-151.

WAYNE, E. J. (1960). Clinical and metabolic studies in thyroid disease. *Brit. med. J.* **1**, 78-90.

WHYBROW, P. C., PRANGE, A. J. and TREADWAY, C. R. (1969). Mental changes accompanying thyroid gland dysfunction. *Arch. gen. Psychiat.* **20**, 48-63.

PARATHYROID DISORDERS

Hyperparathyroidism

Primary hyperparathyroidism commonly presents with symptoms referable to the urinary tract (renal calculi or nephrocalcinosis) or with symptoms due to bone disease. Less frequently other physical manifestations such as peptic ulceration or pancreatitis may bring the patient to medical attention. But in addition non-specific symptoms such as lassitude, weakness and anorexia and mild mental disturbances such as anxiety, depression and impairment of concentration and of memory commonly occur. Thus Karpati and Frame (1964) noted "nervousness", "irritability" and "tension" in about one third of their series of 33 cases; of 34 patients studied by Henson (1966) seven were depressed, while among the 54 patients in the series reported by Petersen (1968) 36 showed some affective disturbance and 12 complained of impairment of memory. Furthermore, notable improvement in the mental state, particularly as regards symptoms of depression and lack of energy is frequently reported by such patients after parathyroidectomy (Watson, 1968; Anderson, 1968). In most cases, the mental disturbances are relatively unimportant when compared with the patients' other symptoms, but sometimes they are the only manifestations of the disease. Boonstra and Jackson (1965), for example, have reported one patient with hyperparathyroidism who complained only of nervousness, depression and fatigue, and another whose presenting symptoms were mood variation with depression, weight loss and constipation. Of 200 patients studied by Watson (1968) eight presented as a psychiatric problem, while Thorén and Werner (1969) have also noted that the first manifestations of hyperparathyroidism are sometimes mental disturbances such as confusion, agitation, nervousness, apathy, depression and retardation.

Hypercalcaemic Crisis

Most patients with hyperparathyroidism have serum calcium levels less than 15 mg/100 ml (7·5 mEq/1), the normal range being 9·0-11·0 mg/100 ml (4·5-5·5 mEq/1), and severe psychiatric disturbances are uncommon. In a small proportion of cases however the serum calcium level may rise suddenly to as much as 20 mg/100 ml (10 mEq/1) or more, with the production of a toxic confusional state. These hypercalcaemic crises seem to occur particularly during immobilization of the patient which leads to an increase in the resorption of calcium from the bones. They are characterized by muscular weakness, nausea and vomiting, drowsiness and confusion and subsequently stupor. Lemann and Donatelli (1964) reviewed 42 cases of hyperparathyroidism complicated by hypercalcaemic crisis and noted that mental confusion was prominent in 57 per cent, and other reviewers (Payne and Fitchett, 1965; MacLeod and Holloway, 1967) have also emphasized the frequent occurrence of mental changes. Sometimes, though rarely, hyperparathyroidism may present with prominent mental symptoms due to such a crisis (Andersson and Lindholm, 1967; Bartlett, 1967; Marks, 1968; Condon, Granville, Jordan and Helgason, 1968). There is good evidence that the confusion is directly related to the hypercalcaemia. EEG abnormalities, particularly generalized slowing of activity, have been noted when the serum calcium level is very high (Moure, 1967; Allen and Singer, 1970), and after treatment there is a return to normal which matches both the improvement in the mental state and the fall in serum calcium concentration. Furthermore, similar toxic confusional states may arise in association with hypercalcaemia due to conditions other than hyperparathyroidism. Rogers (1968) has recorded the development of hypercalcaemia (serum calcium 16·4 mg/100 ml) following prolonged treatment of hypoparathyroidism by dihydrotachysterol (A.T.10); the patient was confused and drowsy and was experiencing auditory hallucinations and expressing paranoid delusions, but recovered completely within a few days when the drug was withdrawn and the serum calcium fell to normal. Hypercalcaemia associated with malignant disease in the absence of bone metastases may also cause the patient to become confused. This complication appears to be due to the production, by the tumour, of a parathyroid hormone-like substance, and removal of the tumour both reduces the serum calcium and markedly improves the mental state (Bourne, Tremblay and Ansell, 1964; O'Grady, Morse and Lee, 1965; Strickland, Bold and Medd,

1967; Omenn, Roth and Baker, 1969). Although almost any malignant neoplasm may cause this type of hypercalcaemia, hypernephromata and bronchial carcinomas account for 60 per cent of cases (Lafferty, 1966). Other causes of hypercalcaemic crisis with mental dysfunction have been reviewed by Clunie, Gunn and Robson (1967) and include Vitamin D intoxication, multiple myeloma and leukaemia.

Other Mental Disorders in Hyperparathyroidism

Severe mental disturbance other than that associated with a hypercalcaemic crisis is rare in hyperparathyroidism and when it occurs it is often difficult to determine whether or not the endocrine disorder is responsible. Anderson (1968) has reported three patients who were frankly psychotic before para-thyroidectomy, with gross thought disorder and intermittent paranoia and disorientation; post-operatively there was no improvement in their mental state and the hyperparathyroidism and psychosis were probably coincidental. However, a number of examples of an apparently functional type of mental disorder probably due to a moderate degree of hypercalcaemia have been reported. Agras and Oliveau (1964) have described a patient with well-marked depressive and paranoid symptoms and a history of intermittent mental disturbance for some years previously. The serum calcium concentration was found to be 14 mg/100 ml and within 48 hours of the removal of a parathyroid adenoma, there was a notable improvement in the mental state; three months later the patient was more cheerful and amiable than for many years. Agras and Oliveau reviewed previously published case reports and found only five similar cases of hyperparathyroidism associated with a psychosis and a clear sensorium; all these patients were severely depressed, often with paranoid features. A few further cases have since been reported:

(a) Reilly and Wilson (1965) described a patient who had been mentally ill with a paranoid schizophrenia-like disorder for six years before hyperpara-thyroidism was diagnosed; after parathyroidectomy some improvement in the mental state was noted.

(b) Marks (1968) reported a patient who had been in a mental institution with a delusional psychosis for 19 years before hyperparathyroidism was diagnosed; following operation the mental state was considered to be "reasonably normal".

(c) Karpati and Frame (1964) have recorded three other possible examples, all of whom improved mentally when their hyperparathyroidism was treated; one had had depression for several years, another gave a two-year history of agitated depression, tremulousness and anxiety, and the third presented with notable obsessive-compulsive symptoms.

(d) An elderly woman with mental disturbance of one month's duration was admitted to hospital in a catatonic state. The serum calcium concentration was 14·6 mg/100 ml, and after removal of a parathyroid adenoma there was a slow improvement in the mental state (Hockaday, Keynes and McKenzie, 1966).

Hypercalcaemia not due to hyperparathyroidism may also give rise to an apparently functional type of mental disorder, and Anderson, Cooper and Naylor (1968) have reported two patients with high serum calcium concentrations due to Vitamin D intoxication who were admitted to psychiatric hospital with severe depression. There was a very prompt improvement in the mental state when the drug was withdrawn. Both patients had had episodes of depression prior to starting treatment with Vitamin D suggesting that they were predisposed to react to the intoxication in the way that they did.

Mental Disorder after Parathyroidectomy

Post-operatively, the serum calcium concentration falls rapidly, often to levels below the normal range. This is, in part, due to temporary hypoparathyroidism consequent on the handling of the normal glands at operations, but it also occurs because, with the correction of the hyperparathyroid state, new bone formation increases markedly and calcium is actively taken up from the blood. This latter phenomenon of so-called "hungry bones" occurs particularly where there has been severe bone disease. Mental abnormalities due to the hypocalcaemia are common, especially tearfulness and depression, and these often respond immediately to the intravenous administration of calcium (Davies and Friedman, 1966). Depression is so common after parathyroidectomy that Dent (1962) advises warning all patients of the possibility. Objective evidence of post-operative mild depression and of slight impairment in learning ability has been obtained by Christie-Brown (1968) who administered a battery of psychological tests to six hyperparathyroid patients before and four days after parathyroidectomy; no similar mental disturbances were noted in a control group of six euthyroid patients undergoing thyroidectomy.

During the first few days after parathyroidectomy the serum magnesium level tends to fall below the normal range of 1·7 to 2·3 mg/100 ml (1·4 to 1·9 mEq/1), possibly a manifestation of "hungry bones", (Heaton and Pyrah, 1963). Rarely, this is associated with mental changes, particularly agitation, aggressiveness and irritability (Davies and Friedman, 1966), and a few examples of severe mental disorder due to hypomagnesaemia have been reported:

(a) Potts and Roberts (1958) have described a patient who, after parathyroidectomy, became mentally confused. The serum magnesium concentration was 0·78 mg/100 ml and the patient's mental state improved after the administration of magnesium, having failed to benefit from treatment with calcium.

(b) Five days after parathyroidectomy a patient became depressed, irritable and hostile; the serum magnesium level was 1·2 mg/100 ml and there was a striking improvement after intravenous infusion of magnesium (Hanna, Harrison, Macintyre and Fraser, 1960).

(c) A patient reported by Jacobs and Merritt (1966) became "overtly psychotic with agitation and paranoid delusions" five days after parathyroidectomy, and there was a dramatic recovery within a few hours of correction of the hypomagnesaemia.

(*d*) Seven days after operation, a patient described by Davies and Friedman (1966) developed signs of tetany and had bouts of depression. These disturbances responded to injections of calcium. Later, in spite of continued administration of calcium, the patient became excited and "completely irrational". At that time the serum magnesium concentration was 0·8 mg/100 ml and improvement occurred with magnesium therapy.

REFERENCES

AGRAS, S. and OLIVEAU, D. C. (1964). Primary hyperparathyroidism and psychosis. *Canad. med. Ass. J.* **91**, 1366-1367.

ALLEN, E. M. and SINGER, F. R. (1970). Electroencephalographic abnormalities in hypercalcemia. *Neurology (Minneap.)* **20**, 15-22.

ANDERSON, D. C., COOPER, A. F. and NAYLOR, G. J. (1968). Vitamin D intoxication with hypernatraemia, potassium and water depletion, and mental depression. *Brit. med. J.* **4**, 744-746.

ANDERSON, J. (1968). Psychiatric aspects of primary hyperparathyroidism. *Proc. roy. Soc. Med.* **61**, 1123-1124.

ANDERSSON, L. and LINDHOLM, T. (1967). Less common manifestations of hyperparathyroidism. *Acta med. scand.* **182**, 411-418.

BARTLETT, W. C. (1967). Acute hyperparathyroid crisis. *Amer. J. Surg.* **114**, 796-799.

BOONSTRA, C. E. and JACKSON, C. E. (1965). Hyperparathyroidism detected by routine serum calcium analysis. *Ann. intern. Med.* **63**, 468-474.

BOURNE, H. H., TREMBLAY, R. E. and ANSELL, J. S. (1964). Stupor, hypercalcemia and carcinoma of the renal pelvis. *New Engl. J. Med.* **271**, 1005-1006.

CHRISTIE-BROWN, J. R. W. (1968). Mood changes following parathyroidectomy. *Proc. roy. Soc. Med.* **61**, 1121-1123.

CLUNIE, G. J. A., GUNN, A. and ROBSON, J. B. (1967). Hyperparathyroid crisis. *Brit. J. Surg.* **54**, 538-541.

CONDON, R. E., GRANVILLE, G. E., JORDAN, P. H. and HELGASON, A. H. (1968). Hypercalcemic crisis and intractable gastrointestinal ulceration in a patient with endocrine polyglandular syndrome. *Ann. Surg.* **167**, 185-190.

DAVIES, D. R. and FRIEDMAN, M. (1966). Complications after parathyroidectomy. *J. Bone Jt. Surg.* **48-B** 117-126.

DENT, C. E. (1962). Some problems of hyperparathyroidism. *Brit. med. J.* **2**, 1419-1425; 1495-1500.

HANNA, S., HARRISON, M., MACINTYRE, I. and FRASER, R. (1960). The syndrome of magnesium deficiency in man. *Lancet*, **2**, 172-176.

HEATON, F. W. and PYRAH, L. N. (1963). Magnesium metabolism in patients with parathyroid disorders. *Clin. Sci.* **25**, 475-485.

HENSON, R. A. (1966). The neurological aspects of hypercalcaemia; with special reference to primary hyperparathyroidism. *J. roy. Coll. Phycns Lond.* **1**, 41-50.

HOCKADAY, T. D. R., KEYNES, W. M. and McKENZIE, J. K. (1966). Catatonic stupor in elderly woman with hyperparathyroidism. *Brit. med. J.* **1**, 85-87.

JACOBS, J. K. and MERRITT, C. R. (1966). Magnesium deficiency in hyperparathyroidism. Case report of toxic psychosis. *Ann. Surg.* **163**, 260-262.

KARPATI, G. and FRAME, B. (1964). Neuropsychiatric disorders in primary hyperparathyroidism. *Arch. Neurol. (Chic.)* **10**, 387-397.

LAFFERTY, F. W. (1966). Pseudohyperparathyroidism. *Medicine (Baltimore)*, **45**, 247-260.

LEMANN, J. and DONATELLI, A. A. (1964). Calcium intoxication due to primary hyperparathyroidism. A medical and surgical emergency. *Ann. intern. Med.* **60**, 447-461.

MACLEOD, W. A. J. and HOLLOWAY, C. K. (1967). Hyperparathyroid crisis. A collective review. *Ann. Surg.* **166**, 1012-1015.

MARKS, C. (1968). Hyperparathyroidism and its clinical effects. *Amer. J. Surg.* **116**, 40-48.

MOURE, J. M. B. (1967). The electroencephalogram in hypercalcemia. *Arch. Neurol. (Chic.)* **17**, 34-51.

O'GRADY, A. S., MORSE, L. J. and LEE, J. B. (1965). Parathyroid hormone-secreting renal carcinoma associated with hypercalcemia and metabolic alkalosis. *Ann. intern. Med.* **63**, 858-868.

OMENN, G. S., ROTH, S. I. and BAKER, W. H. (1969). Hyperparathyroidism associated with malignant tumours of non-parathyroid origin. *Cancer (Philad.)*, **24**, 1004-1012.

PAYNE, R. L. and FITCHETT, C. W. (1965). Hyperparathyroid crisis. Survey of the literature and a report of two additional cases. *Ann. Surg.* **161**, 737-747.

PETERSEN, P. (1968). Psychiatric disorders in primary hyperparathyroidism. *J. clin. Endocr.* **28**, 1491-1495.

POTTS, J. T. and ROBERTS, B. (1958). Clinical significance of magnesium deficiency and its relation to parathyroid disease. *Amer. J. med. Sci.* **235**, 206-219.

REILLY, E. L. and WILSON, W. P. (1965). Mental symptoms in hyperparathyroidism. (A report of three cases.) *Dis. nerv. Syst.* **26**, 361-363.

ROGERS, H. M. (1968). Acute psychosis associated with hypercalcemia: a complication in the treatment of hypoparathyroidism. *Sth. med. J. (Bgham, Ala.)* **61**, 94-95.

STRICKLAND, N. J., BOLD, A. M. and MEDD, W. E. (1967). Bronchial carcinoma with hypercalcaemia simulating cerebral metastases. *Brit. med. J.* **3**, 590-592.

THORÉN, L. and WERNER, I. (1969). Hyperparathyreoidism. Clinical observations in a series of 85 patients. *Acta chir. scand.* **135**, 395-401.

WATSON, L. (1968). Clinical aspects of hyperparathyroidism. *Proc. roy. Soc. Med.* **61**, 1123.

Hypoparathyroidism

Overt Hypoparathyroidism

Parathyroid deficiency is characterized by tetany, epilepsy, eczema and occasionally by raised intracranial pressure and papilloedema, all of which respond to treatment with calcium salts, calciferol or dihydrotachysterol. The diagnosis is based on the demonstration of hypocalcaemia associated with a raised serum inorganic phosphorus concentration, in the absence of renal or bone disease (rickets or osteomalacia). The most common cause is accidental damage to or removal of parathyroid tissue during thyroidectomy; 2 to 3 per cent of all patients undergoing thyroidectomy develop this complication, which is permanent in about two-thirds of cases. There may be a latent period after operation before symptoms of hypocalcaemia appear, and the diagnosis may be delayed for many years. Hypoparathyroidism may also occur after surgical treatment of parathyroid disease, but occasionally it develops, usually during childhood, without apparent cause (idiopathic hypoparathyroidism). Two further conditions of some interest to the psychiatrist, both

very rare, are pseudohypoparathyroidism and pseudo-pseudohypoparathyroidism. The former presents as a hypocalcaemic state similar to that of
idiopathic hypoparathyroidism, but differing in that parathyroid function is
normal; the defect in pseudohypoparathyroidism seems to be an insensitivity
of the target organs to the action of parathyroid hormone. This condition is
associated with various structural abnormalities such as shortness of stature
and calcification of the soft tissues, and sometimes with mental deficiency.
Pseudo-pseudohypoparathyroidism is characterized by these abnormalities of
pseudohypoparathyroidism but without any associated change in serum
calcium or inorganic phosphorus concentrations.

Denko and Kaelbling (1962) have reviewed the psychiatric aspects of these
conditions. Table 7.4 summarizes their observations on 343 previously
published cases. They found that intellectual impairment was very rare in
post-operative (surgical) hypoparathyroidism, but that it was the most
common mental abnormality in the other three conditions. They noted that
treatment often improved intellectual function particularly in idiopathic

Table 7.4

PSYCHIATRIC ABNORMALITIES IN ASSOCIATION WITH IDIOPATHIC AND
SURGICAL HYPOPARATHYROIDISM, PSEUDOHYPOPARATHYROIDISM, AND
PSEUDO-PSEUDOHYPOPARATHYROIDISM
(Denko and Kaelbling, 1962)

	Number of instances reported with :			
Type of psychiatric disturbance	*Idiopathic hypopara-thyroidism*	*Surgical hypopara-thyroidism*	*Pseudo-hypopara-thyroidism*	*Pseudo-pseudo-hypopara-thyroidism*
Intellectual impairment	50	4	49	11
Organic brain syndrome	43	50	2	0
Psychosis ("functional")	9	20	0	0
Pseudo-neurosis	20	13	0	3
Unclassifiable	37	22	10	0
Total	159	109	61	14

hypoparathyroidism. Confusional states or dementia-like conditions ("organic
brain syndrome") occurred frequently in surgical and idiopathic cases, the
majority improving when the serum calcium level was raised to normal.
Neurotic disorders and non-specific disturbances of behaviour in the absence
of any evidence of an organic reaction were, however, also common and
apparently functional psychoses (manic-depressive or schizophrenic) occurred
in a number of patients.

Since publication of the review by Denko and Kaelbling (1962) further
examples of psychiatric disorder in association with hypoparathyroidism
have been reported:

(a) Blanchard (1962), Petch (1963) and Bull and Dillihunt (1965) have each
described cases of hypoparathyroidism presenting with epilepsy and mental
disturbance arising 27 to 33 years after thyroidectomy. Two of these patients

were forgetful and had other symptoms suggestive of dementia while the third had been mildly depressed and nervous. All had serum calcium levels of less than 6·0 mg/100 ml and treatment with calcium salts and calciferol led to immediate improvement, both of the epilepsy and of the mental disturbances.

(b) Six weeks after undergoing partial thyroidectomy, a woman developed an illness characterized by severe depression, confusion, gross impairment of memory, epilepsy and tetany. The serum calcium concentration was 4·4 mg/ 100 ml. Treatment of the hypoparathyroidism led to a rapid clearing of the confusion and a slower improvement of the depression (Clark, Davidson and Ferguson, 1962).

(c) A patient described by Fourman, Davis, Jones et al. (1963) became severely depressed six years after thyroidectomy and failed to respond to treatment until the hypocalcaemia was corrected by the administration of calcium salts and calciferol; a similar case of depression due to hypoparathyroidism has been reported by Dent and Friedman (1964).

(d) Cases of idiopathic hypoparathyroidism, presenting with intellectual deterioration, epilepsy and affective disturbance, sometimes of many years' duration, have been reported by Rose and Vas (1966), by Daniolos (1967), by Fonseca and Calverly (1967) and by Hossain (1970). Treatment with calcium salts and calciferol, in these cases, led to an increase in serum calcium concentration and to considerable improvement in the mental state.

(e) Dimich, Bedrossian and Wallach (1967) have reported a series of 33 patients with hypoparathyroidism. No mental abnormality was noted among the 23 cases arising after operation, but of 10 patients with idiopathic disorders, two gave a history of previous admission to psychiatric hospital, three were mentally subnormal and three had abnormal personality traits such as irascibility and hypochondriasis.

(f) Of 43 patients with post-operative hypoparathyroidism studied by O'Malley and Kohler (1968), 12 (28 per cent) presented with mental symptoms, namely anxiety (7 cases), psychosis (3 cases) and depression (2 cases).

Partial Hypoparathyroidism

Fourman and his colleagues have asserted that after thyroidectomy there is commonly some impairment of parathyroid function, not associated, in normal circumstances, with low levels of serum calcium (Davis, Fourman and Smith, 1961; Jones and Fourman, 1963b; Fourman et al., 1963). The condition is diagnosed by observing a greater than normal fall in serum calcium when the patient is deprived of calcium, either by restricting the dietary intake and administering oral sodium phytate, or by the intravenous administration of a chelating agent such as ethylenediamine tetra-acetic acid (EDTA) (Smith, Davis and Fourman, 1960; Jones and Fourman, 1963a). Davis et al. (1961) found abnormal responses to phytate administration in 24 per cent of post-thyroidectomy cases, while Friis and Hahnemann (1964) noted that 50 per cent of their series of similar patients responded abnormally; in another series reported by Jones and Fourman (1963b), a number of thyroidectomized patients were given EDTA, and 28 per cent became hypocalcaemic.

The importance of this condition to the psychiatrist is that it is alleged to be associated with mental symptoms in the majority of cases. Thus of 46 patients with this syndrome of partial hypoparathyroidism studied by Fourman *et al.* (1963), 26 were depressed and 20 of these improved after treatment with calcium and Vitamin D. Other symptoms include headache, abdominal pain, paraesthesiae and ectodermal lesions such as brittle nails, dry skin and loss of hair. Furthermore, Fourman, Rawnsley, Davis *et al.* (1967) have shown, in a cross-over trial, that calcium citrate 15 G daily administered to such patients is more beneficial than placebo.

There is however some doubt concerning both the existence of partial hypoparathyroidism as a definite entity, and its clinical significance. First, John and Wills (1964) were unable to demonstrate that deprivation of calcium commonly caused a fall in the serum calcium level of thyroidectomized patients, and secondly, careful double-blind studies by Rose (1963) and by Stowers, Michie and Frazer (1967) failed to show that calcium had any beneficial effect on such patients. Nevertheless, the fact that overt hypoparathyroidism is undoubtedly associated with mental disorder makes it advisable to look for evidence of parathyroid deficiency in all psychiatric patients with a history of thyroidectomy.

REFERENCES

BLANCHARD, B. M. (1962). Focal hypocalcaemic seizures 33 years after thyroidectomy. *Arch. intern. Med.* **110**, 382-385.

BULL, D. M. and DILLIHUNT, R. C. (1965). Hypoparathyroidism presenting with convulsions 28 years after thyroidectomy. *J. Amer. med. Ass.* **193**, 308-309.

CLARK, J. A., DAVIDSON, L. J. and FERGUSON, H. C. (1962). Psychosis in hypoparathyroidism. *J. ment. Sci.* **108**, 811-815.

DANIOLOS, D. P. (1967). Idiopathic hypoparathyroidism. Report of a case. *Minn. Med.* **50**, 1083-1087.

DAVIS, R. H., FOURMAN, P. and SMITH, J. W. G. (1961). Prevalence of parathyroid insufficiency after thyroidectomy. *Lancet*, **2**, 1432-1435.

DENKO, J. D. and KAELBLING, R. (1962). The psychiatric aspects of hypoparathyroidism. *Acta psychiat. scand.* Supplement 164.

DENT, C. E. and FRIEDMAN, M. (1964). A comparison between A.T.10 and pure dihydrotachysterol in controlling hypoparathyroidism. *Lancet*, **2**, 164-168.

DIMICH, A., BEDROSSIAN, P. B. and WALLACH, S. (1967). Hypoparathyroidism. Clinical observations in 34 patients. *Arch. intern. Med.* **120**, 449-458.

FONSECA, O. A. and CALVERLEY, J. R. (1967). Neurological manifestations of hypoparathyroidism. *Arch. intern. Med.* **120**, 202-206.

FOURMAN, P., DAVIS, R. H., JONES, K. H., MORGAN, D. B. and SMITH, J. W. G. (1963). Parathyroid insufficiency after thyroidectomy. Review of 46 patients with a study of the effects of hypocalcaemia on the electro-encephalogram. *Brit. J. Surg.* **50**, 608-619.

FOURMAN, P., RAWNSLEY, K., DAVIS, R. H., JONES, K. H. and MORGAN, D. B. (1967). Effect of calcium on mental symptoms in partial hypoparathyroid insufficiency. *Lancet*, **2**, 914-915.

FRIIS, T. and HAHNEMANN, S. (1964). Latent parathyroid insufficiency following thyroidectomy. *Acta med. scand.* **176**, 711-719.

HOSSAIN, M. (1970). Neurological and psychiatric manifestations in idiopathic hypoparathyroidism: response to treatment. *J. Neurol. Neurosurg. Psychiat.* **33**, 153-156.

JOHN, H. T. and WILLS, M. R. (1964). Parathyroid insufficiency after subtotal thyroidectomy. *Brit. J. Surg.* **51**, 586-589.

JONES, K. H. and FOURMAN, P. (1963a). Edetic acid test of parathyroid insufficiency. *Lancet*, **2**, 119-121.

JONES, K. H. and FOURMAN, P. (1963b). Prevalence of parathyroid insufficiency after thyroidectomy. *Lancet*, **2**, 121-124.

O'MALLEY, B. W. and KOHLER, P. O. (1968). Hypoparathyroidism. *Postgrad. Med.* **44**, No. 4, 71-75.

PETCH, C. P. (1963). Hypoparathyroidism presenting with convulsions twenty-seven years after thyroidectomy. *Lancet*, **2**, 124.

ROSE, G. A. and VAS, C. J. (1966). Neurological complications and electroencephalographic changes in hypoparathyroidism. *Acta neurol. scand.* **42**, 537-550.

ROSE, N. (1963). Investigation of post-thyroidectomy patients for hypoparathyroidism. *Lancet*, **2**, 116-118.

SMITH, J. W. G., DAVIS, R. H. and FOURMAN, P. (1960). Calcium deprivation in hypoparathyroidism. A method of diagnosis using sodium phytate. *Lancet*, **2**, 510-514.

STOWERS, J. M., MICHIE, W. and FRAZER, S. C. (1967). A critical evaluation of the trisodium-edetate test for hypoparathyroidism after thyroidectomy. *Lancet*, **1**, 124-127.

SYSTEMIC LUPUS ERYTHEMATOSUS

Systemic lupus erythematosus (SLE) is a disease of connective tissue in which lesions may occur in almost any part of the body. The clinical manifestations include arthritis, rashes, nephritis, hepatitis, endocarditis, lymphadenopathy and splenomegaly, and symptoms referable to the cardiovascular, respiratory, nervous, gastrointestinal and haemopoietic systems. Laboratory diagnosis is based on the demonstration of antinuclear antibodies in the blood, which in particular cause characteristic abnormalities in the neutrophil leucocytes, the so-called LE cell phenomenon. Psychiatric abnormalities, usually in association with lesions of the central nervous system, are common; post-mortem examination of patients with mental disturbance usually shows macroscopic and microscopic changes in the brain, particularly micro-infarcts and other vascular and peri-vascular abnormalities (Johnson and Richardson, 1968).

Fessel and Solomon (1960), reviewing the earlier literature, found reports of 227 patients with SLE and mental disorder and they estimated that mental disturbance occurs in about 22 per cent of all patients with SLE. More recent studies are summarized in Table 7.5. The variation in incidence among the different series is probably due to the exclusion of milder mental disorders by some authors; indeed, Johnson and Richardson (1968) state that if the confusion accompanying fever and the anxiety or despondency accompanying any chronic debilitating disease are considered, almost all patients with SLE would be found to be mentally disturbed at some time during the course of the illness. Severe mental disturbance may occasionally be the presenting symptom, as in a case described by Stern and Robbins (1960). This however must occur very rarely and Fessel and Solomon (1960) could find only six examples

Table 7.5

INCIDENCE OF PSYCHIATRIC DISTURBANCE IN SLE

Authors	Number of patients	% Incidence mental disorder
Medical Research Council (1961)	107	8
Dubois and Tuffanelli (1964)	520	12
Berry and Hodges (1965)	38	26
O'Connor and Musher (1966)	150	51
Guze (1967)	101	12
Johnson and Richardson (1968)	24	33
Heine (1969)	38	37

among 227 cases of SLE complicated by psychosis. However, mental symptoms commonly occur early in the illness and may form part of the presenting condition, as in 14 per cent of 42 patients reported by Meislin and Rothfield (1968).

The type of mental disturbance varies considerably. Most commonly the clinical picture is that of an acute organic syndrome, characterized by confusion, disorientation and memory impairment associated with visual and auditory hallucinations and delusions, generally of a persecutory nature. Of 77 patients with SLE and mental disturbance reported by O'Connor and Musher (1966), 52 (67 per cent) had this type of mental disturbance, and it was also the most common psychosis observed by Stern and Robbins (1960). Much less common is dementia ("chronic brain syndrome") but Lief and Silverman (1960) have reported one example and Johnson and Richardson (1968) have cited others. Severe affective disorders—usually depressive, but sometimes manic—and schizophreniform psychoses, in the absence of any symptoms suggestive of an organic reaction also occur. Heine (1969) has described five patients with purely depressive mental symptoms, while Guze (1967) reported ten episodes of affective disturbance and five of schizophrenia among 101 patients with SLE. In the series of eight mentally disturbed patients reported by Johnson and Richardson (1968) there was one episode of severe depression associated with a suicidal attempt, one of hypomania and two of schizophrenia.

The mental disturbance in SLE is usually transient, ranging in duration from a few days to several months, and patients may have more than one psychotic episode during the course of the illness. In any patient with multiple episodes, the clinical picture is not necessarily constant; Johnson and Richardson (1968) give details of a young woman who on at least five occasions during her illness, showed gross mental disturbances lasting for some days or weeks and on each occasion the symptomatology was different.

Treatment of SLE often includes the administration of glucocorticoids or corticotrophin in high dosage, and this sometimes causes mental disturbances which may not be distinguishable from those complicating the disease itself. Hence in many cases the possible aetiological role of steroid treatment has to be considered, particularly since psychosis due to SLE often responds to an increase in the dose of the drugs, whereas steroid psychoses may only improve if the dose is reduced. Soffer, Elster and Hamerman (1954) observed that seven of ten patients with SLE complicated by psychiatric disturbance showed improvement in their mental state when treatment with steroids was started, and Johnson and Richardson (1968) refer to a number of other studies which have shown that all types of mental disorder (organic, schizo-phrenic or affective) due to SLE may benefit from steroid therapy. Various observations indicate that mental symptoms in SLE are more commonly due to the disease than to treatment. Of 97 published reports of SLE and psychosis reviewed by Fessel and Solomon (1960), the mental disturbance was associated with steroid therapy in 27 cases only. Similarly, in only three of 26 comparable patients studied by Stern and Robbins (1960) could steroids be implicated in the aetiology of the mental disturbance, and in only one of these cases were the authors completely satisfied that this treatment was responsible. O'Connor and Musher (1966) observed that only seven of 52 psychotic patients with SLE became mentally disturbed within two weeks of starting steroid treatment or of increasing the dose and moreover that of 12 patients who first showed mental symptoms while taking steroids only three had recurrences when steroid therapy was reintroduced. Hence, from the practical point of view, it seems reasonable to reduce the steroid dosage only where there is clear evidence that the drug is responsible for the mental disturbance. In all other cases (particularly where the psychiatric symptoms appear while the patient is receiving small doses or at the same time as an increase in activity of the disease) the dose should be increased and the effect on the mental state observed; if this aggravates the mental disorder, the dose should be reduced to the previous level and then decreased further over the course of a few days (Medical Research Council, 1961). Treatment with immuno-suppressive drugs may sometimes benefit the mental disturbance. Brook (1969) has reported such a case, of an 11-year-old girl with SLE who developed delusions, hallucinations, disorientation and memory defect two weeks after starting treat-ment with prednisone; increasing the dose of the steroid was without effect on the mental state, but changing the treatment to cyclophosphamide was followed within one week by a reversion of the mental state to normal. Whatever the aetiology of the mental disturbance non-specific methods of treatment such as phenothiazines or ECT may be used if they are indicated by the symptomatology.

REFERENCES

BERRY, R. G. and HODGES, J. H. (1965). Nervous system involvement in systemic lupus erythematosus. *Trans. Amer. neurol. Ass.* **90**, 231-233.
BROOK, C. G. D. (1969). Psychosis in systemic lupus erythematosus (SLE) and the response to cyclophosphamide. *Proc. roy. Soc. Med.* **62**, 912.

DUBOIS, E. L. and TUFFANELLI, D. L. (1964). Clinical manifestations of systemic lupus erythematosus. Computer analysis of 520 cases. *J. Amer. med. Ass.* **190**, 104-111.

FESSEL, W. J. and SOLOMON, G. F. (1960). Psychosis and systemic lupus erythematosus. A review of the literature and case reports. *Calif. Med.* **92**, 266-270.

GUZE, S. B. (1967). The occurrence of psychiatric illness in systemic lupus erythematosus. *Amer. J. Psychiat.* **123**, 1562-1570.

HEINE, B. E. (1969). Psychiatric aspects of systemic lupus erythematosus. *Acta psychiat. scand.* **45**, 307-326.

JOHNSON, R. T. and RICHARDSON, E. P. (1968). The neurological manifestations of systemic lupus erythematosus. *Medicine (Baltimore)*, **47**, 337-369.

LIEF, V. F. and SILVERMAN, T. (1960). Psychosis associated with lupus erythematosus disseminatus. A report of three cases. *Arch. gen. Psychiat.* **3**, 608-611.

MEDICAL RESEARCH COUNCIL (1961). Treatment of systemic lupus erythematosus with steroids. *Brit. med. J.* **2**, 915-920.

MEISLIN, A. G. and ROTHFIELD, N. (1968). Systemic lupus erythematosus in childhood. Analysis of 42 cases with comparative data on 200 adult cases followed concurrently. *Pediatrics*, **42**, 37-49.

O'CONNOR, J. F. and MUSHER, D. M. (1966). Central nervous system involvement in systemic lupus erythematosus. A study of 150 cases. *Arch. Neurol. (Chic.).* **14**, 157-164.

SOFFER, L. J., ELSTER, S. K. and HAMERMAN, D. J. (1954). Treatment of acute disseminated lupus erythematosus with corticotropin and cortisone. *Arch. intern. Med.* **93**, 503-514.

STERN, M. and ROBBINS, E. S. (1960). Psychoses in systemic lupus erythematosus. *Arch. gen. Psychiat.* **3**, 205-212.

ACUTE INTERMITTENT PORPHYRIA

Acute intermittent porphyria (AIP) is a metabolic disorder inherited as a Mendelian dominant characteristic, in which large amounts of porphyrin precursors are produced in the liver and excreted in the urine. The symptoms of the disease are abdominal (intermittent attacks of abdominal pain, often colicky with vomiting and constipation); neurological (peripheral neuropathy and bulbar palsies with consequent dysphagia, dysphonia and respiratory paralysis); and psychiatric. The psychiatric manifestations, discussed in detail below, are often prominent, and sometimes, as in 14 per cent of the series of 69 patients reviewed by Markovitz (1954), they are the presenting symptoms. Porphyrin metabolism and the clinical aspects of the porphyrias have been reviewed recently by Tschudy (1969).

The diagnosis is made by examining the urine for the presence of porphyrins or of their precursors, delta-aminolaevulinic acid and porphobilinogen. These compounds, although constantly present in the urine of porphyrics in relapse, are pharmacologically inactive and they are not responsible for the symptoms. Freshly voided urine is usually unremarkable in colour, but sometimes it is red, resembling port; the presence of porphyrins can however be detected by their bright-red fluorescence in ultra-violet light and because on exposure to ordinary light the urine slowly turns dark brown or black.

Urinary porphobilinogen may be detected by the Watson-Schwartz test (Watson and Schwartz, 1941; Watson, 1964) which can be carried out in the ward side-room. This test is based on the observation that porphobilinogen reacts with Ehrlich's aldehyde reagent (p-dimethylaminobenzaldehyde in hydrochloric acid) to form a red complex not extractable by chloroform. (In contrast, other compounds, notably urobilinogen, which form a red complex with Ehrlich's aldehyde reagent, are more soluble in chloroform than in water.) The test consists of mixing, in a test-tube, 3 ml of freshly voided urine with an equal volume of Ehrlich's reagent and then with 6 ml of a saturated solution of sodium acetate. Chloroform (5 ml) is then added and the reagents thoroughly shaken. The mixture is then allowed to separate (chloroform is denser than water) and the presence of porphobilinogen indicated by a reddening (varying from pink to deep red, according to the concentration) of the aqueous phase. Fresh urine should always be used because on rare occasions the reaction is inhibited in stale specimens. Positive results almost invariably indicate porphyria (usually AIP but sometimes variegate porphyria where the manifestations of AIP are associated with skin changes), and a negative result makes it extremely unlikely that any florid symptoms are due to the disease. Between attacks, smaller amounts of porphobilinogen can usually be detected in the urine, but a negative result does not entirely rule out the possibility of latent disease. Rarely, substances which produce a reaction with Ehrlich's reagent similar to that of porphobilinogen, are found in association with other disorders; these colour-complexes are however soluble in n-butanol whereas colour due to porphobilinogen is not. Watson, Bossenmaier and Cardinal (1961) have therefore introduced a modification of the original Watson-Schwartz test in which, after extraction with chloroform, the aqueous phase is separated and mixed thoroughly with n-butanol; a red coloration of the aqueous (denser) phase then indicates the presence of porphobilinogen. Fine and Kaplan (1966) have described a patient whose condition was diagnosed as AIP on the basis of a positive classical Watson-Schwartz test, but whose urine proved negative after n-butanol extraction and who, in fact, was suffering from carcinoma of the colon. Townsend (1964), using the modified method, tested the urine of 1000 unselected patients and noted no false positive reactions, although before extraction with n-butanol, 59 samples gave weakly positive results.

There is some suggestion that patients receiving phenothiazine drugs may give positive reactions with Ehrlich's reagent (Jancar and Philpot, 1965; Wetterberg, 1967; Reio and Wetterberg, 1969). Wetterberg (1967) reported that of 1907 patients in mental hospitals in North Sweden (where there is a high prevalence of AIP), 9 per cent showed the presence of porphobilinogen-like substances in the urine. Further study showed that only three patients were suffering from AIP and that the false-positive reactors tended to be those patients who were receiving high dosage phenothiazine preparations. Reio and Wetterberg (1969) have suggested that dyes used to colour this type of drug may be responsible sometimes for these false-positive results.

Psychiatric Manifestations

Estimates of the incidence of mental disturbance in AIP vary (Table 7.6) but this is due, at least in part, to wide variation in the severity and form of the mental symptoms.

Table 7.6

INCIDENCE OF MENTAL DISTURBANCE IN ACUTE INTERMITTENT PORPHYRIA

Authors	*No. of cases*	*Incidence of mental disturbance* (%)
Markovitz (1954)	69	80
Waldenström (1957)	233	44
Goldberg and Rimington (1962)	50	58
Wetterberg (1967)	95	24

Markovitz (1954) reviewed 64 previously published cases and five new ones and found that mental changes had been noted in 80 per cent. He classified these changes as follows:

(*a*) Hallucinations, delirium, confusion or seizures (in 52 per cent of the series)

(*b*) Hysteria, depression, schizophrenia or paranoia (26 per cent)

(*c*) Irritability or restlessness (40 per cent).

Goldberg and Rimington (1962) noted mental symptoms in 29 (58 per cent) of their 50 cases and they graded the disturbances as follows:

(*a*) Depressed, nervous, hysterical, lacrimose or "peculiar"—14 cases (of whom one presented with depression and was treated initially as a psychiatric problem);

(*b*) Confused, hallucinated, disorientated or with personality change— 9 cases;

(*c*) Legally certified (as insane)—6 cases.

Of 40 patients whose mental state was studied during an attack of AIP by Stein and Tschudy (1970), 16 had hallucinations or mental confusion; 7 remained chronically depressed after a bout of illness and 4 (one of whom later committed suicide) required confinement in a psychiatric hospital. Ridley (1969) found a very high incidence of mental disturbance among 25 porphyric patients with neuropathy; 25 of 29 episodes of neuropathy in these patients were associated with mental symptoms such as insomnia with alarming nightmares, confusion, hallucinations, depression, delusions and emotional disturbance.

Some idea of the wide variety of abnormal mental phenomena observed has been given by Ackner, Cooper, Gray and Kelly (1962) and by Kaelbling, Craig and Pasamanick (1961). Table 7.7 summarizes the psychiatric symptoms of 12 patients studied by Ackner *et al.* (1962); the mental disorder was very mild in two patients (cases 9 and 10) and severe enough to warrant admission to a psychiatric hospital in three instances (cases 1, 2 and 5), but only one patient in the series (case 7) presented as a pure psychiatric problem. Kaelbling *et al.* (1961) tested the urine of 2500 unselected psychiatric patients for porphobilinogen, of whom 35 gave positive results. Only 12 patients had the clinical features of porphyria; four of these had been diagnosed as schizophrenic, one as neurotic and seven as having an organic mental reaction.

Hysterical symptoms are often prominent and sometimes, as in 5 of the 25 patients described by Ridley (1969) a diagnosis of hysteria is made before the true nature of the disorder is recognized. This is perhaps understandable

Table 7.7

MENTAL DISTURBANCES IN 12 PATIENTS WITH ACUTE INTERMITTENT PORPHYRIA
(Ackner *et al.*, 1962)

Case no.	Mental disturbances
1	Delirium
2	Depression and attempted suicide
3	Hysteria, paranoia and hallucinations
4	Depression and anxiety
5	Depression, confusion, hallucinations, delusions and hysteria
6	Severe confusion
7	Confusion
8	Confusion
9	Mild depression and irritability
10	Mild depression and tearfulness
11	Depression
12	Depression and confusion

because the symptoms are often very unusual; thus, the abdominal pain is very frequently extremely severe and the patient may scream and adopt unusual postures, yet any abdominal physical signs may be quite unlike those found in the more common medical or surgical disorders (Waldenström, 1957).

A further factor contributing to the wide variation in psychiatric symptomatology may be that the mental and physical disturbances have different aetiologies. Wetterberg (1967) has found some evidence for this in a genetic study. His propositi were of two types: (*A*) 20 patients with AIP who were also mentally disturbed and (*B*) 20 similar patients without mental disorder. While the incidence of porphyria was similar among the sibs of the two groups, mental disturbance was much more common in the sibs of type A propositi. Moreover, although mental illness was most common in those sibs who showed evidence of porphyria, sibs free of the disease also tended to be mentally disturbed if they were related to type A propositi. Wetterberg interpreted these findings as indicating that the biochemical disturbance of AIP is responsible for mental illness in about 70 per cent of cases only, and that in the remaining 30 per cent the mental disorder, though also genetically determined, is transmitted independently of the porphyria. Wetterberg has further suggested that the two types of mental illness can be distinguished clinically; that due to porphyria is characterized by transitory confusional states, visual hallucinations, signs of neurological disturbance and relatively little in the way of depressive symptoms.

Treatment

Although the psychiatrist is likely to seek the help of the physician in treatment, he should be aware of the methods used, which have been reviewed by Goldberg (1968). Analgesics (pethidine or morphine) are often required, but oral promazine 25 to 50 mg three or four times daily is frequently effective in relieving the pain and at the same time it may benefit the mental state. With severe psychiatric disturbance, parenterally administered promazine in 100 to 200 mg doses should be given. There are two complications of which the psychiatrist should be aware. First, a proportion of patients develop hyponatraemia which is sometimes due to inappropriate secretion of anti-diuretic hormone, in which case it can be treated by water restriction; Stein and Tschudy (1970) have reported two such cases where the severe mental disturbance responded to treatment of the hyponatraemia. Secondly, respiratory paralysis may occur, and if severe will require mechanical assistance of respiration. Although treatment is at present symptomatic Atsmon and Blum (1970) have described a patient with variegate porphyria whose symptoms included mental confusion and hallucinations and whose condition responded dramatically to treatment with propranolol, 100 mg every 4 hours. Flacks (1970), however, has reported a similar case who failed to respond to much lower doses of propranolol.

Various drugs may precipitate attacks of porphyria or aggravate the condition and the following are contra-indicated: barbiturates, sulphonamides, oestrogens (including oral contraceptive agents), chloroquine, griseofulvin, and possibly dichloralphenazone ("Welldorm") and methyldopa.

REFERENCES

ACKNER, B., COOPER, J. E., GRAY, C. H. and KELLY, M. (1962). Acute porphyria. A neuropsychiatric and biochemical study. *J. psychosom. Res.* 6, 1-24.

ATSMON, A. and BLUM, I. (1970). Treatment of acute porphyria variegata with propranolol. *Lancet*, 1, 196-197.

FINE, M. H. and KAPLAN, A. I. (1966). False-positive reactions for porphobilinogen. Detection by butanol extraction and report of a case. *J. Amer. med. Ass.* 197, 584-586.

FLACKS, L. M. (1970). Propranolol in acute porphyria. *Lancet*, 1, 363.

GOLDBERG, A. (1968). Diagnosis and treatment of the porphyrias. *Proc. roy. Soc. Med.* 61, 193-196.

GOLDBERG, A. and RIMINGTON, C. (1962). *Diseases of Porphyrin Metabolism.* Springfield, Ill.

JANCAR, J. and PHILPOT, G. R. (1965). Porphobilinogen-like chromogens in urine of epileptics. *Brit. med. J.* 1, 1498.

KAELBLING, R., CRAIG, J. B. and PASAMANICK, B. (1961). Urinary porphobilinogen. Results of screening 2500 psychiatric patients. *Arch. gen. Psychiat.* 5, 494-508.

MARKOVITZ, M. (1954). Acute intermittent porphyria: a report of five cases and a review of the literature. *Ann. intern. Med.* 41, 1170-1188.

REIO, L. and WETTERBERG, L. (1969). False porphobilinogen reactions in the urine of mental patients. *J. Amer. med. Ass.* 207, 148-150.

RIDLEY, A. (1969). The neuropathy of acute intermittent porphyria. *Quart. J. Med.* **38**, 307-333.

STEIN, J. A. and TSCHUDY, D. P. (1970). Acute intermittent porphyria: a clinical and biochemical study of 46 patients. *Medicine (Baltimore)*, **49**, 1-16.

TOWNSEND, J. D. (1964). An evaluation of a recent modification of the Watson-Schwartz test for porphobilinogen. *Ann. intern. Med.* **60**, 306-307.

TSCHUDY, D. P. (1969). Porphyrin metabolism and the porphyrias. In *Duncan's Diseases of Metabolism. Volume I. Genetics and Metabolism.* 6th edition. (Editor, Bondy, P. K.) Chapter 11, pp. 600-635. Philadelphia.

WALDENSTRÖM, J. (1957). The porphyrias as inborn errors of metabolism. *Amer. J. Med.* **22**, 758-773.

WATSON, C. J. (1964). Porphyrin metabolism. In *Diseases of Metabolism* (Editor, Duncan, G. G.) 5th edition. Chapter 11, pp. 850-887. Philadelphia.

WATSON, C. J., BOSSENMAIER, I. and CARDINAL, R. (1961). Acute intermittent porphyria. Urinary porphobilinogen and other Ehrlich reactors in diagnosis. *J. Amer. med. Ass.* **175**, 1087-1091.

WATSON, C. J. and SCHWARTZ, S. (1941). A simple test for urinary porphobilinogen. *Proc. Soc. exp. Biol. (N.Y.)* **47**, 393-394.

WETTERBERG, L. (1967). *A Neuropsychiatric and Genetical Investigation of Acute Intermittent Porphyria.* Stockholm.

CHAPTER 8

ORGANIC BRAIN DISEASE

Psychological Tests of Organic Brain Disease. Hydrocephalic Dementia. Korsakoff's Psychosis and Related Conditions.

PSYCHOLOGICAL TESTS OF ORGANIC BRAIN DISEASE

INTELLECTUAL disability due to brain damage may be detected by the use of certain psychological tests. The sensitivity of these tests is, however, not very great and in general they can only confirm clinical judgment, although on occasions where there is a discrepancy between diagnosis and test results, the latter may prompt the psychiatrist to review his opinion. Psychological investigation is, however, of considerable value in research where quantification of any deficit is desirable. In this chapter only a few of the tests used are described and the reader is referred to recent reviews of the wide range of investigations now available (e.g. by Yates, 1967; and by Zimet and Fishman, 1970).

Use of Intelligence Tests

A simple determination of the level of intelligence (e.g. by means of the Wechsler Adult Intelligence Scale, the Mill Hill Vocabulary Scale or Raven's Progressive Matrices) is sometimes helpful in diagnosing intellectual deterioration, particularly where the patient's score can be compared with that of a similar test administered before the onset of the illness. Allowance must be made for any decline due to normal ageing which may have occurred between the two investigations. Very often, however, there has been no previous assessment, but even so some idea of the premorbid level may be obtained from the patient's past achievements and from his academic and occupational history. Demented patients who are suffering from some progressive cerebral disorder will show a decline in their scores with time and in equivocal cases it is worth repeating the test at intervals.

Comparison of the scores on different intelligence tests has been used to diagnose deterioration. It has been asserted that verbal ability is less affected by brain damage than other intellectual functions, and that vocabulary test scores give a better indication of the premorbid level than scores on tests of performance. But although most normal individuals tend to have similar performance and verbal intelligence quotients (I.Q.), quite wide discrepancies between the two may occur in the absence of brain damage. Thus about 1 in 20 normal subjects will have a verbal I.Q. which exceeds the performance I.Q. by at least 16 points (Field, 1960; Fisher, 1960). Moreover, in clinical practice verbal-performance differences are of limited value in detecting brain damage, and significant discrepancies were found in only 32 per cent of patients with

240

organic cerebral disease studied by Orme, Lee and Smith (1964) and in only 19 per cent of similar patients investigated by Bolton, Britton and Savage (1966). In addition significant differences may be found in functional mental disorder, as in 39 per cent of chronic schizophrenics tested by Orme *et al.* (1964).

Wechsler's deterioration index (Wechsler, 1958) is based on the observation that scores on the subtests of the Wechsler Adult Intelligence Scale (WAIS) decline with age and that the amount of the decrement varies with the subtest. Those which show little loss with age (the "Hold" tests) are Vocabulary, Information, Object Assembly and Picture Completion while those which show the steepest decline (the "Don't Hold" tests) are Digit Span, Similarities, Digit Symbol and Block Design. Wechsler assumed that the intellectual deterioration of dementia was qualitatively similar to that seen in normal ageing, and hence that the difference between the scores on the two sorts of subtest would indicate the severity of the dementia. Wechler's deterioration index is:

$$\frac{\text{Sum of ``Hold'' test scores} - \text{Sum of ``Don't Hold'' test scores}}{\text{Sum of ``Hold'' test scores}}$$

It has been shown to correlate significantly with the degree of cerebral atrophy determined by air encephalography (McFie, 1960; Gonen, 1970) but in clinical practice it is not a particularly useful measure. Of 47 brain-damaged patients studied by Bolton *et al.* (1966) this test correctly identified only 40 per cent, while Bersoff (1970) has found it to be of little value in distinguishing organic from functional psychoses.

New Word Learning

Walton and Black (1957) found that the ability to learn the meanings of unfamiliar words was impaired in subjects with generalized brain damage and they devised a reliable test of diagnostic value, the Modified Word Learning Test (MWLT). The procedure, as described by Walton and Black is as follows: The subject is given the Terman-Merrill vocabulary test (which lists words in order of increasing difficulty) until he is unable to give the meanings of 10 consecutive words. The essence of the test is to determine the ease or difficulty with which the meanings of these 10 unfamiliar words are learnt. The subject is given the definitions of these words and he is then tested to determine whether he now knows their meaning. The procedure of defining the words and then asking the patient to do so is repeated until he can define six of the ten correctly. (On each run-through the wording of the definitions given by the examiner is varied so as to avoid rote-learning). The score (Walton, White, Black and Young, 1959) depends on the number of times that the definitions have to be given to the subject before he achieves the criterion, and varies from 10 when he can define six words correctly after the first set of definitions to zero when the criterion is not reached after 10 presentations. (This method of scoring is however not that originally described by Walton and Black in 1957 and at present both the original and revised systems are in use. To avoid confusion only the revised system described above will be referred to here). On this scoring system, early validation studies showed that normal subjects and patients with functional mental disorder could be clearly distinguished from patients with unequivocal evidence of brain damage. All normal or functional cases scored 6 or more and of 78 patients with generalized cortical damage, 82 per cent scored 5 or less (Walton et al., 1959).

The value of the test as a diagnostic instrument was further investigated by Walton and Black (1959) and by Walton and Mather (1961). In these two studies, over 100 psychiatric patients were examined and again a cut-off score of 6 correctly identified all the patients later diagnosed independently as suffering from a functional disorder, and more than 80 per cent of those later diagnosed as having generalized cortical damage. Further evidence of the validity of the test has been adduced by White and Knox (1965) who investigated a series of 76 elderly subjects from the general population and 90 psychiatric patients suspected of having a dementing illness. The latter showed a much higher incidence of difficulty in learning than the former, and high scores were particularly common among patients with EEG evidence of generalized cortical disease. Furthermore, Bolton, Savage and Roth (1967) have shown that the scores on the MWLT correlate well with those on the Inglis Paired-Associate Learning Test which also discriminates between brain damaged patients and others (see below).

Various modifications of Walton and Black's original test have been introduced. Orme et al. (1964) used the Mill Hill Vocabulary Scale instead of the Terman-Merrill test; Kendrick, Parboosingh and Post (1965) also used the Mill Hill Vocabulary Scale, but in addition they standardized the definitions given to the patients; and Hetherington (1967) used neologisms instead of ordinary meaningful words. These investigators have confirmed Walton and Black's original finding that a high proportion of brain-damaged individuals show impairment of new word learning, but also that a proportion of functionally disturbed patients give abnormally high scores. Orme et al. (1964) found impaired learning in 81 per cent of brain-damaged subjects, but 70 per cent of chronic schizophrenics and 22 per cent of patients with other functional mental disorder also scored high. Kendrick et al. (1965) studied 100 elderly subjects (normal, depressed or brain-damaged) and found that there was no overlap in the scores obtained by normal persons and brain-damaged patients, but that 11 of the 68 depressed individuals gave scores suggesting cerebral damage. Bolton et al. (1967) also found that the test classified correctly all the normal elderly subjects and 71 per cent of the brain-damaged patients in their series, but that 29 per cent of patients with affective disorder and 23 per cent of schizophrenics were misclassified.

The abnormality of learning in depression has been investigated further (Post, 1966; Kendrick, 1967; Kendrick and Post, 1967). It tends to occur in elderly patients of low intelligence where the affective disturbance is severe and associated with prominent delusions and where there are clinical features suggestive of dementia, such as disorientation, confusion, perplexity and subjective difficulties in memory or thinking. Recovery from the depression is associated with the disappearance of these clinical features of "pseudo-dementia" and with a return to normal of learning ability. Such transient cognitive deficiency during depression does not seem to portend the development of dementia, but may be due to a temporary lowering of the level of arousal (Hemsi, Whitehead and Post, 1968).

New word learning depends also to some extent on general intelligence. Walton et al. (1959) administered the MWLT to 45 mentally subnormal patients and noted that 19 gave scores suggestive of brain damage while Bolton et al. (1967) found a significant negative correlation between impairment of learning and intelligence test scores. Hence the results of learning tests administered to patients of low previous intelligence should be interpreted cautiously.

Paired-Associate Learning

Inglis (1959) devised the Paired-Associate Learning Test (PALT) as a sensitive indicator of memory impairment independent of the level of general intellectual functioning. The test material consists of three pairs of words which the patient is required to learn to associate, and is in two forms:

Form A		Form B	
Stimulus	*Response*	*Stimulus*	*Response*
Cabbage	Pen	Flower	Spark
Knife	Chimney	Table	River
Sponge	Trumpet	Bottle	Comb

The tester reads aloud the three pairs of words and explains to the subject what is required of him. He then gives, one by one in random order, the first words of the pairs (the stimulus words) and waits for the subject to make the appropriate response, or if he fails to do so, the tester gives the correct answer. The stimulus words are presented until the subject is able to give three correct consecutive replies to each. If this criterion is not reached after presenting each stimulus word thirty times, the test is stopped. The score varies with the number of times the material has to be presented and the higher the score, the greater the learning difficulty.

Inglis (1959) administered the test to 18 elderly London patients with clinically evident memory disorder and to 18 subjects of the same age and verbal intelligence whose memory was intact. All the patients scored more than 30 (mean, 59·0) while all the controls scored less than 30 (mean, 13·0). A very similar result was obtained in a comparable study by Caird, Sanderson and Inglis (1962) on a Canadian population.

Parsons (1965) tested 214 subjects over the age of 65 years (a random sample of the elderly population of Swansea living in their own homes) and found a highly significant correlation between the test scores and previously assessed degree of memory impairment (Table 8.1). Evidence that the test is a valid one has also been provided by Bolton *et al*. (1967) and by Kendrick *et al*. (1965) who found a highly significant statistical correlation between test

Table 8.1

SCORES ON PAIRED-ASSOCIATE LEARNING TEST AND CLINICAL ASSESSMENT
OF MEMORY IMPAIRMENT
(Parsons, 1965)

Clinical assessment	Number of subjects	Mean PALT score
Normal memory	141	17·4
Slightly impaired memory	48	23·1
Definitely forgetful	19	42·3
*Demented	6	81·2

* i.e. cognitive impairment of such a degree as to render self-care impossible.

scores on the PALT and the MWLT. Kendrick *et al*. (1965) suggest that both types of test measure short-term memory, but Newcombe and Steinberg (1964) observed that the PALT was the better indicator of brain damage.

A much simplified version of the PALT, devised by Isaacs and Walkey (1964) has been recently tested by Priest, Tarighati and Shariatmadari (1969) who administered it to 17 patients with organic mental disturbance and to 34 patients with functional disorders. While the test scores were significantly different in the two groups of patients, there was a very considerable overlap, such that when Isaacs and Walkey's cut-off point was applied, 41 per cent of the functionally disordered patients and 12 per cent of the brain damaged patients were misclassified. Advantages of this test, however, are that it is extremely easy to administer and to score and that it is readily accepted by patients.

Memory-for-Designs Test

This test, developed by Graham and Kendall (1960) involves the reproduction by the patient of simple geometrical designs from memory. The test material comprises 15 cards, each with a different straight-line design, and these are exposed, one at a time for five seconds, to the subject who is then asked to reproduce them. Scoring of each reproduction depends on how much it departs from the original. Graham and Kendall (1960) found that the scores of 243 brain damaged patients were significantly higher than those of non-brain damaged subjects, but that these "raw" scores varied with age and intelligence. Graham and Kendall therefore advocated using scores corrected to eliminate any effect of these variables, but even so there was a considerable overlap between the two groups and the test misclassified over 30 per cent of brain damaged patients and 5 per cent of non-brain damaged subjects. Thus scores in the normal range tend to indicate the absence of cerebral disease, but high scores may have no pathological significance and a similar conclusion has been drawn by Turland and Steinhard (1969) and by Alexander (1970)

A further limitation of the test is that normal elderly subjects (particularly females) may give high scores (Kendall, 1962; Davies, 1967). But in spite of these drawbacks, it has the advantage of being simple to administer and score and of correlating better with clinical diagnosis than many other tests of brain damage (Korman and Blumberg, 1963; Brilliant and Gynther, 1963; Anglin, Pullen and Games, 1965).

REFERENCES

ALEXANDER, D. A. (1970). The application of the Graham-Kendall memory-for designs test to elderly normal and psychiatric groups. *Brit. J. soc. clin. Psychol.* **9**, 85-86.

ANGLIN, R., PULLEN, M. and GAMES, P. (1965). Comparison of two tests of brain damage. *Percept. mot. Skills*, **20**, 977-980.

BERSOFF, D. N. (1970). The revised deterioration formula for the Wechsler Adult Intelligence Scale: a test of validity. *J. clin. Psychol.* **26**, 71-73.

BOLTON, N., BRITTON, P. G. and SAVAGE, R. D. (1966). Some normative data on the WAIS and its indices in an aging population. *J. clin. Psychol.* **22**, 184-188.

BOLTON, N., SAVAGE, R. D. and ROTH, M. (1967). The modified word learning test and the aged patient. *Brit. J. Psychiat.* **113**, 1139-1140.

BRILLIANT, P. J. and GYNTHER, M. D. (1963). Relationship between performance on three tests for organicity and selected patient variables. *J. cons. Psychol.* **27**, 474-479.

CAIRD, W. K., SANDERSON, R. E. and INGLIS, J. (1962). Cross-validation of a learning test for use with elderly psychiatric patients. *J. ment. Sci.* **108**, 368-370.

DAVIES, A. D. M. (1967). Age and the memory-for-designs test. *Brit. J. soc. clin. Psychol.* **6**, 228-233.

FIELD, J. G. (1960). Two types of tables for use with Wechsler's intelligence scales. *J. clin. Psychol.* **16**, 3-7.

FISHER, G. M. (1960). A correlated table for determining the significance of the difference between verbal and performance I.Q.'s on the WAIS and the Wechsler-Bellevue. *J. clin. Psychol.* **16**, 7-8.

GONEN, J. Y. (1970). The use of Wechsler's deterioration quotient in cases of diffuse and symmetrical cerebral atrophy. *J. clin. Psychol.* **26**, 174-177.

GRAHAM, F. K. and KENDALL, B. S. (1960). Memory-for-designs test: revised general manual. *Percept. mot. Skills*, **11**, 147-188.

HEMSI, L. K., WHITEHEAD, A. and POST, F. (1968). Cognitive functioning and cerebral arousal in elderly depressives and dements. *J. psychosom. Res.* **12**, 145-156.

HETHERINGTON, R. (1967). A neologism learning test. *Brit. J. Psychiat.* **113**, 1133-1137.

INGLIS, J. (1959). A paired-associate learning test for use with elderly psychiatric patients. *J. ment. Sci.* **105**, 440-443.

ISAACS, B. and WALKEY, F. A. (1964). A simplified paired-associate test for elderly hospital patients. *Brit. J. Psychiat.* **110**, 80-83.

KENDALL, B. S. (1962). Memory-for-designs performance in the seventh and eighth decades of life. *Percept. mot. Skills*, **14**, 399-405.

KENDRICK, D. C. (1967). A cross-validation study of the use of the SLT and DCT in screening for diffuse brain pathology in elderly subjects. *Brit. J. med. Psychol.* **40**, 173-178.

KENDRICK, D. C., PARBOOSINGH, R-C. and POST, F. (1965). A synonym learning test for use with elderly psychiatric subjects: a validation study. *Brit. J. soc. clin. Psychol.* **4**, 63-71.

KENDRICK, D. C. and POST, F. (1967). Differences in cognitive status between healthy, psychiatrically ill and diffusely brain-damaged elderly subjects. *Brit. J. Psychiat.* **113**, 75-81.

KORMAN, M. and BLUMBERG, S. (1963). Comparative efficiency of some tests of cerebral damage. *J. cons. Psychol.* **27**, 303-309.

McFIE, J. (1960). Psychological testing in clinical neurology. *J. nerv. ment. Dis.* **131**, 383-393.

NEWCOMBE, F. and STEINBERG, B. (1964). Some aspects of learning and memory function in older psychiatric patients. *J. Geront.* **19**, 490-493.

ORME, J. E., LEE, D. and SMITH, M. R. (1964). Psychological assessments of brain damage and intellectual impairment in psychiatric patients. *Brit. J. soc. clin. Psychol.* **3**, 161-167.

PARSONS, P. L. (1965). Mental health of Swansea's old folk. *Brit. J. prev. soc. Med.* **19**, 43-47.

POST, F. (1966). Somatic and psychic factors in the treatment of ederly psychiatric patients. *J. psychosom. Res.* **10**, 13-19.

PRIEST, R. G., TARIGHATI, Sh. and SHARIATMADARI, M. E. (1969). A brief test of organic brain disease. Validation in a mental hospital population. *Acta psychiat. scand.* **45**, 347-354.

TURLAND, D. N. and STEINHARD, M. (1969). The efficiency of the memory-for-designs test. *Brit. J. soc. clin. Psychol.* **8**, 44-49.

WALTON, D. and BLACK, D. A. (1957). The validity of a psychological test of brain damage. *Brit. J. med. Psychol.* **30**, 270-279.

WALTON, D. and BLACK, D. A. (1959). The predictive validity of a psychological test of brain damage. *J. ment. Sci.* **105**, 807-810.

WALTON, D. and MATHER, M. D. (1961). A further study of the predictive validity of a psychological test of brain damage. *Brit. J. med. Psychol.* **34**, 73-75.

WALTON, D., WHITE, J. G., BLACK, D. A. and YOUNG, A. J. (1959). A modified word-learning test: a cross-validation study. *Brit. J. med. Psychol.* **32**, 213-220.

WECHSLER, D. (1958). *The Measurement and Appraisal of Adult Intelligence* (4th Edition). Baltimore.

WHITE, J. G. and KNOX, S. J. (1965). Some psychological correlates of age and dementia. *Brit. J. soc. clin. Psychol.* **4**, 259-265.

YATES, A. J. (1967). Psychological deficit. *Ann. Rev. Psychol.* **17**, 111-144.

ZIMET, C. N. and FISHMAN, D. B. (1970). Psychological deficit in schizophrenia and brain damage. *Ann. Rev. Psychol.* **21**, 113-154.

HYDROCEPHALIC DEMENTIA

Dementia may be associated with enlargement of the ventricles of the brain in two circumstances. First, where there is a primary brain disorder such as cerebral arteriosclerosis or Alzheimer's disease, or indeed any other widespread degenerative condition of the cerebral hemispheres, with consequent passive dilatation of the ventricles (hydrocephalus *ex vacuo*). Secondly, the ventricles may distend because of increased intraventicular pressure and lead to dementia because of the consequent impairment of brain function. In this latter condition of obstructive hydrocephalus the ventricles may be in communication with the subarachnoid space (communicating hydrocephalus) or there may be a block between the two (non-communicating hydrocephalus). The distinction between hydrocephalus *ex vacuo* and communicating obstructive hydrocephalus is very important in that in the latter condition notable improvement in all the symptoms (including those of the dementia) may occur after operative relief of the raised intraventricular pressure. Measurement of the pressure of the cerebrospinal fluid should, in theory, differentiate the two conditions, but the situation is complicated by the fact that there have been a number of recent reports of obstructive hydrocephalus associated with apparently normal pressures (McHugh, 1964; Adams, Fisher, Hakim et al. 1965). The differentiation of this "normal pressure" hydrocephalus from cerebral atrophy is sometimes difficult, particularly since the hydrocephalus may arise without demonstrable cause. The distinction is, however, very important because operation may improve the condition as dramatically as in cases of classical obstructive hydrocephalus, and it seems likely that many patients with normal pressure hydrocephalus in the past have been wrongly diagnosed as cerebral atrophy.

The Diagnosis of Hydrocephalic Dementia

Clinical Features

The symptomatology of normal pressure hydrocephalus arising in adult life has been described by McHugh (1964), by Adams et al. (1965) and by Adams (1966) and further reports consistent with the observations of these workers have been published by McHugh (1966), Hogan and Woolsey (1966), Breig, Ekbom, Greitz and Kugelberg (1967), Hill, Lougheed and Barnett (1967) Weiss and Raskind (1968), Glasaeur, Alker, Leslie and Nicol (1968), Lin, Goodkin, Tong et al. (1968), Baska, Williamson and Ziegler (1968), Ojemann, Fisher, Adams et al. (1969), Braham, Front, Sarova-Pinhas et al. (1969) and Lethlean and Gye (1969).

Intellectual deterioration, with mild to severe memory impairment (particularly for recent events), disorientation, apathy and psychomotor retardation, is extremely common and is probably present to some degree in all cases. Of 50 published reports reviewed by Hogan and Woolsey (1966) 29 showed evidence of dementia and in four this was the only presenting condition (Table 8.2). Difficulty and unsteadiness in walking are other early symptoms and these may occur before any obvious mental change (Messert and Baker, 1966), while incontinence of urine (Adams, 1966), headache (Hogan and Woolsey, 1966), epileptic fits (Nag and Falconer, 1966; Weiss and Raskind, 1968), impotence (Wilkinson, LeMay and Drew, 1966) and akinetic mutism (Messert, Henke and Langheim, 1966) have also been reported.

Abnormal neurological signs are not usually very pronounced, but commonly there is some evidence of pyramidal tract involvement (increased deep reflexes, particularly in the legs and sometimes bilateral extensor plantar responses) and less often extrapyramidal signs or tremor (Adams, 1966; Hill et al., 1967).

Although there are similarities between the symptoms and signs of hydrocephalus and of cortical atrophy, Adams (1966) points out that differentiation

I

may be possible on clinical grounds. He suggests that hydrocephalus should be suspected in patients whose impairment of memory, psychomotor retardation, disturbance of gait and incontinence of urine have occurred early in

Table 8.2

SYMPTOMS OF HYDROCEPHALUS IN 50 ADULT PATIENTS
(Hogan and Woolsey, 1966)

Symptoms	No. of patients
None	4
Headache alone	6
Dementia alone	4
Gait disturbance alone	5
Headache and dementia	8
Headache and gait disturbance	6
Gait disturbance and dementia	11
Headache, dementia and gait disturbance	6
	50

their illness, where there has been rapid development of the condition over the course of a few weeks or months and where the symptoms tend to fluctuate in severity.

Aetiology

Investigation may reveal an obvious obstruction to the flow of the CSF, such as stenosis or occlusion of the aqueduct of Sylvius (Foltz, 1963; McHugh, 1964; Wilkinson *et al.*, 1966; Nag and Falconer, 1966) or a tumour in the third ventricle (McHugh, 1966; Adams, 1966). In other cases the condition arises after meningitis (Hogan and Woolsey, 1966) or much more commonly as the aftermath of a subarachnoid haemorrhage which may be spontaneous or traumatic (Foltz and Ward, 1956; Hogan and Woolsey, 1966; Hill *et al.*, 1967; Bannister, Gilford and Kocen, 1967; Theander and Granholm, 1967; Weiss and Raskind, 1968) and here the obstruction is probably within the arachnoid villi and is due to organization of the subarachnoid exudate (Ellington and Margolis, 1969). Breig *et al.* (1967) have reported three cases where the hydrocephalus was attributed to pressure on the floor of the third ventricle by an abnormally long basilar artery. In a proportion of patients however there is no obvious cause for the hydrocephalus. Of 50 published cases reviewed by Hogan and Woolsey (1966) no discernible cause was found in 11 (22 per cent) while in 33 per cent of the 22 patients in the two more recent series reported by Bannister *et al.* (1967) and by Hill *et al.* (1967), the aetiology was similarly obscure.

Air Encephalography

Communicating hydrocephalus is most easily demonstrated by radiological examination of the head after introducing air into the lumbar subarachnoid space. The essential findings are dilatation of the whole ventricular system (including the third ventricle, the aqueduct and the fourth ventricle), and absence of air over the convexity of the hemispheres. A little air may find its way into the cortical subarachnoid spaces, particularly in the subfrontal region and over the insular cortex (Bannister et al., 1967; Hill et al., 1967), but the appearances are usually quite distinct from those of cerebral atrophy where the dilated cortical subarachnoid channels fill very easily. A further difference between the two conditions is that ventricular enlargement is a late manifestation of cerebral atrophy and it is then associated with profound dementia, whereas in hydrocephalus the ventricles distend early at a time when mental changes may be relatively mild (Adams et al., 1965; McHugh, 1966). Moreover, in cerebral atrophy the enlargement may be asymmetrical and tends to affect the bodies of the lateral ventricles more than the temporal horns (Sjaastad, Skalpe and Engeset, 1969).

A major disadvantage of air encephalography is that it often causes immediate, though usually only temporary, deterioration in the patient's condition, presumably because of disturbances of the intracranial pressures (Hill et al., 1967; Bannister et al., 1967). Impairment of consciousness proceeding to coma may occur and immediate surgical decompression may be necessary. Bannister et al. (1967) have also pointed out that after air encephalography in patients with hydrocephalus, the very slow reabsorption of air from the ventricles may delay operative treatment because of the risk of air embolism.

Isotope Ventriculography and Encephalography

Human serum albumin labelled with radioactive material introduced into the cerebrospinal fluid is absorbed slowly and its distribution within the head may be determined by the use of external scintillation detectors. The material may be injected directly into the ventricles and their size assessed (Di Chiro, 1964; Overbeek, 1968; Brocklehurst, 1968) or the radioactivity of successive samples of ventricular fluid may be measured and the rate of clearance, which is very much slower than in normal hydrocephalus, may be estimated (Killeffer, Crandall and Abbott, 1968). It is generally easier however to introduce radio-iodinated human serum albumin by lumbar intrathecal injection (Di Chiro, 1964; Bannister et al., 1967; Glasaeur et al., 1968; Lin et al., 1968; Patten and Benson, 1968) and to determine its distribution within the head by external scanning. In normal subjects and in patients with cerebral atrophy, isotope encephalography reveals detectable radioactivity over the cerebral cortex within a few hours, and at no time is activity found within the ventricles. In contrast, in patients with communicating hydrocephalus radioactivity is detected only within the ventricles and none over the cortex. Bannister et al. (1967), using these criteria, could clearly differentiate communicating hydrocephalus from cerebral atrophy. They suggest that isotope encephalography has advantages over air encephalography, particularly because it does not appear to interfere with cerebrospinal fluid hydrodynamics and consequently there is no immediate deterioration in the patient's condition. Isotope encephalography is however sometimes followed by aseptic meningitis (Detmer and Blacker, 1965; Nicol, 1967) and since the hazard from radiation is not known with certainty, the investigation should probably be restricted, at present, to elderly demented subjects. The use of human serum albumin labelled with radioactive technetium may be associated with less radiation risk, since this isotope has a shorter half-life than radioactive iodine and its emission is less destructive (Di Chiro, Ashburn and Briner, 1968).

Cerebrospinal Fluid

In many cases of obstructive hydrocephalus when there is no obvious cause, examination of the CSF shows no abnormality, but in other cases there may be an increase in the number of cells and amount of protein, depending on the nature of the responsible lesion. Sometimes the CSF pressure is raised but more commonly it is in the high normal range (i.e. 150-200 mm water). Hogan and Woolsey (1966) reviewed data on CSF pressure in 35 published cases of adult hydrocephalus and noted that in 22 patients the pressure was normal. Occasionally the pressure is elevated early in the course of the illness but falls to normal later (Adams, 1966), or the increase may be intermittent (McHugh, 1964) but there are cases where there is no evidence that the CSF pressure has ever been above normal. In such circumstances it is difficult to understand how the ventricles can remain distended or how reduction of pressure can lead to clinical improvement. Hakim and Adams (1965) have invoked Pascal's Law (i.e. Force exerted = Pressure × Area of walls) and have suggested that a given intraventricular pressure exerts more force when the ventricles are dilated than when of normal size. Geschwind (1968) however, has challenged this explanation and has argued that a reduction in the tensile strength of the walls of the ventricles is initially responsible for the expansion, and that the physical properties of the white matter surrounding the ventricles may be affected by raised intraventricular pressure thus allowing further distension. Greitz (1969) hypothesises that atrophic changes within the brain decrease the resistance to expansion and that the expansion itself produces further ischaemic atrophy, thus aggravating the situation. That there may be such a complex interaction between cerebral atrophic changes and cerebrospinal fluid hydrodynamics is supported by the experience of Appenzeller and Salmon (1967) and of Salmon (1969) who noted marked improvement in the mental state of a number of patients with senile and presenile dementia following surgical decompression of their enlarged ventricles.

Whatever the mechanism, there is now little doubt that normal CSF pressure does sometimes cause distension of the ventricles and that in these cases reduction of the pressure is of benefit to the patient. The distinction between high pressure and normal pressure hydrocephalus is therefore at the present time largely of theoretical importance.

Angiography

In obstructive hydrocephalus carotid arteriography may show an abnormal upward sweep and displacement of the anterior cerebral arteries due to distension of the lateral ventricles. In contrast, these changes are not observed in cerebral atrophy and hence this investigation may be helpful in making the correct diagnosis (McHugh, 1964, 1966; Adams et al., 1965; Glasaeur et al., 1968).

Electroencephalography

EEG abnormalities are frequently found in obstructive hydrocephalus, most commonly diffuse theta or delta waves (i.e. less than 7 cycles per second) and a tendency to photic following at 5 to 20 flashes per second. Even early hydrocephalus is associated with minor abnormalities of this type (Adams, 1966) and this contrasts with the findings in Alzheimer's disease where the early changes are confined to a reduction in alpha activity and where diffuse delta and theta waves are not seen until the condition is well advanced (Gordon and Sim, 1967).

Treatment of Hydrocephalic Dementia

As has already been pointed out, measures taken to reduce intraventricular pressure may greatly improve the clinical condition of patients with obstructive hydrocephalus. Until recently the most common neurosurgical procedure was drainage of the ventricles into the basal cisterns (Torkildsen's operation) but nowadays ventriculo-atrial drainage, involving the shunting of ventricular CSF via non-return valves into the venous blood stream is the treatment of choice in most cases. Reports of the efficacy of such operations vary. Immediate dramatic improvement has been observed by Foltz and Ward (1956), Wilkinson et al. (1966), Adams (1966), Weiss and Raskind (1968) and Greitz, Grepe, Kalmér and Lopez (1969) in patients with dementia, and by Theander and Granholm (1967) in patients with Korsakoff's syndrome. More commonly, improvement occurs over the course of a few weeks, and excellent results have been noted by McHugh (1966), Hogan and Woolsey (1966), Baska et al. (1968), Glasaeur et al. (1968) and Lethlean and Gye (1969). Hill et al. (1967) found a moderate degree of recovery in 6 of their 12 patients after shunt operation, but none became completely normal mentally. Adams (1966) found that the mental disability improved more rapidly than did the disturbance of gait while Bannister et al. (1967) observed that the degree of improvement was inversely proportional to the duration of the disorder. Nag and Falconer (1966) noted that ventriculocisternal shunt had no effect on their patients' epilepsy although other symptoms tended to improve. Ojemann et al. (1969) have reported their experience of 28 patients treated operatively and have noted that the best results are seen in patients with the typical clinical syndrome and who show complete obstruction of CSF flow in the basal cisterns. That improvement is related to reduction of intraventricular pressure is indicated first by post-operative demonstration of a decrease in ventricular size (Hogan and Woolsey, 1966; Weiss and Raskind, 1968; Glasaeur *et al.* 1968; Greitz *et al.* 1969) and secondly by the observation that if the implanted valve ceases to function, the condition of the patient deteriorates until the valve is replaced (Glasaeur *et al.* 1968; Baska *et al.* 1968). Greitz *et al.* (1969) have noted a post-operative increase in cerebral blood flow which also correlates with the patient's improvement.

Repeated removal of lumbar cerebrospinal fluid reduces the pressure in the ventricular system and may improve the symptoms of obstructive hydro-cephalus, and this may enable the clinician to predict a good response to ventriculo-atrial drainage, but a shunt operation may succeed where repeated lumbar puncture has failed (Adams *et al.* 1965; Hill *et al.* 1967). McHugh (1966) observed a remarkable temporary improvement in the mental state of a patient immediately after a single lumbar puncture, but this must be a rather rare phenomenon.

REFERENCES

ADAMS, R. D. (1966). Further observations on normal pressure hydrocephalus. *Proc. roy. Soc. Med.* **59**, 1135-1140.
ADAMS, R. D., FISHER, C. M., HAKIM, S., OJEMANN, R. G. and SWEET, W. H. (1965). Symptomatic occult hydrocephalus with "normal" cerebrospinal fluid pressure. A treatable syndrome. *New Engl. J. Med.* **273**, 117-126.
APPENZELLER, O. and SALMON, J. H. (1967). Treatment of parenchymatous degeneration of the brain by ventriculo-atrial shunting of the cerebrospinal fluid. *J. Neurosurg.* **26**, 478-482.
BANNISTER, R., GILFORD, E. and KOCEN, R. (1967). Isotope encephalography in the diagnosis of dementia due to communicating hydrocephalus. *Lancet*, **2**, 1014-1017.
BASKA, R. E., WILLIAMSON, W. P. and ZIEGLER, D. K. (1968). Symptomatic occult hydrocephalus: a case report and review. *Sth. med. J. (Bgham, Ala.)* **61**, 249-252.
BRAHAM, J., FRONT, D., SAROVA-PINHAS, I., KOSARY, I. Z. and CZERNIAK, P. (1969). Brain atrophy, hydrocephalus and dementia in adults. *Israel J. med. Sci.* **5**, 1213-1218.
BREIG, A., EKBOM, K., GREITZ, T. and KUGELBERG, E. (1967). Hydrocephalus due to elongated basilar artery. A new clinico-radiological syndrome. *Lancet*, **1**, 874-875.
BROCKLEHURST, G. (1968). Use of radio-iodinated serum albumin in the study of cerebrospinal fluid flow. *J. Neurol. Neurosurg. Psychiat.* **31**, 162-168.
DETMER, D. E. and BLACKER, H. M. (1965). A case of aseptic meningitis secondary to intrathecal injection of I^{131} human serum albumin. *Neurology (Minneap.)* **15**, 642-643.
DI CHIRO, G. (1964). New radiographic and isotopic procedures in neurological diagnosis. *J. Amer. med. Ass.* **188**, 524-529.
DI CHIRO, G., ASHBURN, W. L. and BRINER, W. H. (1968). Technetium Tc 99m serum albumin for cisternography. *Arch. Neurol. (Chic.)* **19**, 218-227.
ELLINGTON, E. and MARGOLIS, G. (1969). Block of arachnoid villus by subarachnoid haemorrhage. *J. Neurosurg.* **30**, 651-657.
FOLTZ, E. L. (1963). Discussion on "Hydrocephalus after subarachnoid haemorrhage" *J. Neurosurg.* **20**, 1047-1048.

FOLTZ, E. L. and WARD, A. A. (1956). Communicating hydrocephalus from subarachnoid bleeding. *J. Neurosurg.* **13**, 546-566.

GESCHWIND, N. (1968). The mechanism of normal pressure hydrocephalus. *J. neurol. Sci.* **7**, 481-493.

GLASAEUR, F. E., ALKER, G. J., LESLIE, E. V. and NICOL, C. F. (1968). Isotope cisternography in hydrocephalus with normal pressure. *J. Neurosurg.* **29**, 555-561.

GORDON, E. B. and SIM, M. (1967). The E.E.G. in presenile dementia. *J. Neurol. Neurosurg. Psychiat.* **30**, 285-291.

GREITZ, T. (1969). Effect of brain distension on cerebral circulation. *Lancet*, **1**, 863-865.

GREITZ, T. V. B., GREPE, A. O. L., KALMÉR, M. S. F. and LOPEZ, J. (1969). Pre- and post-operative evaluation of cerebral blood flow in low pressure hydrocephalus. *J. Neurosurg.* **31**, 644-651.

HAKIM, S. and ADAMS, R. D. (1965). The special clinical problem of symptomatic hydrocephalus with normal cerebrospinal fluid pressure. Observations on cerebrospinal fluid hydrodynamics. *J. neurol. Sci.* **2**, 307-327.

HILL, M. E., LOUGHEED, W. M. and BARNETT, H. J. M. (1967). A treatable form of dementia due to normal-pressure, communicating hydrocephalus. *Canad. med. Ass. J.* **97**, 1309-1320.

HOGAN, P. A. and WOOLSEY, R. M. (1966). Hydrocephalus in the adult. *J. Amer. med. Ass.* **198**, 524-528.

KILLEFFER, F. A., CRANDALL, P. H. and ABBOTT, M. (1968). [131]ISHA ventricular clearance in evaluation of symptomatic occult hydrocephalus. *Bull. Los Angeles neurol. Soc.* **33**, 129-135.

LETHLEAN, K. and GYE, R. (1969). Dementia in the adult due to occult hydrocephalus. *Proc. Aust. Ass. Neurol.* **5**, 13-18.

LIN, J. P-T., GOODKIN, R., TONG, E. C. K., EPSTEIN, F. J. and VINCIGUERRA, E. (1968). Radioiodinated serum albumin (RISA) cisternography in the diagnosis of incisural block and occult hydrocephalus. *Radiology*, **90**, 36-41.

McHUGH, P. R. (1964). Occult hydrocephalus. *Quart. J. Med.* **33**, 297-308.

McHUGH, P. R. (1966). Hydrocephalic dementia. *Bull N. Y. Acad. Med.* **42**, 907-917.

MESSERT, B. and BAKER, N. H. (1966). Syndrome of progressive spastic ataxia and apraxia associated with occult hydrocephalus. *Neurology (Minneap.)*, **16**, 440-442.

MESSERT, B., HENKE, T. K. and LANGHEIM, W. (1966). Syndrome of akinetic mutism associated with occult hydrocephalus. *Neurology (Minneap.)*, **16**, 635-649.

NAG, T. K. and FALCONER, M. A. (1966). Non-tumoral stenosis of the aqueduct in adults. *Brit. med. J.* **2**, 1168-1170.

NICOL, C. F. (1967). A second case of aseptic meningitis following isotope cisternography using I[131] human serum albumin. *Neurology (Minneap.)*, **17**, 199-200.

OJEMANN, R. G., FISHER, C. M., ADAMS, R. D., SWEET, W. H. and NEW, P. F. J. (1969). Further experience with "normal" pressure hydrocephalus. *J. Neurosurg.* **31**, 279-294.

OVERBEEK, W. J. (1968). Isotope investigation of hydrocephalus. *Psychiat. Neurol. Neurochir. (Amst.)* **71**, 99-103.

PATTEN, D. H. and BENSON, D. F. (1968). Diagnosis of normal-pressure hydrocephalus by RISA cisternography. *J. nucl. Med.* **9**, 457-461.

SALMON, J. H. (1969). Senile and presenile dementia. Ventriculoatrial shunt for symptomatic treatment. *Geriatrics*, **24**, No. 12, 67-72.

SJAASTAD, O., SKALPE, I. O. and ENGESET, A. (1969). The width of the temporal horn in the differential diagnosis between pressure hydrocephalus and hydrocephalus ex vacuo. *Neurology (Minneap.)*, **19**, 1087-1093.

THEANDER, S. and GRANHOLM, L. (1967). Sequelae after spontaneous subarachnoid haemorrhage, with special reference to hydrocephalus and Korsakoff's syndrome. *Acta neurol. scand.* **43**, 479-488.

WEISS, S. R. and RASKIND, R. (1968). "Normal pressure" hydrocephalus treated by ventriculo-atrial shunt. Report of three cases and suggestions for study. *Int. Surg.* **50**, 340-349.

WILKINSON, H. A., LEMAY, M. and DREW, J. H. (1966). Adult aqueductal stenosis. *Arch. Neurol. (Chic.)* **15**, 643-648.

KORSAKOFF'S PSYCHOSIS AND RELATED CONDITIONS

The characteristic feature of the amnestic syndrome is a severe impairment of memory due to organic brain disease in the absence of any generalized intellectual deterioration, impairment of consciousness or inattentiveness. Most commonly it occurs as the aftermath of Wernicke's encephalopathy, due to thiamine deficiency (Korsakoff's psychosis, Wernicke–Korsakoff syndrome) but clinically similar conditions occur with other types of brain disease and these will also be discussed here.

The Wernicke-Korsakoff Syndrome

Wernicke's Encephalopathy

Descriptions of this condition have changed little since Wernicke's original account in 1881 (translated recently by Brody and Wilkins, 1968) which reported two cases in association with chronic alcoholism and one consequent on pyloric obstruction. Recent reports include those by Frantzen (1966) and by Biemond (1969).

The symptoms and signs characteristic of the disorder appear usually after a period of persistent vomiting. The initial neurological disturbance is a coarse nystagmus, soon followed by ophthalmoplegia with bilateral external rectus palsies, paralysis of vertical or horizontal conjugate gaze and sometimes paralysis of the other external ocular muscles. Irregularity of the pupils and typical Argyll Robertson changes have been reported. Retinal haemorrhages are common and papilloedema with impairment of visual acuity occurs occasionally. A prominent feature is ataxia, mainly of the trunk and due to cerebellar damage or vestibular paresis, and to a lesser extent of the limbs when it is due to the commonly associated peripheral neuropathy. From the earliest stages, mental changes may be noted, particularly apathy followed by impairment of consciousness, disorientation, memory disturbances and confabulation, but sometimes the mental state is more like that of delirium tremens with general excitement and visual hallucinations. The symptoms and signs of 20 cases reported by Biemond (1969) are set out in Table 8.3.

The principal neuropathological changes are neuronal degeneration and haemorrhage in the thalamus, hypothalamus, midbrain and mammillary bodies, similar to those observed in experimentally induced thiamine deficiency in animals.

Wernicke's encephalopathy is most commonly associated with chronic alcoholism, but other causes of thiamine deficiency are sometimes responsible, and these include prolonged starvation (Frantzen, 1966; Drenick, Joven and Swendseid, 1966), vitamin B deficiency in an otherwise adequate diet (de Wardener and Lennox, 1947; Cruickshank, 1950) hyperemesis gravidarum

Table 8.3

SIGNS OF WERNICKE'S ENCEPHALOPATHY
(20 cases, Biemond, 1969)

Signs	No. of patients	Per cent
Mental disturbance	20	100
Nystagmus	18	90
Polyneuritis	17	85
Oculomotor disturbances	13	65
Ataxia	10	50
Retinal haemorrhages	6	30

(Chaturachinda and McGregor, 1968; Biemond, 1969) and gastric disease such as carcinoma of the stomach, achalasia of the cardia and pyloric obstruction (Campbell and Russell, 1941; Biemond, 1969). It has also been reported in association with pernicious anaemia (Campbell and Russell, 1941) and as a complication of chronic haemodialysis for renal failure (Lopez and Collins, 1968). In Biemond's (1969) series of 20 patients the aetiology was:

Alcoholism	10 cases
Hyperemesis gravidarum	7 cases
Carcinoma pylorus	1 case
Cardiospasm	1 case
Self-imposed malnutrition	1 case

Untreated, most patients with Wernicke's encephalopathy die, but the administration of vitamin B preparations (including, of course, thiamine) leads to a rapid improvement in the ocular symptoms and mental confusion. Unless this treatment is given early, however, recovery from the acute illness is likely to be followed by permanent impairment of memory. Cole, Turner, Frank et al. (1969) noted an improvement in the extraocular paralysis within a few hours of administering thiamine intravenously, and that in the absence of liver disease, 10 mg thiamine was effective. Hepatic disease interferes with the utilization of thiamine and hence much higher doses (250 mg daily or more) should be given as a routine. Since these patients may lack other vitamins it seems better to administer multi-vitamin preparations (e.g. high-potency "Parenterovite") rather than thiamine on its own.

Korsakoff's Psychosis

The symptomatology of Korsakoff's psychosis has been reviewed by Lewis (1961), Victor (1964), Talland (1965) Willanger (1966) and Biemond (1969).

Memory Disturbances

The principal abnormality in the mental state is a gross impairment of memory, which is of two types. Firstly, there is an inability to lay down new memories such that the patient has complete amnesia for events after the onset of the illness. Often this disturbance is so severe that items may not be recalled after the passage of only a few minutes. Associated with this defect is an inability to learn new material. Very short-term memory is however unaffected and hence the patient can usually reproduce a short series of numbers immediately after presentation (i.e. the "digit span" is normal). The second type of memory impairment is a retrograde amnesia for events before the onset of the illness, which may extend backwards for days, weeks, months or even years. Hence patients with Korsakoff's psychosis may remember events in early life but be unable to recall more recent happenings. Emotional factors determine to some extent what is remembered and what is forgotten, and these catathymic influences may be responsible for the almost invariable denial of excessive drinking in cases with an alcoholic aetiology and may explain why forgotten memories may sometimes be recovered after the administration of intravenous sodium amylobarbitone. Insight is always impaired, often to the point of complete unawareness of any memory defect. The patient is usually calm and apathetic; less often he is euphoric. The amnesia contrasts strikingly with the usually excellent preservation of other intellectual functions, and long-established skills such as those involved in speaking, writing, calculating and spelling are unaffected.

Distortion of Time Sense

Patients with Korsakoff's psychosis are disoriented in time and are unable to give the date accurately and consistently. They underestimate time intervals, particularly that which has elapsed since the onset of the illness and they have great difficulty in placing past events in their correct order of occurrence. (This disruption of the temporal frame of reference may be the basis for confabulation—see below). Commonly, these patients cannot state their own age correctly or can only do so after considerable thought and calculation.

Confabulation

In the early stages of the disorder, particularly where the cause is alcoholism, the patient commonly gives a reasonably coherent, but quite false, account of recent events, especially in relation to his personal activities; as the disease becomes more chronic this confabulation is less evident. No adequate explanation for this phenomenon exists, but it has been proposed that it may be purposive, to avoid the embarrassment associated with forgetting, or to please the examiner, or that it may be the result of suggestion. But examination of the content of these false memories often shows that they consist of confused fragments of past experience and a more likely explanation is that they are secondary to the breakdown in the patient's temporal frame of reference; that is to say, confabulations are bits of real memories recalled by the patient but which are fused and referred by him to the amnesic period instead of to their correct time in the past.

Results of Psychological Testing

Many of these clinical findings have been confirmed in the psychological laboratory. General intelligence (as measured, for example, by the Wechsler Adult Intelligence Scale) is normal or only very slightly impaired, but tests of memory show gross deficiency in the capacity to reproduce correctly test material such as drawings and narrative passages, and estimates of the duration of short periods of time are less accurate among patients with Korsakoff's psychosis than among normal subjects. Very short term memory (tested by estimation of the digit span) is unaffected (Victor, Talland and Adams, 1959; Malerstein and Belden, 1968). Talland (1965) noted that eyeblink conditioning, using a buzzer as the conditioned stimulus and a puff of air on the cornea as the unconditioned stimulus, occurred more slowly than normal, while extinction was extremely rapid, consistent with the defect in learning which these patients show.

Neuropathological Findings

Although the pathological lesions in Korsakoff's psychosis are widespread, the most constant changes are found first in the mammillary bodies which are often macroscopically small and which almost always show atrophy and gliosis on histological examination, and secondly in the thalamus, which shows subacute and chronic degenerative changes. Similar lesions are common in the periventricular and periaqueductal grey matter, and less frequently in other parts of the brain-stem and in the cerebellum. The distribution of these changes is identical to that seen in Wernicke's encephalopathy (Malamud and Skillicorn, 1956; Victor, 1964). Although the consensus is that the amnesia is due to the mammillary body lesions, Victor (1964) has suggested that bilateral damage to the dorsomedial nuclei of the thalamus is of greater importance and he states that the mammillary bodies may be severely affected in the absence of memory disturbance.

REFERENCES

BIEMOND, A. (1969). Wernicke's encephalopathy and Korsakow's syndrome. *Psychiat. clin.* (*Basel*), **2**, 146-166.

BRODY, I. A. and WILKINS, R. H. (1968). Wernicke's encephalopathy. *Arch. Neurol.* (*Chic.*) **19**, 228-238.

CAMPBELL, A. C. P. and RUSSELL, W. R. (1941). Wernicke's encephalopathy: the clinical features and their probable relationship to Vitamin B deficiency. *Quart. J. Med.* **10**, 41-64.

CHATURACHINDA, K. and McGREGOR, E. M. (1968). Wernicke's encephalopathy and pregnancy. *J. Obstet. Gynaec. Brit. Cwlth.* **75**, 969-971.

COLE, M., TURNER, A., FRANK, O., BAKER, H. and LEEVY, C. M. (1969). Extraocular palsy and thiamine therapy in Wernicke's encephalopathy. *Amer. J. clin. Nutr.* **22**, 44-51.

CRUICKSHANK, E. K. (1950). Wernicke's encephalopathy. *Quart. J. Med.* **19**, 327-338.

DE WARDENER, H. E. and LENNOX, B. (1947). Cerebral beriberi (Wernicke's encephalopathy) *Lancet*, **1**, 11-17.

DRENICK, E. J., JOVEN, C. B. and SWENDSEID, M. E. (1966). Occurrence of acute Wernicke's encephalopathy during prolonged starvation for the treatment of obesity. *New Engl. J. Med.* **274**, 937-939.
FRANTZEN, E. (1966). Wernicke's encephalopathy. 3 cases occurring in connection with severe malnutrition. *Acta neurol. scand.* **42**, 426-441.
LEWIS, A. (1961). Amnesic syndromes. The psychopathological aspect. *Proc. roy. Soc. Med.* **54**, 955-961.
LOPEZ, R. I. and COLLINS, G. H. (1968). Wernicke's encephalopathy. A complication of chronic hemodialysis. *Arch. Neurol. (Chic.)* **18**, 248-259.
MALAMUD, N. and SKILLICORN, S. A. (1956). Relationship between the Wernicke and the Korsakoff syndrome. *Arch. Neurol. Psychiat. (Chic.)* **76**, 585-596.
MALERSTEIN, A. J. and BELDEN, E. (1968). WAIS, SILS and PPVT in Korsakoff's syndrome. *Arch. gen. Psychiat.* **19**, 743-750.
TALLAND, G. A. (1965). *Deranged Memory*. New York.
VICTOR, M. (1964). Observations on the amnestic syndrome in man and its anatomical basis. In *Brain Function, Volume II. RNA and Brain Function, Memory and Learning* (Editor Brazier, M. A. B.), pp. 311-340. Berkeley.
VICTOR, M., TALLAND, G. A. and ADAMS, R. D. (1959). Psychological studies of Korsakoff's psychosis: I. General intellectual functions. *J. nerv. ment. Dis.* **128** 528-537.
WILLANGER, R. (1966). The amnestic syndrome in the early phase of Wernicke's encephalopathy. *Acta neurol. scand.* **42**, 442-454.

Other Causes of the Amnestic Syndrome

Symonds (1966), in a comprehensive review of disorders of memory, has suggested that the term Korsakoff's psychosis should be reserved for the typical amnestic syndrome following Wernicke's encephalopathy due to thiamine deficiency. Identical mental states with gross impairment of memory in the absence of dementia, however, occur in association with various brain lesions particularly in the hippocampus and hypothalamus, and these are sometimes loosely referred to as Korsakoff's psychosis or Korsakoff-like conditions.

Temporal Lobe Disorders

Bilateral hippocampal damage commonly causes the amnestic syndrome. In particular, acute necrotizing encephalitis affecting the temporal lobes is sometimes followed by a Korsakoff-like state. Rose and Symonds (1960) reported four such cases where recovery from the acute phase of an encephalitis of indefinite aetiology left the patients with permanent defects in recent memory and with retrograde amnesia for some years before the illness but without any generalized intellectual deterioration. Their symptomatology differed from patients with Korsakoff's psychosis in that there was no tendency to confabulate and in that they showed insight. More recently, cases of acute necrotizing encephalitis due to infection with herpes simplex virus have been reported as leading to a similar chronic mental state (Drachman and Adams, 1962; Leider, Magoffin, Lennette and Leonards, 1965; Starr and Phillips, 1968; Glaser and Pincus, 1969). The early diagnosis of herpes simplex encephalitis has practical importance since this condition may respond to treatment with idoxyuridine, an analogue of thymidine which inhibits DNA synthesis and the growth of DNA viruses such as herpes (Nolan, Carruthers and Lerner, 1970). The illness presents with fever, headache and mental confusion; physical examination usually shows no specific abnormalities, but the EEG is always abnormal, often with temporal lobe foci on one or both sides and the CSF usually contains increased white cells and protein. Biopsy of the temporal lobe, which shows intra-nuclear inclusion bodies, is essential for early diagnosis, and waiting to demonstrate a rise in serum antibody titre may delay treatment too long (Campbell, 1969; Adams, 1969). Subacute encephalitis of unspecified aetiology affecting mainly the temporal lobes has also been reported to give rise to the amnestic syndrome, from which the patient may recover completely (Himmelhoch, Pincus, Tucker and Detre, 1970).

Encephalitis affecting the temporal lobes has been reported in association with malignant neoplasms, particularly carcinoma of the bronchus (Brierley, Corsellis, Hierons and Nevin, 1960; Yahr, Duvoisin and Cowen, 1965; Corsellis, Goldberg and Norton, 1968). In these cases the amnestic syndrome may be the first sign of the disorder, and the neoplasm may not give rise to other symptoms for many months. Korsakoff-like states have also been described in association with other bilateral affections of the temporal lobes. In particular, infarction of the hippocampi due to occlusion of both posterior cerebral arteries has been implicated (Victor, Angevine, Mancall and Fisher, 1961; DeJong, Itabashi and Olson, 1969), while Victor (1964) has described a patient with a severe memory disorder who, at autopsy, was found to have Alzheimer's disease with pathological changes most marked in the hippocampal regions.

Further evidence that bilateral lesions of the temporal and hippocampal structures may cause the amnestic syndrome derives from observations on the effects of temporal lobectomy in man, usually undertaken to treat temporal lobe epilepsy. Scoville and Milner (1957) found that of 10 patients who had undergone bilateral medial temporal lobe resections, three immediately developed severe defects in recent memory, and five others were affected to a moderately severe degree but could still retain some impressions of new places and names. At operation, the uncus, amygdala and hippocampus had been removed on both sides, but Scoville and Milner attributed the memory disturbance to the hippocampal destruction since the degree of memory impairment appeared to be proportionate to the extent of the hippocampal lesions. Terzian and Ore (1955) have described a similar case where permanent loss of memory occurred after bilateral temporal lobe resection, while Whitty and Lewin (1960) observed transient Korsakoff-like states following bilateral cingulectomy.

Occasionally, patients with temporal lobe epilepsy who have undergone unilateral temporal lobectomy are left with persistent amnesia (Walker, 1957; Penfield and Milner, 1958). In most cases this can be attributed to the existence of damage in the opposite hippocampus, so that operation leaves the patient with little or no functioning hippocampal tissue on either side. Lesser degrees of memory impairment after unilateral operation have also been described by Serafetinides and Falconer (1962) and here too the defect was most prominent in patients with co-existing damage on the unoperated side. However, Dimsdale, Logue and Piercy (1964) have reported an example of the amnestic syndrome following unilateral temporal lobectomy where extensive investigation had failed to reveal any contralateral lesion. That unilateral disease may sometimes cause profound disturbance of memory is further illustrated by a patient described by Smith and Smith (1966) who had a malignant temporal lobe astrocytoma presenting as a Korsakoff-like state.

Psychological testing of patients with severe memory disturbance due to hippocampal disease gives results very similar to those found in Korsakoff's psychosis, i.e. little or no impairment of general intelligence, normal ultra-short-term (digit span) memory, and inability to lay down new memory traces or to learn new material (Drachman and Arbit, 1966).

Anoxia

Survivors of attempted hanging sometimes develop symptoms of the amnestic syndrome immediately after regaining consciousness. Berlyne and Strachan (1968) have reviewed the literature and have reported a new example who showed the characteristic defects of recent memory and learning together with slight general intellectual loss. The syndrome may also follow cardiac arrest (McNeill, Tidmarsh and Rastall, 1965), carbon monoxide poisoning and other causes of cerebral anoxia, and is probably due to selective damage of the hippocampal structures, which appear to be particularly vulnerable to deprivation of oxygen.

Hypothalamic Disease

Cerebral tumours in the region of the hypothalamus may cause the syndrome. Williams and Pennybacker (1954) found that of 180 patients with verified intracranial lesions, memory impairment was most common when the floor and walls of the third ventricle were involved. Four patients—three with craniopharyngiomata and the other with a third ventricle tumour—had typical amnestic states. Palmai, Taylor and Falconer (1967) have described a patient with a craniopharyngioma presenting with the amnestic syndrome, and have summarized the clinical features of 13 previously reported cases. In addition to memory disturbance, these patients showed symptoms of hypothalamic dysfunction (somnolence, reversal of sleep rhythm, changes in libido, polydipsia, polyphagia and amenorrhoea) of raised intracranial pressure, and impairment of vision due to involvement of the optic pathways. In those cases presenting with mental changes and minimal endocrine disturbance, the correct diagnosis was usually much delayed, and Palmai *et al.* suggest that patients with Korsakoff-like states who give no history of alcoholism or past anoxia should be investigated to demonstrate or exclude a hypothalamic neoplasm. The amnesia of these patients is probably due to interference by the tumour with mammillary body function.

In tuberculous meningitis derangement of memory sometimes occurs, probably because of a predilection of the tuberculous exudate to involve the basal meninges in the region of the third ventricle. Williams and Smith (1954) described 19 patients with tuberculous meningitis who developed the amnestic syndrome. Typically, the disturbances in memory were preceded by drowsiness, confusion, disorientation and incontinence and were associated with little loss of general intelligence. All the patients in Williams and Smith's series recovered apart from persistent and complete amnesia for the illness, although a few continued to complain of mild forgetfulness.

The hippocampi are connected to the mammillary bodies by the fornix system, and it is tempting to conclude from a knowledge of the causes of the amnestic syndrome that memory is dependent on the integrity of these pathways. Certainly, section of both fornices does sometimes cause the syndrome (Sweet, Talland and Ervin, 1959), supporting this contention, but more often it is without effect on memory (Victor, 1964) and hence it is not possible to make any simple proposition concerning the anatomical basis of memory or of amnestic conditions.

Subarachnoid Haemorrhage

Walton (1953) described a series of 312 cases of spontaneous subarachnoid haemorrhage, of whom six developed a Korsakoff-like state, usually some hours or days after the bleed. Alcoholism appeared to predispose to this complication which was noted in two of the three alcoholics in the entire series. In all cases the memory defect was transient, clearing up completely after periods ranging from a few days to several months, similar to the course of the amnestic syndrome when it follows severe head injury.

Obstructive hydrocephalus, as has been noted earlier in this chapter, may follow subarachnoid haemorrhage and Theander and Granholm (1967) have reported four patients with this condition whose mental state was identical to that seen in Korsakoff's psychosis. All four were treated by a shunt operation, after a period of observation had shown no indication of any spontaneous improvement, and the condition of three of them benefited markedly.

There is some suggestion that rupture of aneurysms of the anterior cerebral and anterior communicating arteries is particularly likely to interfere with memory. Höök and Norlén (1964) and Logue, Durward, Pratt et al. (1968) have described a number of patients with ruptured aneurysms in these situations and Logue et al. suggest that the memory defect is related to their close proximity to the base of the third ventricle. Amnesia may appear for the first time following operative treatment of anterior communicating artery aneurysms. Lindqvist and Norlén (1966) found that 17 of 33 patients were affected post-operatively and that in 11 cases the memory disorder improved markedly within six months, but that the condition in five patients appeared to be permanent. Talland, Sweet and Ballantine (1967) have reported two similar cases where permanent amnesic states occurred after surgical treatment of anterior communicating artery aneurysms.

REFERENCES

ADAMS, J. H. (1969). Acute necrotizing encephalitis. In *Current Problems in Neuropsychiatry* (Editor Herrington, R. N.). British Journal of Psychiatry Special Publication No. 4, pp. 35-39. Ashford.

BERLYNE, N. and STRACHAN, M. (1968). Neuropsychiatric sequelae of attempted hanging. *Brit. J. Psychiat.* **114**, 411-422.

BRIERLEY, J. B., CORSELLIS, J. A. N., HIERONS, R. and NEVIN, S. (1960). Subacute encephalitis of later adult life mainly affecting the limbic areas. *Brain*, **83**, 357-368.

CAMPBELL, A. M. G. (1969). Herpes encephalitis I. The clinical picture. *Postgrad. med. J.* **45**, 382-385.

CORSELLIS, J. A. N., GOLDBERG, G. J. and NORTON, A. R. (1968). "Limbic encephalitis" and its association with carcinoma. *Brain*, **91**, 481-496.

DEJONG, R. N., ITABASHI, H. H. and OLSON, J. R. (1969). Memory loss due to hippocampal lesions. Report of a case. *Arch. Neurol. (Chic.)* **20**, 339-348.

DIMSDALE, H., LOGUE, V. and PIERCY, M. (1964). A case of persisting impairment of recent memory following right temporal lobectomy. *Neuropsychologia*, **1**, 287-298.

DRACHMAN, D. A. and ADAMS, R. D. (1962). Herpes simplex and acute inclusion-body encephalitis. *Arch. Neurol. (Chic.)* **7**, 45-63.

DRACHMAN, D. A. and ARBIT, J. (1966). Memory and the hippocampal complex. *Arch. Neurol. (Chic.)* **15**, 52-61.

GLASER, G. H. and PINCUS, J. H. (1969). Limbic encephalitis *J. nerv. ment. Dis.* **149**, 59-67.

HIMMELHOCH, J., PINCUS, J., TUCKER, G. and DETRE, T. (1970). Sub-acute encephalitis: behavioural and neurological aspects. *Brit. J. Psychiat.* **116**, 531-538.

HÖÖK, O. and NORLÉN, G. (1964). Aneurysm of the anterior communicating artery. *Acta neurol. scand.* **40**, 219-240.

LEIDER, W., MAGOFFIN, R. L., LENNETTE, E. H. and LEONARDS, L. N. R. (1965). Herpes-simplex-virus encephalitis. *New Engl. J. Med.* **273**, 341-347.

LINDQVIST, G. and NORLÉN, G. (1966). Korsakoff's syndrome after operation on ruptured aneurysm of the anterior communicating artery. *Acta psychiat. scand.* **42**, 24-34.

LOGUE, V., DURWARD, M., PRATT, R. T. C., PIERCY, M. and NIXON, W. L. B. (1968). The quality of survival after rupture of an anterior cerebral aneurysm. *Brit. J. Psychiat.* **114**, 137-160.

MCNEILL, D. L., TIDMARSH, D. and RASTALL, M. L. (1965). A case of dysmnesic syndrome following cardiac arrest. *Brit. J. Psychiat.* **111**, 697-699.

NOLAN, D. C., CARRUTHERS, M. M. and LERNER, A. M. (1970). Herpes virus Hominis encephalitis in Michigan. *New Engl. J. Med.* **282**, 10-13.

PALMAI, G., TAYLOR, D. C. and FALCONER, M. A., (1967). A case of craniopharyngioma presenting as Korsakov's syndrome. *Brit. J. Psychiat.* **113**, 619-623.

PENFIELD, W. and MILNER, B. (1958). Memory defect produced by bilateral lesions in the hippocampal zone. *Arch. Neurol. Psychiat. (Chic.)* **79**, 475-497.

ROSE, F. C. and SYMONDS, C. P. (1960). Persistent memory defect following encephalitis. *Brain*, **83**, 195-212.

SCOVILLE, W. B. and MILNER, B. (1957). Loss of recent memory after bilateral hippocampal lesions. *J. Neurol. Neurosurg. Psychiat.* **20**, 11-21.

SERAFETINIDES, E. A. and FALCONER, M. A. (1962). Some observations on memory impairment after temporal lobectomy for epilepsy. *J. Neurol. Neurosurg. Psychiat.* **25**, 251-255.

SMITH, R. A. and SMITH, W. A. (1966). Loss of recent memory as a sign of focal temporal lobe disorder. *J. Neurosurg.* **24**, 91-95.

STARR, A. and PHILLIPS, L. (1968). An analysis of impaired memory following herpes simplex encephalitis. *Trans. Amer. neurol. Ass.* **93**, 286-287.

SWEET, W. H., TALLAND, G. A. and ERVIN, F. R. (1959). Loss of recent memory following section of fornix. *Trans. Amer. neurol. Ass.* **84**, 76-78.

SYMONDS, C. (1966). Disorders of memory. *Brain*, **89**, 625-644.

TALLAND, G. A., SWEET, W. H. and BALLANTINE, H. T. (1967). Amnesic syndrome with anterior communicating artery aneurysm. *J. nerv. ment. Dis.* **145**, 179-192.

TERZIAN, H. and ORE, G. D. (1955). Syndrome of Klüver and Bucy reproduced in man by bilateral removal of the temporal lobes. *Neurology (Minneap.)*, **5**, 373-380.

THEANDER, S. and GRANHOLM, L. (1967). Sequelae after spontaneous subarachnoid haemorrhage with special reference to hydrocephalus and Korsakoff's syndrome. *Acta neurol. scand.* **43**, 479-488.

VICTOR, M. (1964). Observations on the amnestic syndrome in man and its anatomical basis. In *Brain Function, Volume II. RNA and Brain Function, Memory and Learning* (Editor, Brazier, M. A. B.), pp. 311-340. Berkeley.

VICTOR, M., ANGEVINE, J. B., MANCALL, E. I. and FISHER, C. M. (1961). Memory loss with lesions of hippocampal formation. *Arch. Neurol. (Chic.)* **5**, 244-263.

WALKER, A. E. (1957). Recent memory impairment in unilateral temporal lesions. *Arch. Neurol. Psychiat. (Chic.)* **78**, 543-552.

WALTON, J. N. (1953). The Korsakov syndrome in spontaneous subarachnoid haemorrhage. *J. ment. Sci.* **99**, 521-530.

WHITTY, C. W. M. and LEWIN, W. (1960). A Korsakoff syndrome in the post-cingulectomy confusional state. *Brain*, **83**, 648-653.

WILLIAMS, M. and PENNYBACKER, J. (1954). Memory disturbances in third ventricle tumours. *J. Neurol. Neurosurg. Psychiat.* **17**, 115-123.

WILLIAMS, M. and SMITH, H. V. (1954). Mental disturbances in tuberculous meningitis. *J. Neurol. Neurosurg. Psychiat.* **17**, 173-182.

YAHR, M. D., DUVOISIN, R. C. and COWEN, D. (1965). Encephalopathy associated with carcinoma. *Trans. Amer. neurol. Ass.* **90**, 80-84.

Transient Amnesia in Alcoholism

Alcoholics not infrequently experience episodes of amnesia lasting a few hours, usually during a bout of heavy drinking. They are not associated with loss of consciousness and therefore the term "blackout" which is often applied to them, particularly by the patients themselves, is unsuitable. Goodwin, Crane and Guze (1969a, b) studied 100 alcoholic subjects without other psychiatric disorder or evidence of brain damage and noted that 64 admitted to having had one or more episodes of amnesia without loss of consciousness for at least part of a drinking bout. Comparison of these 64 patients with the remaining 36 who had not had this experience showed that amnesias were significantly more common in patients who drank most heavily, whose drinking occurred in discrete bouts and who showed loss of control (i.e. inability to drink socially). They were also more common in patients with a past history of head injury leading to unconsciousness.

Amnesias first appeared late in the course of the illness, well after symptoms of physical dependence had been noted (Table 8.4), and they almost invariably occurred only while large amounts of alcohol, particularly spirits, were being consumed.

Goodwin *et al.* (1969*b*) have delineated two types of amnesia with possibly different aetiologies. First, there may be a complete and permanent ("*en bloc*") loss of memory for a period usually of a few hours but sometimes for as long as several days—with sudden onset and sudden recovery. Such

Table 8.4

ONSET OF VARIOUS MANIFESTATIONS OF ALCOHOLISM AMONG 100 PATIENTS
(Goodwin *et al.*, 1969*a*)

Disturbance	Mean age at onset (years)	Proportion affected (per cent)
Frequent drunkenness	27	98
Weekend drunkenness	28	82
Morning drinking	31	84
"Benders'	31	76
Neglecting meals	32	86
"Shakes"	33	88
Job loss from drinking	33	69
Separation or divorce from drinking	34	44
Amnesic episodes	35	64
Joined Alcoholics Anonymous	36	39
Hospitalized for drinking	37	100
Delirium tremens	38	45

episodes were reported by 36 of Goodwin *et al.*'s 100 alcoholics. Most commonly these patients gave a history of waking from sleep with no memory for the events of the previous evening, but 12 patients had experiences which terminated while fully conscious, that is, they suddenly found themselves in strange circumstances unable to recollect what had happened during the previous few hours. Behaviour during these amnesic periods tends to be very similar to that during bouts of heavy drinking for which memory is intact, but there is a tendency for patients to travel long distances as in fugue states. Following an amnesic episode some patients are alarmed and fearful lest they have done someone serious harm and they may make enquiries concerning their behaviour, or they may be so frightened by the experience that they abstain from alcohol thereafter. With continued drinking however amnesias become more frequent and the patient is less concerned by them (Kessel and Walton, 1965).

The second type of alcoholic amnesia described by Goodwin *et al.* (1969*b*) is of a fragmentary kind, where the patient does not realize that events have been forgotten until he is told about them later. These forgotten memories tend to return with time, and this recall may be facilitated by further drinking. A further difference between this fragmentary type of memory loss and "*en bloc*" amnesia is that the former tend to occur earlier in the course of alcoholism.

REFERENCES

GOODWIN, D. W., CRANE, J. B. and GUZE, S. B. (1969a). Alcoholic "blackouts": a review and clinical study of 100 alcoholics. *Amer. J. Psychiat.* **126**, 191-198.
GOODWIN, D. W., CRANE, J. B. and GUZE, S. B. (1969b). Phenomenological aspects of the alcoholic "blackout". *Brit. J. Psychiat.* **115**, 1033-1038.
KESSEL, N. and WALTON, H. (1965). *Alcoholism.* Harmondsworth.

Transient Global Amnesia

In 1964, Fisher and Adams reported 17 patients who developed severe disturbances of memory of sudden onset, gradually recovering after a short period—usually a few hours. Other examples of this condition—"transient global amnesia"—have also been described by Bender (1960), Shuttleworth and Morris (1966) Bolwig (1968) and Brain (1969). During the episode there is evidence of a serious defect in short-term memory and of a retrograde amnesia for a variable period before the onset of the attack; the patient is perplexed, often realizes that his mental function is deficient and he may be disoriented in time and place. There is however no suggestion of any impairment of consciousness or of general intellectual ability; digit span and arithmetical calculation are unaffected and neurological examination shows no abnormality. On recovery, the patient cannot remember what happened during or shortly before the attack, but apart from this amnesia there are no permanent sequelae. Recurrences, however, have been reported.

The aetiology of transient global amnesia is unknown. It occurs only in middle-aged and elderly persons and may be precipitated by bathing in cold water or by sexual intercourse. The consensus is that it is not an hysterical phenomenon and that it is probably due to transient ischaemia of those brain structures concerned with memory.

REFERENCES

BENDER, M. B. (1960). Single episode of confusion with amnesia. *Bull. N. Y. Acad. Med.* **36**, 197-207.
BOLWIG, T. G. (1968). Transient global amnesia. *Acta neurol. scand.* **44**, 101-106.
BRAIN, R. (1969). Disorders of memory. In *Recent Advances in Neurology and Neuropsychiatry*, 8th Edition (Editors Brain, R. and Wilkinson, M.). London.
FISHER, C. M. and ADAMS, R. D. (1964). Transient global amnesia. *Acta neurol. scand.* Supplement 9.
SHUTTLEWORTH, E. C. and MORRIS, C. E. (1966). The transient global amnesic syndrome. *Arch. Neurol. (Chic.)*, **15**, 515-520.

CHAPTER 9

PSYCHIATRIC ASPECTS OF PREGNANCY AND THE PUERPERIUM

Termination of Pregnancy. Contraception. Sterilization. Post-partum Mental Disorders.

TERMINATION OF PREGNANCY

Legal, Moral and Ethical Aspects of Abortion

Legal Considerations

In Great Britain before 1968

UNTIL 1968 the law in England and Wales was based first on Section 58 of the Offences against the Person Act of 1861, which made punishable any unlawful attempt to procure an abortion, and secondly on Section 1 of the Infant Life (Preservation) Act of 1929 which allowed abortion only if done in good faith for the purpose of preserving the life of the mother. A change in the interpretation of these laws resulted from the precedent set by *Rex v. Bourne* in 1938. Mr Aleck Bourne, a distinguished gynaecological surgeon, was prosecuted because he had aborted a girl aged 14 years who had conceived as the result of rape. Mr Bourne informed the Attorney-General of what he had done and he was charged with procuring an abortion. He was acquitted after Mr Justice Macnaghten directed the jury that since it was lawful to terminate a pregnancy to preserve the life of the mother, it was lawful to induce an abortion "if the probable consequence of the continuance of the pregnancy will be to make the woman a physical or mental wreck" (British Medical Journal, 1938). As a result of this decision abortion became legal in England and Wales where there was a serious medical (physical or mental) indication.

Scottish law differed from that in England and Wales until 1968. Under the common law of Scotland it was possible "for a doctor acting in good faith to perform a therapeutic abortion, where after a careful study of all the circumstances of the case, and after due consultation with colleagues, he decides that the disadvantages of continuing the pregnancy are greater than those of ending it" (Baird, 1967).

The Abortion Act, 1967

In April 1968 the Abortion Act became effective in England, Wales and Scotland and made abortion legal "if two registered medical practitioners are of the opinion, formed in good faith:

(*a*) that the continuance of the pregnancy would involve risk to the life of the pregnant woman or of injury to the physical or mental health of the

266

pregnant woman or any existing children of her family, greater than if the pregnancy were terminated;
or

(b) that there is a substantial risk that if the child were born it would suffer from such physical or mental abnormalities as to be seriously handicapped.

"In determining whether the continuance of a pregnancy would involve such risk of injury as is mentioned in paragraph (a) . . ., account may be taken of the pregnant woman's actual or reasonably foreseeable environment."

In addition, the Act (i) stipulates that abortion must normally be carried out in a National Health Service hospital or other approved place, (ii) makes provision for immediate termination where the operation is necessary to save the life of the mother or to prevent grave permanent injury to her physical or mental health and (iii) allows for conscientious objection by the doctor, but places the burden of proof of conscientious objection on the doctor himself. Figure 9.1 shows Certificate A on which the opinion of the two medical practitioners is given.

The Medical Defence Union (1968), the Medical Protection Society (1968) and the Abortion Law Reform Association (1968) have commented on some of the implications of the Act. Two of their observations are of particular interest to the psychiatrist. First, abortion may be carried out if the social and economic consequences of continued pregnancy are thought likely to have an adverse effect on the health of the mother or of her existing offspring, and that in determining what the effect might be, the marital status and intelligence of the woman may be taken into consideration. Secondly, abortion is legal if serious consideration has to be given to the possibility that the child will be unable to lead an independent life when of an age to do so. Thus if there seems to be a serious risk that the child will be affected by an inherited psychiatric condition such as Huntington's chorea or phenylketonuria, abortion may be carried out. Moreover the Abortion Law Reform Association (1968) suggests that if it is thought that the child will develop with a severe mental handicap because of its upbringing by a psychopathic mother abortion would be legal. No mention is made, however, of other serious inherited mental disorders such as schizophrenia or manic-depressive psychosis but abortion might be legal where there is a strong family history of these conditions and particularly where both parents are affected. In such circumstances it would seem reasonable, before abortion is undertaken, to obtain specialist genetic opinion concerning the risk to the child.

United States of America

Although each State has its own laws on abortion, until 1967 legislation generally allowed abortion only when continuation of the pregnancy threatened the life of the mother, but a few States permitted it on strict medical grounds. In recent years, however, the laws have been more liberally

IN CONFIDENCE   Certificate **A**

Not to be destroyed within three years of the date of operation

ABORTION ACT 1967

Certificate to be completed before an abortion is
performed under Section 1(1) of the Act

I,..

(Name and qualifications of practitioner in block capitals)

of ....

....

(Full address of practitioner)

and I, ...

(Name and qualifications of practitioner in block capitals)

of ....

....

(Full address of practitioner)

hereby certify that we are of the opinion, formed in good faith, that in the case of................

....

(Full name of pregnant woman in block capitals)

of ....

....

(Usual place of residence of pregnant woman in block capitals)

(Ring appropriate number(s))

1. the continuance of the pregnancy would involve risk to the life of the pregnant woman greater than if the pregnancy were terminated;

2. the continuance of the pregnancy would involve risk of injury to the physical or mental health of the pregnant woman greater than if the pregnancy were terminated;

3. the continuance of the pregnancy would involve risk of injury to the physical or mental health of the existing child(ren) of the family of the pregnant woman greater than if the pregnancy were terminated;

4. there is a substantial risk that if the child were born it would suffer from such physical or mental abnormalities as to be seriously handicapped.

This certificate of opinion is given before the commencement of the treatment for the termination of pregnancy to which it refers.

Signed ....

                                    Date..

Signed ....

                                    Date..

Figure 9.1 On completion this certificate should be sent to the gynaecologist terminating the pregnancy, who is required by law to keep it for three years after the operation.

interpreted and therapeutic abortions have been undertaken more frequently. In 1967, Colorado, North Carolina and California passed laws allowing termination of pregnancy in cases of incest and rape (including statutory rape, i.e. felonious intercourse) and where there is a serious risk that continuation of the pregnancy would impair the physical or mental health of the mother. In Colorado and North Carolina, but not in California, the new laws allow abortion if there is a risk of serious physical deformity or mental retardation in the child. Laws passed in 1968 and 1969 in the States of Georgia, Maryland, New Mexico, Arkansas, Kansas and Oregon are basically similar to those of Colorado, except that incest is not an indication in Georgia or Maryland and abortion for statutory rape is not allowed in Maryland (Ingram, 1969). The law in the U.S.A. is, however, still changing and during 1970 the States of Hawaii, Maryland and New York abolished almost all restrictions.

Other Countries

Legislation on abortion varies very considerably throughout the world, and Roemer (1967) has reviewed the situation. She lists five major indications for legal abortion:

1. When the mother's life is in danger (as in Western Australia, Venezuela, Chile and France)
2. When there is a risk to the mental or physical health of the mother (as in Switzerland, Honduras and Syria)
3. When there is a risk that the child will be abnormal (as in Sweden)
4. When the pregnancy has resulted from rape or incest (as in Denmark and Mexico)
5. Where the social circumstances (living conditions, economic responsibilities, number of existing children, etc.) make it undesirable for the mother to have any further children (as in Japan, Poland, Czechoslovakia and Yugoslavia).

In the Scandinavian countries the social circumstances may be taken into consideration in deciding whether abortion on medical grounds should be undertaken, but the social circumstances themselves cannot be the only reasons for termination.

Apart from the above type of legislation which allows legal abortion in certain circumstances, there is a total ban on abortion in some countries such as Italy, while in Russia, Hungary and Rumania, abortion can be obtained on demand. Abortion on demand in Hungary has led to the situation where, in 1965, there were 135 legal abortions for every 100 live births (Potts, 1967).

Morals and Abortion

While there is very considerable variation in the moral attitude of individuals to abortion, most religious authorities condemn it to a greater or lesser extent. The Roman Catholic Church takes the most unyielding viewpoint, that no woman should be aborted; it asserts that the foetus has the full rights of human existence from the moment of conception and that it is morally wrong and forbidden by divine law to take an innocent human life. Hence abortion is considered immoral even when its purpose is to save the life of the mother because it is thought to be less of an evil that both mother and child should die than that the child should be murdered (Zalba, 1966).

Vere (1967) presents the Protestant point of view which does not accept the Roman Catholic dogma that the foetus has a soul, but nevertheless regards every abortion as an evil which should only be permitted when a greater evil would result from continuation of the pregnancy.

The Jewish attitude (Jakobovits, 1959; Goldman, 1969) maintains that up to the moment that labour starts, the foetus is part of the mother, and that it is therefore morally permissible to terminate the pregnancy on medical grounds or possibly for some other grave reason. During labour the child has more rights and its destruction can only be undertaken to save the life of the mother; but in these circumstances it is obligatory to kill the child if the life of the mother can be saved only by doing so. After delivery of the head the child may be killed only if both the mother *and* the child would otherwise die. Only when the infant is one month of age is its life considered as inviolable as that of an adult.

Medical Ethics and Abortion

The accepted code of behaviour within the medical profession comprises certain rules concerning the relationship of the doctor to his patients, to his colleagues and to members of other professions. The British Medical Association (1965) has summarized the ethical duties of doctors. The basis of these ethics is the Hippocratic oath, dating from the 5th century B.C. which includes a promise not to abort—"I will give no deadly poison to anyone if asked, nor suggest any such counsel; and in like manner I will not give to a woman a pessary to induce abortion". A modern restatement of the Hippocratic oath, the Declaration of Geneva, was produced in 1947 by the World Medical Association; it asks doctors to "maintain the utmost respect for human life from the time of conception".

In 1967, shortly before the Abortion Act became law, the British Medical Association declared that "artificial termination of pregnancy is permissible only when it is in the interests of the health of the mother or where there is a risk of serious abnormality of the foetus" (British Medical Association, 1967). In making this declaration, the B.M.A. indicated that termination for certain other reasons such as risk to the health of the existing children might be unethical even though legal under the new Act.

Although the British Medical Association did not change its views with the passing of the Abortion Act, the General Medical Council has altered its attitudes to the ethics of abortion to conform with the new law. The G.M.C. has the legal authority in Great Britain to investigate complaints against doctors, to adjudicate on charges of "infamous conduct in a professional respect" and to erase the names of those found guilty from the Medical Register. Until the Abortion Act became law the G.M.C. always regarded induced non-therapeutic abortion as "so grave an offence as to lead almost invariably to erasure of the doctor's name from the Register", but in 1968 it decided to regard "as a serious matter the termination of pregnancy if done in circumstances which contravene the law" (British Medical Journal, 1968). A similar sequence of events has recently occurred in Canada; in 1969 the Canadian criminal code was amended to permit abortion if the mental or physical health of the mother was in danger, and in 1970 the Canadian Medical Association removed abortion from its list of unethical practices. It seems possible therefore that future legislation making the abortion laws even more liberal than now may further alter the ethical position of the medical profession.

REFERENCES

ABORTION LAW REFORM ASSOCIATION (1968). *A Guide to the Abortion Act, 1967*, London.
BAIRD, D. (1967). Sterilization and therapeutic abortion in Aberdeen. *Brit. J. Psychiat.* **113**, 701-709.
BRITISH MEDICAL ASSOCIATION (1965). *Members Handbook*. London.
BRITISH MEDICAL ASSOCIATION (1967). Annual Report of Council 1966-67. *Brit. med. J. Supplement.* **2**, 66.
BRITISH MEDICAL JOURNAL (1938). Charge of procuring abortion: Rex v. Bourne. *Brit. med. J.* **2**, 199-205.
BRITISH MEDICAL JOURNAL (1968). G. M. C. and Abortion Act, 1967. *Brit. med. J.* **2**, 185.
GOLDMAN, M. J. (1969). Abortion: Jewish law and the law of the land. *Illinois med. J.* **135**, 93-95.
INGRAM, J. I. (1969). Changing aspects of abortion law. *Amer. J. Obstet. Gynec.* **105**, 35-42.
JAKOBOVITS, I. (1959). *Jewish Medical Ethics*. New York, N.Y.
MEDICAL DEFENCE UNION (1968). *Memoranda on the Abortion Act 1967 and the Abortion Regulations, 1968*. London.
MEDICAL PROTECTION SOCIETY (1968). *Abortion Act 1967. Comments and Advice*. London.
POTTS, M. (1967). Legal abortion in Eastern Europe. *Eugen. Rev.* **59**, 232-250.
ROEMER, R. (1967). Abortion law: the approaches of different nations. *Amer. J. publ. Hlth.* **57**, 1906-1922.
VERE, D. W. (1967). Why the preservation of life? In *Ethical Responsibility in Medicine* (Editors Edmunds, V. and Scorer, C. G.). Edinburgh.
ZALBA, M. (1966). The Catholic Church's viewpoint on abortion. *Wld. med. J.* **13**, 88-93.

Psychiatric Indications for Termination of Pregnancy

A few medical conditions, such as Eisenmenger's syndrome, thyrotoxic heart disease with cardiac failure and diabetic nephropathy are associated, in pregnancy, with such high maternal morbidity and mortality rates that the pregnancy should always be terminated (British Medical Association Committee on Therapeutic Abortion, 1968). There are however no psychiatric conditions which carry a similar absolute indication to terminate, and indeed no mental disorder is so aggravated by pregnancy that it would be right to advise an unwilling patient that she must be aborted for the sake of her

health. The psychiatric indications for abortion are therefore closely dependent on legislation and vary from country to country. Ethical and moral
issues may also influence the decision to terminate. But ethics and morals
seem to be of less importance than the law; in Poland, Czechoslovakia and
Hungary, where the vast majority of the population is Roman Catholic, and
the Church influential, more than 1 in 5 of all pregnant women have a legal
abortion (Potts, 1967).

The influence of legislation on possible psychiatric indications is shown by
comparing American statistics on abortion before and after legal change.
Tietze (1968) obtained data on all the therapeutic abortions carried out in
some 300 hospitals in the United States during the period 1963-65 (i.e. before
any legal reform). There were a total of 2,007 therapeutic abortions, corresponding to a rate of 1·9 per 1000 deliveries and of these, 34 per cent were
induced on psychiatric grounds, 27·2 per cent because of physical disease and
21·7 per cent because of possible congenital deformity of the child due to
maternal rubella. Similar findings were noted in more limited surveys on
therapeutic abortions in Columbus, Ohio, during 1949-65 (Copeland and
Essig, 1969) and in St Louis, Missouri, during 1955-64 (Simon, Senturia and
Rothman, 1967). In Columbus there were 1·3 therapeutic abortions per 1000
deliveries and in 29·7 per cent the indications were psychiatric while in St
Louis, 34·8 per cent were induced on psychiatric grounds. During the first
year after the introduction of the 1967 abortion laws in Colorado and
California, there were respectively 11·6 and 11·2 therapeutic abortions per
1000 live births in these States; the indication was psychiatric in 71·2 per cent
of the cases in Colorado, and in 86·8 per cent in California (Droegemueller,
Taylor and Drose, 1969; Thurstone, 1969). Diggory, Peel and Potts (1970)
have compared British data before and after the Abortion Act of 1967 came
into operation on April 27th 1968. Table 9.1 shows the steady increase in the

Table 9.1

THERAPEUTIC ABORTIONS IN ENGLAND AND WALES, 1961-69
(Before April 27th 1968, data are estimates)
(Diggory et al., 1970)

Year	Number of therapeutic abortions
1961	14,280
1962	16,830
1963	16,580
1964	18,300
1965	19,530
1966	21,380
1967	27,200
1968	31,270
1969	53,021

estimated number of therapeutic abortions carried out each year in England
and Wales during the period 1961-1967, with further increases after the
Abortion Act became effective. Table 9.2 gives the grounds for termination
relating to the 65,000 therapeutic abortions carried out during the first

eighteen months of the Act. By far the most common indication is a risk to the physical or mental health of the woman, but the actual numbers aborted on psychiatric grounds are not given.

Table 9.2

THERAPEUTIC ABORTIONS IN ENGLAND AND WALES, APRIL 27TH 1968 TO
OCTOBER 28TH 1969, BY GROUNDS
(Diggory *et al.*, 1970)

Grounds	Number
1. Life of woman	2,664
2. Health of woman	47,127
3. Health of other children	2,610
4. Risk of handicap to child	1,856
5. Life-saving emergency	20
6. Emergency to avoid health damage	53
2. with 4	1,048
3. with others	9,863
Total	65,241

The degree of advancement of pregnancy may also influence a decision on termination. Dilatation of the cervix followed by curettage of the uterus is the simplest procedure but this can be undertaken safely only during the first ten to twelve weeks of pregnancy. Alternatively, during this early period, the contents of the uterus may be aspirated by vacuum suction. When the pregnancy is more than three months advanced the surgeon usually resorts to hysterotomy, a much more difficult procedure, but the introduction into the uterus of an abortifacient paste, or the intra-amniotic injection of hypertonic glucose or saline are possible alternatives (Peel and Potts, 1969; Potts, 1970).

Suicide in Pregnancy

In those parts of the world where abortion may be undertaken only to preserve the life of the mother, the sole psychiatric indication is a substantial risk of suicide if the pregnancy is allowed to proceed. Suicide in pregnancy is however quite rare. Indeed there is some evidence that it is less common during pregnancy than at other times. Rosenberg and Silver (1965) scrutinized the coroners' records of three counties in California for the years 1961 to 1963 and found that out of a total of 207 suicides in women aged 16 to 50 years, only three had been pregnant at the time, whereas the expected number, if suicide and pregnancy were independent, was 17·6. Barno (1967) found that suicide among pregnant women was about one-fortieth as common as among the general female population, but he did not take into account the variation of suicide rate with age. He found only 14 cases of suicide in relation to pregnancy in the State of Minnesota during the 16-year period 1950-65. Of these only four killed themselves during pregnancy and the remainder post partum. None of the women had conceived illegitimately and none had requested a therapeutic abortion. A very low incidence of suicide in pregnancy was also reported by Arthure, Tomkinson, Organe *et al.* (1969) in England

and Wales. During the eleven years 1956-66 only eight suicides during pregnancy were discovered during the course of an enquiry into the causes of maternal deaths, but the authors point out that suicides during early pregnancy were unlikely to come to their attention. Weir (1969) examined the records of the coroners of the London Boroughs and of the City of London for the years 1948-62 and found 51 pregnant suicides. He compared the number of suicides during pregnancy with that to be expected if pregnancy and suicide were independent, and noted that for women below the age of 25 years the risk of suicide was increased during pregnancy while above that age pregnancy seemed to be protective (Table 9.3). Indeed in the older age

Table 9.3

EXPECTED AND OBSERVED NUMBERS OF PREGNANCIES AMONG FEMALE
SUICIDES AGED 15-24 AND AGED 25-44, IN LONDON 1948-62
(Weir, 1969)

	Age 15-24	Age 25-44	Age 15-44
Total number of suicides:	146	866	1012
Number of pregnant suicides:			
Expected:	8·6	41·9	50·5
Observed:	22	29	51

group he found evidence that suicide sometimes occurred because of an inability to become pregnant. For women of both age groups, he noted that the observed number of pregnant suicides was very nearly the same as that expected.

Attempted suicide during pregnancy has also been studied. Otto (1965) found that of 1376 Swedish girls under the age of 21 who had attempted suicide, 78 (5·7 per cent) were pregnant at the time, and of these the unwanted pregnancy was the main reason for the attempt in 34 cases. Whitlock and Edwards (1968) reported a series of 483 attempted suicides among Brisbane women, and of these 30 (6·7 per cent) were pregnant. In only seven per cent of the pregnant women was the pregnancy the main cause of the attempt and 57 per cent wished the pregnancy to go to term.

Threats of suicide if termination is not carried out are not uncommon. Höök (1963) followed up 249 Swedish women who were refused legal abortion, and 14 of these (5·6 per cent) had threatened suicide. At follow up (after at least 7½ years) only three had in fact made suicidal attempts. All three were unsuccessful and none were directly related to the pregnancy or to the refusal. However suicide due to unwanted pregnancy undoubtedly does occur, and in Weir's (1965) series of 65 suicides among pregnant women in London, the pregnancy was considered a contributory cause in most cases, while occasionally there was the clearest evidence (from suicidal notes etc.) that the pregnancy was the major factor. There was no indication that any of these women had requested abortion and had been refused, but there have been a few cases reported where refusal to perform a therapeutic abortion has led to the woman taking her own life. Tylden (1966) has described such a case, of a married woman aged 32 years whose depression became more severe when she became pregnant and whose request for termination was refused; she committed suicide two weeks before the expected date of delivery, while Anderson (1962) has reported a patient who committed suicide one year after her request for abortion was turned down. Assessing the risk of suicide in association with pregnancy is complicated by the fact that attempted suicide does sometimes occur after abortion. Five such cases have been reported by Jansson (1965) and four by Patt, Rappaport and Barglow (1969) where the attempt was made shortly after legal termination, while Pare (1967) has reported a patient who was denied a legal abortion and who killed herself after having an illegal operation.

To summarize, suicidal attempts are not uncommon during pregnancy and sometimes the woman's attitude to the pregnancy is responsible for the attempt. Suicide itself however is uncommon, but it does sometimes occur in relation to the unwanted pregnancy, and occasionally it follows refusal of a request for legal termination. In considering the risk attention should also be paid to the possibility of suicide or attempted suicide following termination.

Other Indications for Termination

The British Medical Association Committee on Therapeutic Abortion (1968) has listed the following possible psychiatric indications for termination of pregnancy:

1. *Reactive depression*, particularly where there is a risk of suicide or where the mother is in a state of hopeless despair.
2. *Obsessional states* where the pregnancy is clearly aggravating the symptoms.
3. *Schizophrenia* where deterioration has occurred during the pregnancy or in previous pregnancies.
4. *Mental deficiency*, where the strain of an unwanted pregnancy has caused severe disturbance.

In addition, the B.M.A. suggests that anxiety or hysterical reactions to an unwanted pregnancy do not constitute indications for termination unless there are other mental disturbances, and that endogenous depression is not an indication even if precipitated by the realization of an unwanted pregnancy.

As has been pointed out, these indications are not absolute and the social circumstances and the amount of support available to the patient from relatives, friends, social workers and doctors must all be taken into consideration before a decision is made. Furthermore, these indications are likely to change with future changes in the law.

REFERENCES

ANDERSON, E. W. (1962). Psychiatric aspects of abortion. In *Proceedings of the Third World Congress of Psychiatry*. Vol. II, pp. 1170-1174. Toronto.

ARTHURE, H., TOMKINSON, J., ORGANE, G., KUCK, M., ADELSTEIN, A. M. and WEATHERALL, J. A. C. (1969). Report on confidential enquiries into maternal deaths in England and Wales, 1964-66. *Department of Health and Social Security Reports on Public Health and Medical Subjects.* No. 119 H.M.S.O. London.

BARNO, A. (1967). Criminal abortion deaths, illegitimate pregnancy deaths and suicides in pregnancy. Minnesota 1950-1965. *Amer. J. Obstet. Gynec.* **98**, 356-363.

BRITISH MEDICAL ASSOCIATION COMMITTEE ON THERAPEUTIC ABORTION (1968). Indications for termination of pregnancy. *Brit. med. J.* **1**, 171-175.

COPELAND, W. E. and ESSIG, G. F. (1969). Therapeutic abortion. *J. Amer. med. Ass.* **207**, 713-715.

DIGGORY, P., PEEL, J. and POTTS, M. (1970). Preliminary assessment of the 1967 Abortion Act in practice. *Lancet,* **1**, 287-291.

DROEGEMUELLER, W., TAYLOR, E. S. and DROSE, V. E. (1969). The first year of experience in Colorado with the new abortion law. *Amer. J. Obstet. Gynec.* **103**, 694-702.

HÖÖK, K. (1963). Refused abortion. A follow-up study of 249 women whose applications were refused by the National Board of Health in Sweden. *Acta psychiat. scand.* Supplement 168.

JANSSON, B. (1965). Mental disorders after abortion. *Acta psychiat. scand.* **41**, 87-110.

OTTO, U. (1965). Suicidal attempts made by pregnant women under 21 years. *Acta paedopsychiat.* **32**, 276-288.

PARE, C. M. B. (1967). A follow-up study of patients referred for termination of pregnancy on psychiatric grounds. *Brit. J. Psychiat.* Supplement, July 1967, pp. 3-4.

PATT, S. L., RAPPAPORT, R. G. and BARGLOW, P. (1969). Follow-up of therapeutic abortion. *Arch. gen. Psychiat.* **20**, 408-414.

PEEL, J. and POTTS, M. (1969). *Textbook of Contraceptive Practice.* Cambridge.

POTTS, M. (1967). Legal abortion in Eastern Europe. *Eugen. Rev.* **59**, 232-250.

POTTS, M. (1970). Termination of pregnancy. *Brit. med. Bull.* **26**, 65-71.

ROSENBERG, A. J. and SILVER, E. (1965). Suicide, psychiatrists and therapeutic abortion. *Calif. Med.* **102**, 407-411.

SIMON, N. M., SENTURIA, A. G. and ROTHMAN, D. (1967). Psychiatric illnesses following therapeutic abortion. *Amer. J. Psychiat.* **124**, 59-65.

THURSTONE, P. B. (1969). Therapeutic abortion. The experience of San Mateo County General Hospital and the State of California. *J. Amer. med. Ass.* **209**, 229-231.

TIETZE, C. (1968). Therapeutic abortions in the United States. *Amer. J. Obstet. Gynec.* **101**, 784-787.

TYLDEN, E. (1966). Suicide risk in unwanted pregnancy. *Med. Wld. (Lond.)* **104**, No. 1. 25-28.

WEIR, J. G. (1965). Suicide during pregnancy. A study of 65 pregnant suicides in London. In *Proceedings of the Second International Congress of Psychosomatic Medicine in Obstetrics and Gynaecology.*

WEIR, J. G. (1969). Suicide during pregnancy (*Unpublished observations.*)

WHITLOCK, F. A. and EDWARDS, J. E. (1968). Pregnancy and attempted suicide. *Comprehens. Psychiat.* **9**, 1-12.

Psychiatric Consequences of Abortion and of Refusal to Terminate Pregnancy

In recent years a number of investigators have studied the psychological and psychiatric condition of women who have had their pregnancies terminated and of women who have had their request for abortion refused. From these studies it is not possible to reach any general conclusions, first because the indications for therapeutic termination vary from country to country and secondly because the mental state of the woman is very often an important factor in determining the success of her application for abortion. Thus, where mental disturbance is an indication only when very severe, patients who are refused abortion may fare better than those who are aborted, because the former have the greater mental stability. On the other hand, if abortion can be undertaken in the absence of strong psychiatric indications the mental state after termination may be better than that after refusal because in the latter circumstances the woman is subjected to greater stress. In spite of these limitations in the interpretation of results much useful information is now available.

Since suicide and attempted suicide have already been discussed they will not be considered further here.

Effects of Termination of Pregnancy

Minor mental disturbance, particularly feelings of guilt and mild depression are not uncommon after legal abortion. Ekblad (1955) followed up 479 Swedish women who had had a legal abortion on psychiatric grounds and noted that 25 per cent showed some guilt—in 14 per cent it was mild and in 11 per cent more severe. Guilt feelings were more common where there were strong psychiatric indications for the termination or where there was an initial reluctance of the patient to agree to the operation. Arén (1958) found that of 100 Swedish women aborted legally, 48 reported guilt feelings and that in 23 these were severe and interfered with work or sleep. Niswander and Patterson (1967) followed up 116 therapeutic abortions and found that three women seriously regretted the operation while with another three there was some doubt in the patients' minds as to whether or not they should have consented to it. Moderately severe guilt was experienced by 22 per cent of the 46 patients reported by Simon, Senturia and Rothman (1967) and very severe guilt by 13 per cent.

There have been three reports on London women by Pare (1967),* Clark, Forstner, Pond and Tredgold (1968) and by McCoy (1968). Pare (1967) observed that mild feelings of guilt were common among his 53 patients during the two or three weeks following the abortion, but that these rarely lasted for as long as six months. Clark *et al.* (1968) also noted that guilt feelings were short lived and that six months after the operation only three of the 120 women in their series were dissatisfied. Among the 62 women described by McCoy (1968), however, 32 per cent suffered some self reproach immediately after the operation; at follow-up after at least one year, 27 per cent still experienced regrets, which in 14 per cent were severe.

The majority of women appear to be completely satisfied after legal termination and in particular they report an immediate improvement in their

* See also Pare and Raven (1970)

mental state. Of the 116 patients followed up by Niswander and Patterson (1967) 68·1 per cent felt better immediately after operation and 82·8 per cent showed favourable long-term effects. Patt, Rappaport and Barglow (1969) noted that 57 per cent of their patients experienced remission of their psychiatric symptoms immediately after the abortion. Clark *et al.* (1968) observed prompt improvement in 77 per cent of their patients (permanent in 58 per cent and temporary in 19 per cent) while immediate relief of symptoms following the abortion was noted in 50 per cent of the patients reported by Simon *et al.* (1967).

Severe mental disturbance after termination of pregnancy is uncommon but when it does occur it is often difficult to determine if the illness has been precipitated by the operation or if it is a continuation of previous psychiatric disorder. Jansson (1965) has reported a series of 57 patients admitted to psychiatric hospitals in Göteborg within one year of an abortion; most of these patients were depressed. Thirty-four of the abortions were legal and 23 were illegal or spontaneous. From data on the number of legal and other abortions in Göteborg during the same period of time, Jansson calculated that 1·92 per cent of legal abortions subsequently required admission to psychiatric hospital, whereas of those whose abortions were illegal or spontaneous the admission rate was only 0·27 per cent. This difference, highly significant statistically, is to be expected, however, since legal abortion is very often undertaken on psychiatric grounds. Indeed, while 50 per cent of the patients whose abortions were legal had had previous psychiatric care, the corresponding figure for the other patients was only 13·1 per cent. In Jansson's series, the abortion was considered to have been at least partly responsible for the development of the psychiatric disorder in 31 cases (54 per cent) including 15 cases (26 per cent) where it appeared to be the most important factor.

Simon *et al.* (1967) reported that six of their 46 patients were hospitalised for mental disorder after abortion, but that in only one case did the mental illness appear to be directly precipitated by the operation, and these authors conclude that serious psychiatric disorder following termination is usually related to pre-existing psychiatric illness.

Effects of Refusal to Terminate the Pregnancy

Women whose requests for legal abortion are refused may obtain a termination illegally. Of 249 Swedish cases of refused abortion reported by Höök (1963), 50 (20 per cent) had threatened to seek an illegal operation and 28 (11 per cent) put this threat into effect. An even higher incidence of spontaneous or illegally induced abortion has been noted in other series (Table 9.4). Both Höök (1963) and Pare (1967) noted a much lower incidence among those who were married and living with their husbands. Of women whose pregnancies proceeded to term, the majority reared the children themselves and in only a small proportion was the baby adopted or fostered

(Table 9.4). Again there was a difference between married women living with their husbands and other women, in that the former were more likely to keep the child, and in spite of the expected difficulties, to be grateful that the abortion did not take place (Höök, 1963; Pare, 1967; Clark *et al.*, 1968.)

Table 9.4

OUTCOME OF REFUSAL TO TERMINATE PREGNANCY

	Höök (1963)	Pare* (1967)	Clark et al. (1968)	Forssman & Thuwe (1966)
Kept baby	72%	48%	42%	} 65%
Adoption or fostering	13%	15%	17%	
Abortion or stillbirth	15%	38%	41%	35%
Total no. of cases	238	61	93	196

* See also Pare and Raven (1970) who have obtained similar results in a larger series.

Eventually, most women seem to adjust well to the refusal to abort and its consequences. In Höök's (1963) series of 249 women, only 24 per cent were poorly adjusted several years later while Clark *et al.* (1968) noted a deterioration in mental state following refusal in only seven per cent of their cases. Nevertheless serious mental disorder has been reported after refusal to perform a legal abortion. Höök (1963) found that 13 per cent of the women in his series had been unable to work at times because of mental disturbance consequent on the refusal. In Pare's series (1967) of 61 refused abortions there were a number of severe adverse mental reactions including two in previously stable women who had kept their babies, but who developed severe neurotic symptoms consequent on the stress of looking after the child.

The adverse effect on the children born after refusal to terminate has been studied by Forssman and Thuwe (1966). These authors reported a 21-year follow-up of 120 children born to Swedish women who had been refused a therapeutic abortion, and of 120 control children born at the same time. A number of important differences were noted. In particular more of the unwanted children had an insecure home during childhood, and the incidence of mental disturbance requiring psychiatric care and of delinquent or criminal behaviour was much greater among the unwanted than among the controls.

REFERENCES

ARÉN, P. (1958). On legal abortion in Sweden. Tentative evaluation of justification of frequency during last decade. *Acta obstet. gynec. scand.* **37**, Supplement 1.

CLARK, M., FORSTNER, I., POND, D. A. and TREDGOLD, R. F. (1968). Sequels of unwanted pregnancy. A follow-up of patients referred for psychiatric opinion. *Lancet*, **2**, 501-503.

EKBLAD, M. (1955). Induced abortion on psychiatric grounds. A follow-up of 479 women. *Acta psychiat. scand.* Supplement 99.

FORSSMAN, H. and THUWE, I. (1966). One hundred and twenty children born after application for therapeutic abortion refused. Their mental health, social adjustment and educational level up to the age of 21. *Acta psychiat. scand.* **42**, 71-88.

Höök, K. (1963). Refused abortion. A follow-up study of 249 women whose applications were refused by the National Board of Health in Sweden. *Acta psychiat. scand.* Supplement 168.

Jansson, B. (1965). Mental disorders after abortion. *Acta psychiat. scand.* **41**, 87-110.

McCoy, D. R. (1968). The emotional reaction of women to therapeutic abortion and sterilization. *J. Obstet. Gynaec. Brit. Cwlth.* **75**, 1054-1057.

Niswander, K. R. and Patterson, R. J. (1967). Psychological reaction to therapeutic abortion. I. Subjective patient response. *Obstet and Gynec.* **29**, 702-706.

Pare, C. M. B. (1967). A follow-up study of patients referred for termination of pregnancy on psychiatric grounds. *Brit. J. Psychiat.* Supplement, July 1967, pp 3-4.

Pare, C. M. B. and Raven, H. (1970). Follow-up of patients referred for termination of pregnancy. *Lancet,* **1**, 635-638.

Patt, S. L., Rappaport, R. G. and Barglow, P. (1969). Follow-up of therapeutic abortion. *Arch. gen. Psychiat.* **20**, 408-414.

Simon, N. M., Senturia, A. G. and Rothman, D. (1967). Psychiatric illness following therapeutic abortion. *Amer. J. Psychiat.* **124**, 59-65.

CONTRACEPTION

Moral, Ethical and Legal Aspects of Contraception

Moral and Ethical Problems

People vary widely in their attitudes to contraception from those who view coitus as sinful except for the purpose of procreation to those who consider that intercourse without contraception is immoral unless a child is earnestly desired. Draper (1965) has summarized the attitude of the different religions. The Roman Catholic Church bans all methods of contraception except continence and the restriction of intercourse to the infertile period of the menstrual cycle (the "safe period" or "rhythm" method), and this ban was confirmed by *Humanae Vitae*, the Pope's encyclical of 1968. In spite of the Catholic ban, the use of contraceptives by Catholics is very common. In Great Britain only 59·7 per cent of Catholic married couples conform to the Church's teaching—48·4 per cent take no contraceptive precautions and 11·3 per cent use the safe period or practise abstinence (Pierce and Rowntree, 1961).

The Anglican Church's attitude to contraception has changed in the past 50 years. The Lambeth Conference condemned birth control in 1908 and 1920, but took a more liberal view in 1930, and in 1958 it advocated responsible parenthood, placing the responsibility for family planning on the consciences of the parents themselves. More recently, some prominent members of the Church of England have indicated that parents have a positive moral duty to limit the number of their children.

Judaism obliges every married couple to have children (at least one boy and one girl) and forbids the use of contraceptives by men; it allows women to take precautions on medical grounds. Islam has no clear objection to birth control, and favours its use if the health of the woman demands it (Draper, 1965).

The evolution of the attitudes of the medical profession in Great Britain to birth control has been described by Fryer (1965). Until about 1912 advocates of contraception had always been condemned. The most notable example of this antipathy was the action of the General Medical Council in 1887 in finding Dr Henry Albutt guilty of "infamous conduct in a professional respect" after he had published an inexpensive booklet describing contraceptive methods. In 1912 Sir James Barr, in his presidential address to the British Medical Association, criticized those who condemned contraception, thus marking the beginning of a more enlightened era, and the view that giving advice on birth control is against medical ethics is now held by only a very small minority. Indeed in an editorial in the *Lancet* in 1968 regret was expressed at the Roman Catholic Church's continued stand against contraception.

Legal Aspects

Draper (1965) has summarized the legislation of different countries concerning contraception. She notes that there are four different types of law:
1. Those banning the manufacture of contraceptives as in Eire (and in France until 1967, where however condoms have always been permitted on the grounds that they are considered as prophylactics against venereal disease).
2. Those legislating against the sale of contraceptives as in Eire and until recently in certain American States. (In striking contrast, all pharmacists in Sweden are required by law to stock contraceptives.)
3. Those forbidding the advertising of contraceptives as in Belgium, France, Spain, Holland and Eire.
4. Those banning giving advice in birth control methods as in Eire, Spain and Italy. (In Sweden, however, the law requires that the school curriculum must include teaching on birth control.)

In Great Britain there has been no legislation specifically concerned with birth control, but care must be taken in advertising to avoid contravening the Obscene Publications Act of 1857. Most local authorities however forbid the sale of contraceptives from public slot machines and the Television Act of 1954 forbids the advertisement of contraceptives on television. There is now official recognition in Britain of the need for birth control and the Family Planning Act of 1967 encourages Local Authorities to provide family planning clinics as part of their health services (Peel and Potts, 1969).

In the United States, a federal Act of 1873 (the "Comstock Act") forbidding the advertising of contraceptives or sending them through the mails has gradually ceased to be enforced, but some State laws banning contraception were rigidly implemented until recently. The situation in Connecticut until 1965 has been described by Buxton (1964). Because it was illegal to use any drug or instrument to prevent conception or to advise others in their use, Buxton, although Professor of Obstetrics and Gynecology at Yale University School of Medicine, was unable to provide a contraceptive service and some of his patients died as a result. In 1961 the Planned Parenthood League set up a family planning clinic in Connecticut but it was closed after eight days and the Directors of the clinic were arrested and fined. In June 1965, however, the United States Supreme Court ruled that the Connecticut law was unconstitutional. Pilpel (1966) has analysed this ruling and its implications.

REFERENCES

BUXTON, C. L. (1964). Birth control problems in Connecticut. Medical necessity, political cowardice and legal procrastination. *Conn. Med.* **28**, 581-584.
DRAPER, E. (1965). *Birth Control in the Modern World*. London.
FRYER, P. (1965). *The Birth Controllers*. London.
PEEL, J. and POTTS, M. (1969). *Textbook of Contraceptive Practice*. Cambridge.
PIERCE, R. M. and ROWNTREE, G. (1961). Birth control in Britain. Part II. Contraceptive methods used by couples married in the last thirty years. *Popul. Stud.* **15**, 121-160.
PILPEL, H. F. (1966). Birth control and a new birth of freedom. *Ohio St. Law J.* **27**, 679-690.

The Need for Contraception

With advances in the prophylaxis and treatment of disease the expectation of life has increased very considerably and a greater proportion of infants are now surviving to adult life. The biological fertility of the human race is, however, geared to a relatively low survival rate (Parkes, 1965), and Henry (1961) has calculated that in populations where contraceptive precautions are not taken, each woman has on average eight live children. This figure would undoubtedly be higher in countries with good medical services where infertility can be treated and the stillbirth rate markedly reduced. The combined effect of high natural fertility and low mortality has led to the current situation where, unless contraceptive precautions are taken, every married fertile couple will almost inevitably be overwhelmed by the number of children with consequent physical and mental strain, a lowering of the standard of living and general unhappiness. Shapiro (1967) studied 101 families where there were five or more children of school age or under and found that only five of the mothers were not discontented in any way with the number of their children, and that only one (a woman with eight children already) wished for more. Even those mothers who appeared to be coping well with the situation expressed concern, ranging from anxiety to despair, about the continuing pregnancies while those who were not coping were even more distressed. Three mothers had attempted suicide, two had threatened suicide and one was suspected of baby killing.

In addition to the need to limit the size of the family there is also a need to plan the timing of the birth of the children. Gavron (1966) has pointed out that the legal and political emancipation of women in the last fifty years has led to greater opportunities for women to work and to have interests outside the home. This development, together with the increasing use of contraception itself has revolutionized the life of women from one of constant childbearing to one where the family is generally completed within 10 years of marriage. With earlier marriage many women nowadays have had all their children by the age of thirty, and because of the increased expectation of life they can look forward to many years of working and of developing other interests. Gavron (1966) studied 48 middle-class young married women with at least one child under five years of age and 48 similar women who were of working-class. Ninety six per cent had worked before marriage, 86 per cent had continued to work after marriage and 33 per cent continued working—almost invariably in a part-time capacity—after the birth of the first child. Although the majority were unable to work because of their family commitments— Gavron calls them "captive wives"—only eight per cent of middle-class and 12 per cent of working-class women had no desire to return to work when their children were old enough for them to do so. Obtaining emotional and intellectual satisfaction was the principal reason given by those in the middle-class sample for wishing to work, but financial considerations were more important among those of working-class. Clearly the expectation of so many women to be able to finish their childbearing and child rearing at a given age makes the arrival of an unplanned baby particularly disruptive and has increased the need for contraception.

Surveys on married couples in Great Britain have shown that the use of contraceptive methods is increasing. Rowntree and Pierce (1961) interviewed, in 1959-60, a representative sample of the population and noted that those marrying after 1950 had the most favourable attitudes to contraception while those marrying before 1930 were least in favour. Sixty eight per cent of the total sample reported using birth control methods at some time during their marriage, most commonly the use of a sheath or coitus interruptus. Pierce and Rowntree (1961) noted that these findings were similar to those of an American study carried out a few years previously. In a more recent survey reported by Glass (1968), the sample interviewed was representative of British women who had married in 1941 or later and who were 35 years of age or less at the time of marriage. The use of contraceptives was reported by 87·4 per cent of the sample and the proportion of couples using each method is given in Table 9.5.

Table 9.5

METHODS USED BY BRITISH WOMEN WHO HAVE PRACTISED BIRTH CONTROL
(Glass, 1968)

Method	Proportion who have used method at some time (%)
Safe period	11·2
Coitus interruptus	43·4
Sheath	61·2
Oral contraceptive	18·7
Diaphragm	18·4
Intrauterine device	1·6

Another indication of the increasing demand is the remarkable growth in Great Britain of the family planning movement. The first birth control clinic was opened in 1921 and by 1938 there was an annual attendance of 14,000 new patients at the Family Planning Association's 56 clinics. By 1960 there were 340 clinics and 90,000 new patients per year, in 1967 there were 750 clinics with 175,000 new attendances and by June 1970, 1000 clinics were operating. In addition, in recent years family planning clinics have been established by independent organisations, by hospitals and by Local Authorities. In spite of the increasing facilities there is the clearest evidence that the demand for advice and education on contraceptive methods is not being met. Steele (1966) interviewed 100 consecutive patients with threatened or incomplete abortions and found that 50 of the pregnancies were unwanted and that only 15 women were using some sort of contraceptive method. Fraser and Watson (1968) studied 1000 women from the Paddington district of London and 500 from Welwyn Garden City, a new town twenty miles north of London, and noted that 63 per cent of the pregnancies in Paddington and 42 per cent of those in Welwyn were unplanned; in 70 per cent of unplanned pregnancies no contraceptive precautions had been taken. The increasing demand for legal abortion, discussed earlier in this Chapter, is a further indication that contraceptive precautions are not being taken when they should.

While of course psychiatrists and other clinicians are primarily interested in the need for contraception as it directly affects their patients, all doctors are concerned with the tremendous increase in world population that is now occurring, particularly in the developing countries. During 1960-67 the world birth rate was 34 per 1000 of the population and the death rate 15 per 1000 resulting in an annual rate of population increase of about 1·9 per cent (United Nations, 1968). On the basis of this increase the United Nations Department of Economic and Social Affairs has estimated that by the year 2000 the 1965 world population of 3,300 million will have risen to at least 6,100 million (Population Newsletter, 1968). This population explosion is due mainly to the eradication of malaria in developing countries and to the provision of public health services and it can only be controlled by widespread prevention of conception. Even in Britain where birth control methods are extensively used the population is increasing because of the very low death rate, and Baird (1965) has pointed out that unless the average number of children per family is kept below 2·3, the population will continue to increase.

REFERENCES

BAIRD, D. (1965). A fifth freedom? *Brit. med. J.* **2**, 1141-1148.
FRASER, A. C. and WATSON, P. S. (1968). Family planning—a myth? *Practitioner*, **201**, 351-353.
GAVRON, H. (1966). *Captive Wives. Conflicts of Housebound Mothers.* London.
GLASS, D. V. (1968). Contraception in marriage. *Fam. Planning* **17**, 55-56.

HENRY, L. (1961). Some data on natural fertility. *Eugen. Quart.* **8**, 81-91.

PARKES, A. S. (1965). Biological aspects of the control of human fertility. *Practitioner.* **194**, 455-462.

POPULATION NEWSLETTER (1968). April. No. 1 pp. 8-9.

ROWNTREE, G. and PIERCE, R. M. (1961). Birth Control in Britain. Part I. Attitudes and practices among persons married since the first world war. *Popul. Stud.* **15**, 3-31.

SHAPIRO, P. C. (1967). Large families and family planning. *Eugen. Rev.* **59**, 257-262.

STEELE, S. J. (1966). Family planning advice after abortion. *Lancet*, **2**, 742-743.

UNITED NATIONS (1968). *Demographic Yearbook, 1967.* New York.

Attitudes to Contraception

In general, most people who practise contraception value the greater freedom that it gives them and are content with the measures they take. Clearly however this contentment lasts only for as long as the particular method remains effective. The failure rate of a method is expressed as the number of unwanted pregnancies per hundred women-years, i.e. the number of unwanted pregnancies occurring each year among 100 women taking the precaution in question, and it can be calculated from Pearl's formula:

$$\text{Failure rate per 100 women-years} = \frac{\text{Total accidental pregnancies} \times 1200}{\text{Total months of exposure to risk}}$$

The failure rate varies from method to method and Table 9.6 shows that it is lowest with oral contraceptives and highest when spermicidal chemicals,

Table 9.6

CONTRACEPTIVE FAILURE RATES

(Potts and Swyer, 1970)

Method	Pregnancies per 100 women-years of exposure
Sterilization	0·02
Oral contraceptives	0·1
Intrauterine devices	2·0
Condoms and diaphragms	15·0
Spermicides, calendar rhythm and coitus interruptus	25·0

coitus interruptus or the rhythm method are used (Potts and Swyer, 1970). Three types of oral contraceptive preparations are available and they differ in their efficacy. First, and most effective with a negligible failure rate are formulations combining an oestrogen (mestranol or ethinyloestradiol) with a progestogen, and these are taken daily for some twenty-one days in each cycle starting five days after the onset of menstruation. They have a threefold contraceptive action: they inhibit ovulation, alter the mucus of the uterine cervix so as to impede the passage of sperm, and they interfere with the implantation of the fertilized ovum. Secondly the hormones may be given sequentially; an oestrogen tablet is taken daily from the fifth day of the cycle for 11 to 15 days, and then a tablet containing both oestrogen and progestogen is taken daily until the 25th day. These sequential preparations, however, only inhibit ovulation and the conception rate is much higher (about 1·0 per 100 women years) than with the combined formulation. The Committee on Safety of Drugs (1969*a*) has reported on this difference in efficacy between the two types of contraceptive steroids, but points out that sequential preparations are much less likely to fail than barrier or mechanical methods. In a later statement the Committee on Safety of Drugs (1969*b*) referred to data (since published by Inman, Vessey, Westerholm and Engelund, 1970, and by the Committee on Safety of Drugs, 1970) suggesting that the incidence of thromboembolism was highest among women taking tablets containing more than 50 microgrammes of oestrogen and it recommended that these preparations (which include all sequential formulations) should not normally be prescribed. Thirdly, chlormadinone acetate, a progestogen, is effective when taken continuously in low dosage (0·5 mg per day). Since chlormadinone does not interfere with ovulation, the menstrual periods may continue normally, and its contraceptive action is mediated by rendering the cervical mucus hostile to the passage of sperm. The failure rate with chlormadinone is much higher than with other oral contraceptives and rates of over 5 per 100 women-years have been reported (Howard, Elstein, Blair and Morris, 1969; Butler and Hill, 1969). In January 1970 chlormadinone acetate was temporarily withdrawn by the manufacturers because in long-term toxicity trials non-carcinomatous nodules had developed in the mammary glands of beagle bitches.

Most married couples appear to favour the use of contraceptives; 64·5 per cent of those interviewed by Rowntree and Pierce (1961) expressed unqualified approval and only 15·3 per cent were entirely antagonistic, often for religious reasons. Emotional attitudes, other than moral objection, do sometimes prevent people from seeking advice or from being conscientious in the precaution that they have decided to take. Some of the conflicts which may arise over the use of contraceptives have been described by Rowntree and Pierce (1961), Draper (1963, 1965), Lehfeldt and Guze (1966), Shapiro, (1967), Wallach and Garcia (1968) and Molinski (1969). Some husbands and wives feel that it is wrong to enjoy sexual relations when there is no risk of pregnancy, or that guilt over intercourse can only be atoned for by a pregnancy, or that it is unnatural for coitus never to be followed by conception. Birth control may be considered harmful, particularly that it may permanently impair fertility or health, a view fostered by some doctors 50 years ago. There are also those who fear that society may condemn users of contraceptives for indulging in practices which could lead to promiscuity. Some wives regard contraception as a frustration of their biological urge to procreate, while others prefer not to have the responsibility of taking precautions because this conflicts with their desire to be modest and submissive and for their husbands to be dominant. Husbands sometimes use their power to impregnate to their own ends, either to control or punish their wives or to compensate for their inadequacies by proving their potency and virility.

The emotional difficulties experienced by women attending a clinic or their own doctor for contraceptive advice have been described by Draper (1963) and Shapiro (1967). Many women are anxious on such occasions and are embarrassed when questioned about their sexual life or when they are examined internally, and they may fail to keep their appointments, while some men experience embarrassment in buying condoms.

It is therefore not surprising that when patients are given the responsibility of ensuring the success of a contraceptive measure it will occasionally fail. Lehfeldt (1959) has described the "wilful exposure to unwanted pregnancy" by intelligent and well-instructed patients who nevertheless repeatedly use the method incorrectly or inconsistently. The opportunity for patient failure is shared by all the older methods of contraception (i.e. coitus interruptus, the rhythm method and the barrier methods) but is less likely with oral contraceptives. In contrast, the efficacy of intrauterine devices and of sterilizing operations is not dependent on consistent motivation.

Prejudices against individual methods of contraception may lead to failure (Draper, 1965; Lehfeldt and Guze, 1966; Shapiro, 1967). Condoms are sometimes disliked because of their association, in the user's mind, with venereal disease and prostitution, and because they interfere with sensation. Diaphragms may not be tolerated by those women who have an aversion to internal self-examination, and like condoms they tend to interfere with the spontaneity of intercourse. Women who are considering the use of oral contraceptives are sometimes fearful of thromboembolic disease or cancer, but there are now excellent data on the risk of thrombosis which can be presented to the patient and her husband so that they can decide whether or not to use contraceptive steroids. Deep-vein thrombosis or pulmonary embolism, requiring admission to hospital is about nine times more common among users of oral contraceptives than among non-users, while the risk of cerebral arterial thrombosis is about six times as great (Vessey and Doll, 1968; 1969; Doll and Vessey, 1970). Of all women taking oral contraceptives about one in two thousand are admitted annually to hospital with thromboembolic disease, but the annual mortality rate is much less—about 1·3 per 100,000 users in the age group 20 to 34 years and 3·4 per 100,000 users aged 35-44 (Inman and Vessey, 1968). Reference had already been made to the suggestion that there is a higher incidence of thromboembolism among women taking preparations containing more that 50 microgrammes of oestrogen per tablet. However, as Potts and Swyer (1970) have pointed out, the risk of dying from pregnancy and childbirth among women taking oral contraceptives is so low that even though there is a mortality due to thromboembolism, women on oral contraceptives have an overall expectation of life greater than women using other methods of birth control. The reduction in mortality of women taking oral contraceptives is particularly notable in countries where maternal mortality is high.

There is some doubt concerning the risk of cancer among women taking oral contraceptives. Melamed, Koss, Flehinger et al. (1969) found a small but significantly greater prevalence of uterine cervical carcinoma in situ among women on contraceptive steroids than among women using a diaphragm. These authors were however unable to decide in favour of either of the two possible explanations, that barrier methods of contraception decrease the risk of cancer or that oral preparations are carcinogenic.

REFERENCES

BUTLER, C. and HILL, H. (1969). Chlormadinone acetate as oral contraceptive. *Lancet*, **1**, 1116-1119.

COMMITTEE ON SAFETY OF DRUGS (1969a). Sequential oral contraceptives. *Adverse Reaction Series*. No. 8.

COMMITTEE ON SAFETY OF DRUGS (1969b). Oral contraceptives containing oestrogens. *Adverse Reaction Series*. No. 9.

COMMITTEE ON SAFETY OF DRUGS (1970). Combined oral contraceptives. *Brit. med. J.* **2**, 231-232.

DOLL, R. and VESSEY, M. P. (1970). Evaluation of rare adverse effects of systemic contraceptives. *Brit. med. Bull.* **26**, 33-38.

DRAPER, E. (1963). Emotional barriers in the clinics. In *Family Planning in the Sixties*. Appendix 5, pp. 13-23, Family Planning Association, London.

DRAPER, E. (1965). *Birth Control in the Modern World*. London.

HOWARD, G., ELSTEIN, M., BLAIR, M. and MORRIS, N. F. (1969). Low dose continuous chlormadinone acetate as an oral contraceptive. A clinical trial. *Lancet*, **2**, 24-26.

INMAN, W. H. W. and VESSEY, M. P. (1968). Investigation of deaths from pulmonary, coronary and cerebral thrombosis and embolism in women of childbearing age. *Brit. med. J.* **2**, 193-199.

INMAN, W. H. W., VESSEY, M. P., WESTERHOLM, B. and ENGELUND, A. (1970). Thromboembolic disease and the steroidal content of oral contraceptives. A report to the Committee on Safety of Drugs. *Brit. med. J.* **2**, 203-209.

LEHFELDT, H. (1959). Wilful exposure to unwanted pregnancy (WEUP). Psychological explanation for patient failures in contraception. *Amer. J. Obstet. Gynec.* **78**, 661-665.

LEHFELDT, H. and GUZE, H. (1966). Psychological factors in contraceptive failure. *Fertil. and Steril.* **17**, 110-116.

MELAMED, M. R., KOSS, L. G., FLEHINGER, B. J., KELISKY, R. P. and DUBROW, H. (1969). Prevalence rates of uterine cervical carcinoma in situ for women using the diaphragm or contraceptive oral steroids. *Brit. med. J.* **3**, 195-200.

MOLINSKI, H. (1969). Oral contraceptives: emotional forces affecting the attitudes of men and women. *Advanc. Fertil. Contr.* **4**, 17-21.

POTTS, D. M. and SWYER, G. I. M. (1970). Effectiveness and risks of birth-control methods. *Brit. med. Bull.* **26**, 26-32.

ROWNTREE, G. and PIERCE, R. M. (1961). Birth control in Britain. Part I. Attitudes and practices among persons married since the first world war. *Popul. Stud.* **15**, 3-31.

SHAPIRO, P. C. (1967). Large families and family planning. *Eugen. Rev.* **59**, 257-262.

VESSEY, M. P. and DOLL, R. (1968). Investigation of relation between use of oral contraceptives and thromboembolic disease. *Brit. med. J.* **2**, 199-205.

VESSEY, M. P. and DOLL, R. (1969). Investigation of relation between use of oral contraceptives and thromboembolic disease. A further report. *Brit. med. J.* **2**, 651-657.

WALLACH, E. E. and GARCIA, C-R. (1968). Psychodynamic aspects of oral contraception. *J. Amer. med. Ass.* **203**, 927-931.

Mental Effects of Oral Contraceptives

Mild mental symptoms, particularly depression, tiredness, irritability and impairment of libido occur fairly commonly among women taking oral contraceptive preparations. Nilsson, Jacobson and Ingemanson (1967) found that of 281 patients who had been prescribed Anovlar (Schering), more than one quarter experienced such side effects and that about one in seven discontinued taking the drug because they had become intolerable. In a prospective study, Nilsson and Almgren (1968) compared the symptoms of 54 postpartum women taking oral contraceptives with those of 104 controls using other contraceptive methods, and they found that tiredness, emotional lability, irritability, depressed mood, feelings of inferiority, difficulty in working, worry about the future and sleep disturbance were significantly more common among women on the drug. In another study, by Lewis and Hoghughi (1969), it was found that 19 of 50 women taking oral contraceptives were depressed (including six where the depression was severe), whereas among 50 well-matched controls, there was only one instance of severe depression and two of mild depression. Many other studies have also indicated that there is an association between the use of oral contraceptive preparations and psychiatric symptoms (Nilsson and Sölvell, 1967; Kane, Daly, Ewing and Keeler, 1967; Kane, 1968; Grant and Pryse-Davies, 1968; Kane, Treadway and Ewing, 1969; Herzberg and Coppen, 1970). Serious mental disturbance sometimes occurs: attempted suicide has been reported (Grant and Pryse-Davies, 1968; Lewis and Hoghughi, 1969) and on rare occasions psychotic illnesses appear to be precipitated by the use of oral contraceptives (Daly, Kane and Ewing, 1967; Kane, 1969). But oral contraceptives often increase the well-being of the woman. Nilsson, Jacobson et al. (1967) found that 45·3 per cent of their 281 patients reported improvement in their sexual adaptation, usually attributable to feelings of increased security, but sometimes to an increase in libido, while alleviation of premenstrual depression and irritability by oral contraceptives has been noted by Herzberg and Coppen (1970).

Adverse mental reactions to contraceptive steroids occur more commonly in women with a previous history of psychiatric disorder, particularly depression (Lewis and Hoghughi, 1969) or of mental disturbance during a pregnancy (Nilsson, Jacobson et al., 1967), while Herzberg and Coppen (1970) have reported an association between the development of depression and high scores of Neuroticism and Extraversion on the Maudsley Personality Inventory.

The type of preparation and the dosage of the individual steroids also seem to determine the likelihood of mental side-effects. Over a six-year period, Grant and Pryse-Davies (1968) studied 797 women who had received one or more of 34 oral contraceptive preparations, and they recorded the incidences of symptoms such as depression, loss of libido, tiredness and irritability. Table 9.7, which sets out some of their findings, shows that the incidence of depression and loss of libido varied very considerably from one preparation to another and was lowest among patients using sequential formulations. Goldzieher (1968) has also reported that mental side-effects are uncommon among women taking sequential preparations; of more than 9000 patients, only 2·2 per cent complained of nervousness and only 0·9 per cent of depression. Thus, from the psychiatric point of view, sequential contraceptives are to be preferred, but unfortunately they have certain serious disadvantages which limit their usefulness: they have a higher failure rate

Table 9.7

INCIDENCE OF DEPRESSION AND LOSS OF LIBIDO AMONG WOMEN
TAKING ORAL CONTRACEPTIVE AGENTS
(Grant and Pryse-Davies, 1968)

Drug (Trade name)	No. of women studied	Incidence of loss of libido and depression (%)
*Metrulen	25	20
*Metrulen-M *Ovulen-1 mg	30	13
*Demulen	19	21
*Conovid	27	22
*Conovid E *Previson	28	10
*Orthonovin 2 mg *Norinyl-2	55	20
*Lyndiol	28	3
*Lyndiol 2·5	34	26
Primovlar	29	13
Anovlar 21	136	30
Norlestrin	32	25
Minovlar	21	10
*Ovex	57	11
Volidan	85	34
†*C-Quens 21	11	7
†*Sequens	62	
†*Lutestral	25	

* high oestrogen content (> 50 microgrammes)
† sequential preparations (not completely effective as contraceptive)

than the combined regime (Committee on Safety of Drugs, 1969*a*) and they contain more oestrogen than the Committee on Safety of Drugs (1969*b*) considers advisable; in addition, many contain chlormadinone acetate, which is at present suspected of producing long-term breast changes.

The tendency to mental disturbance seems to be related to the oestrogen-progestogen balance of the preparation (Table 9.8). Thus the very low incidence of mental side-effects with sequential preparations is probably related to the fact that they are strongly oestrogenic, while conversely patients taking strongly progestogenic combined formulations such as Orthonovin and Anovlar tend to experience the greatest mental disturbance (Grant and Pryse-Davies, 1968; Lewis and Hoghughi, 1969). Grant and Pryse-Davies (1968) also found that preparations containing ethinyloestradiol produce more disturbance than those containing mestranol (Table 9.8), but West (1968) was unable to confirm this. Dennis and Jeffery (1968) have reported a patient who became depressed while taking a combined preparation and who

Table 9.8

INCIDENCE OF PSYCHOLOGICAL DISTURBANCES AMONG WOMEN USING
VARIOUS TYPES OF ORAL CONTRACEPTIVE
(Grant and Pryse-Davies, 1968)

	Ethinyloestradiol				*Mestranol*			
	Number of women	*Depression and decreased libido (%)*	*Tiredness (%)*	*Irritability (%)*	*Number of women*	*Depression and decreased libido (%)*	*Tiredness (%)*	*Irritability (%)*
Strongly progestogenic combined tablets	214	28	8	5	108	17	10	3
Other combined tablets	420	20	14	9	174	16	8	2
Sequential regimens	201	7	8	5	100	5	8	5

improved when the drug was changed to continuous low-dosage chlormadinone acetate, suggesting perhaps that the latter is less likely to produce adverse mental reactions.

Some psychiatrists (e.g. Murawski, Sapir, Shulman *et al.*, 1968; Orchard, 1969) have asserted that the mental disturbances are psychogenic reactions and related to the conflicts which women may experience when they take effective contraceptive precautions. But similar side-effects have been observed in women who have been prescribed contraceptive steroids as treatment of gynaecological disorders (Scott and Brass, 1966; Nilsson, Jacobson *et al.*, 1967) favouring a biochemical explanation for their occurrence. Two chemical hypotheses have in fact been proposed. First, Grant and Pryse-Davies (1968) have related mood disturbance to changes in monoamine oxidase activity, and secondly the effects of contraceptive steroids on tryptophan metabolism have been implicated. Grant and Pryse-Davies (1968) obtained endometrial biopsies and showed that MAO activity varied with the type of medication that the patient was receiving. They found that strongly progestogenic combined preparations caused a notable increase in endometrial MAO activity during the second half of the menstrual cycle, in contrast to the sequential formulations where MAO activity was low at all times, and they suggest that depression and loss of libido might arise from similarly induced disturbances in MAO activity within the brain. But the endometrial changes may not be typical of the rest of the body; indeed a *decrease* in MAO activity has been observed in the serum of women taking oral contraceptives (Tryding, Nilsson, Tufvesson *et al.*, 1969) and the hypothesis remains unproven.

There is some evidence that contraceptive steroids alter tryptophan metabolism by creating a functional deficiency of pyridoxine, a co-enzyme involved in the conversion of tryptophan to 5-hydroxytryptamine. Oestrogens increase the urinary output of xanthenuric acid and other tryptophan metabolites and these effects are prevented by the concomitant administration of pyridoxine (Rose, 1966; Toseland and Price, 1969). Such alterations in tryptophan metabolism could lead to decreased synthesis of 5-hydroxytryptamine in the brain and consequent mental depression and Winston (1969) has suggested that pyridoxine might be of value in treating steroid-induced mood disturbance; he reports a case where at a dose of 50 mg daily pyridoxine did appear to be of benefit.

REFERENCES

COMMITTEE ON SAFETY OF DRUGS (1969*a*). Sequential oral contraceptives. *Adverse Reaction Series*. No. 8.

COMMITTEE ON SAFETY OF DRUGS (1969*b*). Oral contraceptives containing oestrogens. *Adverse Reaction Series*. No. 9.

DALY, R. J., KANE, F. J. and EWING, J. A. (1967). Psychosis associated with the use of a sequential oral contraceptive. *Lancet*, 2, 444-445.

DENNIS, K. J. and JEFFERY, J. D'A. (1968). Depression and oral contraceptives. *Lancet*, 2, 454-455.

GOLDZIEHER, J. W. (1968). The incidence of side effects with oral or intrauterine contraceptives. *Amer. J. Obstet. Gynec.* 102, 91-94.

GRANT, E. C. G. and PRYSE-DAVIES, J. (1968). Effect of oral contraceptives on depressive mood changes and on endometrial monoamine oxidase and phosphatases. *Brit. med. J.* 3, 777-780.

HERZBERG, B. and COPPEN, A. (1970). Changes in psychological symptoms in women taking oral contraceptives. *Brit. J. Psychiat.* 116, 161-164.

KANE, F. J. (1968). Psychiatric reactions to oral contraceptives. *Amer. J. Obstet. Gynec.* 102, 1053-1063.

KANE, F. J. (1969). Psychosis associated with the use of oral contraceptive agents. *Sth. med. J. (Bgham, Ala)*, 62, 190-192.

KANE, F. J., DALY, R. J., EWING, J. A. and KEELER, M. H. (1967). Mood and behavioural changes with progestational agents. *Brit. J. Psychiat.* 113, 265-268.

KANE, F. J., TREADWAY, C. R. and EWING, J. A. (1969). Emotional change associated with oral contraceptives in female psychiatric patients. *Comprehens. Psychiat.* 10, 16-30.

LEWIS, A. and HOGHUGHI, M. (1969). An evaluation of depression as a side effect of oral contraceptives. *Brit. J. Psychiat.* 115, 697-701.

MURAWSKI, B. J., SAPIR, P. E., SHULMAN, N., RYAN, G. M. and STURGIS, S. H. (1968). An investigation of mood states in women taking oral contraceptives. *Fertil. and Steril.* 19, 50-63.

NILSSON, Å. and ALMGREN, P-E. (1968). Psychiatric symptoms during the postpartum period as related to use of oral contraceptives. *Brit. med. J.* 2, 453-455.

NILSSON, Å., JACOBSON, L. and INGEMANSON, C. A. (1967). Side-effects of an oral contraceptive with particular attention to mental symptoms and sexual adaptation. *Acta obstet. gynec. scand.* 46, 537-556.

NILSSON, L. and SÖLVELL, L. (1967). Clinical studies on oral contraceptives—a randomized, double blind, crossover study of 4 different preparations, Anovlar mite, Lyndiol mite, Ovulen and Volidan. *Acta obstet. gynec. scand.* Supplement 8.

ORCHARD, W. H. (1969). Psychiatric aspects of oral contraceptives. *Med. J. Aust.* **1**, 872-876.

ROSE, D. P. (1966). The influence of oestrogens on tryptophan metabolism in man. *Clin. Sci.* **31**, 265-272.

SCOTT, J. W. and BRASS, P. (1966). Massive norethynodrel therapy in the treatment of endometriosis. *Amer. J. Obstet. Gynec.* **95**, 1166-1167.

TOSELAND, P. A. and PRICE, S. (1969). Tryptophan and oral contraceptives. *Brit. med. J.* **1**, 777.

TRYDING, N., NILSSON, S. E., TUFVESSON, G., BERG, R., CARLSTRÖM, S., ELMFORS, B. and NILSSON, J. E. (1969). Physiological and pathological influences on serum monoamine oxidase level. Effect of age, sex, contraceptive steroids and diabetes mellitus. *Scand. J. clin. Lab. Invest.* **23**, 79-84.

WEST, J. (1968). Mood and the "Pill". *Brit. med. J.* **4**, 187-188.

WINSTON, F. (1969). Oral contraceptives and depression. *Lancet*, **2**, 377.

STERILIZATION

Surgical sterilization is a very effective means of preventing conception and it has the advantage over most other methods in that its efficacy does not depend on the continual vigilance of the patient. The operation, in women, entails dividing the Fallopian tubes and ligating their cut ends. This is most easily undertaken either early in the puerperium when the uterus is large and the tubes readily accessible, or at the same time as hysterotomy or Caesarean section; it can, however, be carried out at any other time. Hysterectomy is sometimes undertaken as a contraceptive measure, particularly where there is a suspicion of uterine disease or where the patient or doctor has religious objections to other methods of birth control. Campbell (1964) has estimated that in 1960 in the United States, six per cent of all hysterectomies were performed solely to prevent further pregnancy.

In the male, the usual sterilization procedure is ligation and division of the vasa deferentia, a relatively simple procedure which can be done as an outpatient under local anaesthesia, although many patients do in fact prefer a general anaesthetic.

Legal and Moral Aspects

In Great Britain, the legality of sterilization performed to prevent conception has never been tested in the courts, and the legal position is therefore uncertain. The Medical Defence Union, however, has stated that there are no grounds for believing that voluntary sterilization is against the law, and conclude that it may be carried out for any indication including medical, socio-economic or psychiatric, or indeed purely to limit the size of the family. Full valid consent of the patient is however necessary and there may be some doubt of the legality of the operation in mentally disturbed or defective persons unless it is undertaken for therapeutic reasons. In order to avoid legal action by the spouse the written consent of both husband and wife should always be obtained (Addison, 1966; 1967).

In the United States medically indicated therapeutic sterilization is legal in all States regardless of how minimal the indication (Gampell, 1964) and apart from Connecticut and Utah where contraceptive sterilization may be undertaken only on grounds of "medical necessity" there are no laws restricting the use of the procedure (Journal of the American Medical Association, 1968).

Moral attitudes to sterilization, like those to contraception in general, vary widely, but with sterilization there is the added problem of whether or not a person has the moral right to deal with his body in any way he chooses. At one extreme is the view of the Roman Catholic Church which condemns contraceptive sterilization, although it allows operative procedures such as hysterectomy and prostatectomy where there is a purely medical indication, even though they render the patient infertile. At the other extreme stand those who argue that any measure which preserves and consolidates the family is morally praiseworthy (Blacker, 1964). The Church of England takes up an intermediate position, and while not condemning sterilization, advocates the use of other contraceptive measures where possible (Church of England National Assembly Board for Social Responsibility, 1962).

REFERENCES

ADDISON, P. H. (1966). Sterilization and the law. *Brit. med. J.* **1**, 1597.

ADDISON, P. H. (1967). Legal aspects of sterilization and contraception. *Med.-leg. J. (Camb.)* **35**, 164-167.

BLACKER, C. P. (1964). Voluntary sterilization: its role in human betterment. *Eugen. Rev.* **56**, 77-80.

CAMPBELL, A. A. (1964). The incidence of operations that prevent conception. *Amer. J. Obstet. Gynec.* **89**, 694-700.

CHURCH OF ENGLAND NATIONAL ASSEMBLY BOARD FOR SOCIAL RESPONSIBILITY (1962). *Sterilization—an Ethical Enquiry.* London.

GAMPELL, R. J. (1964). Legal status of therapeutic abortion and sterilization in the United States. *Clin. Obstet. Gynec.* **7**, 22-36.

JOURNAL OF THE AMERICAN MEDICAL ASSOCIATION (1968). (Editorial) Voluntary male sterilization. *J. Amer. med. Ass.* **204**, 821-822.

Tubal Ligation

Indications

Thompson and Baird (1968) give the following five indications for undertaking sterilization in women:

1. *Medical.*—Serious disease, normally of heart, chest or kidneys, which makes childbearing dangerous to life or health.
2. *Psychiatric.*—Severe mental disturbance necessitating psychiatric treatment, which makes further childbearing inadvisable.
3. *Obstetric.*—History of serious obstetric complications.

4. *Debility and Multiparity*.—Extreme debility characterized by severe anaemia, lassitude, progressive deterioration in wellbeing, and depression, usually associated with rapid childbearing and large family size. Consideration of the social circumstances was of particular importance in this group.

5. *Other*.—Eugenic or social circumstances.

Table 9.9 gives the frequency of each indication in Thompson and Baird's series of 186 patients. Debility and multiparity was the most common indication and was present in 134 cases (71·9 per cent) and only seven (3·8 per cent) patients were sterilized because of severe mental disturbance. These findings are similar to those reported by Blacker and Peel (1969), who obtained data on a large sample of women who had been sterilized during

Table 9.9

INDICATIONS FOR STERILIZATION IN 186 WOMEN
(Thompson and Baird, 1968)

Indication	Number	Per cent
Medical	22	11·8
Medical + Debility and Multiparity	12	6·4
Psychiatric	2	1·1
Psychiatric + Debility and Multiparity	5	2·7
Obstetric	19	10·2
Obstetric + Debility and Multiparity	25	13·4
Debility and Multiparity	92	49·4
Other	9	4·8
Total	186	100·0

1966 in England and Wales. They classified the indications (with relative frequencies in parentheses) as follows:

(*a*) Domestic and family problems, including high parity, marital stress, etc. (49 per cent)

(*b*) In association with termination of pregnancy or with repeated Caesarean section (28 per cent)

(*c*) Physical disease or defect making further pregnancy dangerous to health (16 per cent)

(*d*) Psychiatric (7 per cent).

Psychological Effects

Most follow-up studies have shown that tubal ligation very frequently improves the general health of the woman, the marital relationship (including its sexual aspects) and the socio-economic position of the family (Ekblad, 1961; Adams, 1964; Black and Sclare, 1968; Thompson and Baird, 1968; Whitehouse, 1969). Table 9.10 lists a number of studies where the proportion of women who were completely and permanently satisfied by the operation ranged from 71·8 per cent (McCoy, 1968) to 98·7 per cent (Lu and Chun, 1967). In each series, however, a number of women seriously regretted the operation and wished they had not agreed to it, the incidence ranging from 0·1 per cent (Lu and Chun, 1967) to 15·4 per cent (McCoy, 1968). The reasons given by these women for their change of mind varied. In some there had been a deterioration in the marital relationship, either due to a decrease in the wife's libido or to a loss of interest in the husband who had turned elsewhere for sexual satisfaction. Sometimes the regrets were understandable because of new unforeseen circumstances; one or more of the children may have died and the wife may have wished to replace them or the husband may

Table 9.10

POST-OPERATIVE ATTITUDES OF WOMEN UNDERGOING TUBAL LIGATION

Authors	*Number in series*	*% entirely satisfied*	*% with serious regrets*
Ekblad (1961)	225	77·8	6·7
Adams (1964)	173	88·4	2·9
Kaij and Malmquist (1965)	179	78·7	3·9
Barglow and Eisner (1966)	833	94·0	4·2
Lu and Chun (1967)	1,055	98·7	0·1
Black and Sclare (1968)	168	96·4	3·6
Thompson and Baird (1968)	186	86·5	4·3
McCoy (1968)	39	71·8	15·4
Enoch and Jones (1968)	98	75·5	3·1
Whitehouse (1969)	95	86·3	6·2
Steptoe (1970)	278	98·0	—

have died and on remarriage the woman may have desired further children. Occasionally the maternal instinct seemed frustrated by the operation and Whitehouse (1969) described two such patients who actually increased their family by adoption. Thompson and Baird (1968) reported two women who felt unhappy when their youngest children started going to school and who would have liked to have had further babies. Less intense longing for further children has been noted by Ekblad (1961) who also observed that a small proportion of his patients became unduly fearful for the safety of their existing children. Other patients, particularly those whose religion forbids sterilization, sometimes felt extremely guilty and wished that the operation had not been carried out. Occasionally the reason for the regret was not readily understandable as with a patient of Whitehouse (1969) who felt cheated of the monthly worry that she might be pregnant.

Because the operation is virtually irreversible a number of investigators have attempted to discover those factors associated with a poor outcome. Ekblad (1961) noted that only 50 per cent of women sterilized below the age of 26 years were entirely satisfied with the operation, compared with 83 per cent of those aged 26 years or more, consistent with previous studies which had suggested that regrets were more likely among young women. Although Barglow and Eisner (1966) and Thompson and Baird (1968) found no correlation between age and outcome, many gynaecologists feel unhappy about sterilizing women below the age of 30. With increasing family size the risk of serious regrets diminishes strikingly (Thompson and Baird, 1968) and Ekblad (1961; 1963) found that of 60 childless women only 28 (47 per cent) were completely satisfied with the operation whereas among 213 women with children, 174 (82 per cent) expressed no regrets. Unhappiness about steriliz-ation is also more common where pressure has been applied to the woman to undergo operation; for example where the initiative comes from the doctor rather than from the patient (Whitehouse, 1969), where there are medical, psychiatric or obstetric grounds (Thompson and Baird, 1968), or where sterilization is made a condition of termination of pregnancy (Ekblad, 1961). Other factors producing an unsatisfactory outcome are where the husband has been reluctant to agree to the operation (Whitehouse, 1969), where the patient has an abnormal personality with aggressive, histrionic or immature characteristics and where the marital relationship is poor (Ekblad, 1961). Intelligence does not appear to correlate with outcome, nor apparently does the presence or absence of minor neurotic symptoms.

Pregnancies after tubal ligation have been reported in most series, and this is a cause of an obviously different sort of dissatisfaction. Thompson and Baird (1968) in their series of 186 cases noted three such failures necessitating further operation, and this incidence is similar to that found by other in-vestigators. All sterilizing operations have a failure rate, and this must be pointed out to the patient—indeed even hysterectomy may not prevent conception and subsequent delivery of a live child (Winslow, Strasbaugh and Mervine, 1969).

Although tubal ligation is usually considered to be irreversible, Williams (1969) has pointed out that it is sometimes possible to restore fertility by further operation. He reported four cases where the patency of the Fallopian tubes was re-established by tubo-uterine implantation, resulting in three of the women becoming pregnant and delivering live children. He circulated a questionnaire to gynaecologists in Great Britain and obtained details of a further 42 cases where tubo-uterine implantation had been carried out following sterilization. Eleven (27 per cent) of the women subsequently conceived, but only seven (17 per cent) were delivered of live children, because two had aborted and in two the pregnancy was ectopic. The incidence of ectopic pregnancy is very high following this type of operation and Williams advises that this danger should be pointed out to the patient.

Serious psychiatric disorder seems to be uncommon after tubal ligation. In a series of 1055 patients sterilized in Hong Kong, Lu and Chun (1967) noted only four such instances, an incidence similar to that which exists in the general population. Most other studies have also shown that serious mental disorder is rare, but Ellison (1964) has reported 20 patients where tubal ligation appeared to have precipitated mental disorder severe enough to cause admission to a psychiatric hospital. Sixteen of these patients were depressed (10 with paranoid features), in two the diagnosis was schizophrenia and two patients were suffering from anxiety states. In view of these findings Ellison advises against sterilization in women except where every other method of contraception has been shown to be unsatisfactory, but this is an extreme view with which most clinicians would not agree.

REFERENCES

ADAMS, T. W. (1964). Female sterilization. *Amer. J. Obstet. Gynec.* **89**, 395-401.

BARGLOW, P. and EISNER, M. (1966). An evaluation of tubal ligation in Switzerland. *Amer. J. Obstet. Gynec.* **95**, 1083-1094.

BLACK, W. P. and SCLARE, A. B. (1968). Sterilization by tubal ligation—a follow up study. *J. Obstet. Gynaec. Brit. Cwlth.* **75**, 219-224.

BLACKER, C. P. and PEEL, J. H. (1969). Sterilization of women. *Brit. med. J.* **1**, 566-567.

EKBLAD, M. (1961). The prognosis after sterilization on social-psychiatric grounds. A follow-up study of 225 women. *Acta psychiat. scand.* Supplement 161.

EKBLAD, M. (1963). Social-psychiatric prognosis after sterilization of women without children. A follow up study of 60 women. *Acta psychiat. scand.* **39**, 481-514.

ELLISON, R. M. (1964). Psychiatric complications following sterilization of women. *Med. J. Aust.* **2**, 625-628.

ENOCH, M. D. and JONES, K. (1968). Follow-up of sterilized women. *Lancet*, **1**, 1247-1248.

KAIJ, L. and MALMQUIST, A. (1965). Prognosis after sterilization in connection with parturition. A follow-up study of 179 women. *Acta psychiat. scand.* **41**, 204-217.

LU, T. and CHUN, D. (1967). A long term follow-up study of 1055 cases of post-partum tubal ligation. *J. Obstet. Gynaec. Brit. Cwlth.* **74**, 875-880.

McCOY, D. R. (1968). The emotional reaction of women to therapeutic abortion and sterilization. *J. Obstet. Gynaec. Brit. Cwlth.* **75**, 1054-1057.

STEPTOE, P. C. (1970). Recent advances in surgical methods of control of fertility and infertility. *Brit. med. Bull.* **26**, 60-64.

THOMPSON, B. and BAIRD, D. (1968). Follow up of 186 sterilized women. *Lancet*, **1**, 1023-1027.

WHITEHOUSE, D. B. (1969). Tubal ligation. A follow up study. *Advanc. Fertil. Contr.* **4**, 22-26.

WILLIAMS, G. F. J. (1969). Tubo-uterine implantation—with special reference to reversal of sterilization. *Lancet*. **1**, 825-827.

WINSLOW, H. C., STRASBAUGH, N. and MERVINE, N. D. (1969). Pregnancies following hysterectomy. Review of 100 years' recorded experience and report of a case. *Penn. Med.* **72**, 45-51.

Vasectomy

Vasectomy entails dividing the vasa deferentia and ligating the cut ends (Hanley, 1968). The patient remains fertile for some time after operation because the ejaculate will contain spermatozoa stored pre-operatively, either in the seminal vesicles or elsewhere distal to the site of operation. Contraceptive precautions should therefore be taken until the semen is shown to be azoospermic. Freund and Davis (1969) noted a steady and regular decline in the sperm count in each successive post-operative specimen of semen and observed that after six to ten ejaculations (i.e. within a week or two of operation) the specimens of all the 13 men they studied were free of sperm. Hanley (1968) also points out that the decrease in sperm count is more directly related to the number of post-operative ejaculates than to the time elapsed and suggests explaining this to the patient. Under normal circumstances the first specimen may be examined two months after operation and further specimens tested at monthly intervals; contraceptive precautions should be taken until two successive samples are azoospermic.

The failure rate with vasectomy is low; in a series of 1923 patients reported by Alderman (1968) it was 0·98 per cent. Spontaneous recanalization of the vas does, however, sometimes occur, as in five of 432 patients operated on by Schmidt (1966); other instances have been reported by Bunge (1968) and by Pugh and Hanley (1969). Resection of several centimetres of each vas may reduce the likelihood of spontaneous recanalization, but this makes any future surgical reanastomosis less feasible. Surgeons are therefore now devising other ways to prevent recanalization, for example by folding the cut ends of the vas back on themselves so that they point away from each other (Pugh and Hanley, 1969). With change of circumstances, a proportion of patients wish to have their fertility restored, and request surgical reanastomosis. Phadke and Phadke (1967) have reported 76 such men. In 37 the reanastomosis was requested following remarriage and in 28 following the death of an existing child. In nine cases the indication was a desire for more children while in one it was "psychological" and in another it was "religious". Reanastomosis, on average five years after vasectomy, was undertaken in all these patients, and sperm reappeared in the semen of 83 per cent; at the time of follow-up 55 per cent of the wives had become pregnant.

The vast majority of married couples appear to be well satisfied with vasectomy; Jackson (1969) has reported a follow-up of 1011 men at least one year after operation and in 18 instances only did either the man or his wife express any regrets. Generally, sexual satisfaction tends to improve and sexual intercourse to increase in frequency (Ferber, Tietze and Lewit, 1967; Rodgers and Ziegler, 1968), but 1·48 per cent of the patients in Jackson's (1969) series reported some deterioration in their sexual life. Subtle psychological changes seem to be quite common, however. Ferber et al. (1967) found that most men were reluctant to inform others that they had had the operation, because they feared that it might be thought that they had undergone some form of castration and that their virility had been affected. Ziegler, Rodgers and Kriegsman (1966) and Ziegler, Rodgers and Prentiss (1969) have noted that after vasectomy there is an increased tendency for men to demonstrate their masculinity, presumably a psychological defence against anxiety produced by castration fantasies. Consistent with this is an observation by Beazley and Fraser (1969) that men often refuse to undergo vasectomy because they cannot distinguish between fertility and virility or potency, although they are perfectly agreeable to tubal ligation in their wives. More serious psychological disturbance is uncommon but Schmidt (1966) has reported one patient who complained of post-operative impotence. In the present state of knowledge it would seem reasonable to restrict vasectomy to couples who are judged to be stable, happily married and who already have a family (Hanley, 1968).

REFERENCES

ALDERMAN, P. M. (1968). Vasectomy for voluntary male sterilization. *Lancet*, 2, 1137-1138.

BEAZLEY, J. M. and FRASER, W. J. (1969). Voluntary sterilization. *Lancet*, 2, 531-533.

BUNGE, R. G. (1968). Bilateral spontaneous reanastomosis of the ductus deferens. *J. Urol. (Baltimore)* 100, 762.

FERBER, A. S., TIETZE, C. and LEWIT, S. (1967). Men with vasectomies: a study of medical, sexual and psychosocial changes. *Psychosom. Med.* 29, 354-366.

FREUND, M. and DAVIS, J. E. (1969). Disappearance rate of spermatozoa from the ejaculate following vasectomy. *Fertil. and Steril.* 20, 163-170.

HANLEY, H. G. (1968). Vasectomy for voluntary male sterilization. *Lancet*, 2, 207-209.

JACKSON, L. N. (1969). Vasectomy in the United Kingdom. *Practitioner*, 203, 320-323.

PHADKE, G. M. and PHADKE, A. G. (1967). Experiences in the re-anastomosis of the vas deferens. *J. Urol. (Baltimore)* 97, 888-890.

PUGH, R. C. B. and HANLEY, H. G. (1969). Spontaneous recanalization of the divided vas deferens. *Brit. J. Urol.* 41, 340-347.

RODGERS, D. A. and ZIEGLER, F. J. (1968). Changes in sexual behaviour consequent to use of non-coital procedures of contraception. *Psychosom. Med.* 30, 495-505.

SCHMIDT, S. W. (1966). Technics and complications of elective vasectomy. *Fertil. and Steril.* 17, 467-482.

ZIEGLER, F. J., RODGERS, D. A. and KRIEGSMAN, S. A. (1966). Effect of vasectomy on psychological functioning. *Psychosom. Med.* 28, 50-63.

ZIEGLER, F. J., RODGERS, D. A. and PRENTISS, R. J. (1969). Psychosocial response to vasectomy. *Arch. gen. Psychiat.* 21, 46-54.

POST-PARTUM MENTAL DISORDERS

Prevalence of Puerperal Psychosis

Mental disorders in the puerperium show well-marked variation in their severity. Most are mild and transitory, and only a small minority are extremely severe and require admission to a psychiatric hospital. The latter, known usually as puerperal psychoses, have been studied more intensively and will be considered here while less severe disturbances will be discussed separately later in this chapter.

Estimates of the proportion of puerperal women who develop severe mental disorder necessitating their admission to hospital vary. Vislie (1956) quotes studies where the rates range from 0·8 to 2·5 per 1000 deliveries, and some more recent investigations are listed in Table 9.11.

The study by Hemphill (1952) is particularly worthy of note. He followed up all the women delivered in Bristol during the ten-and-one-half year period January 1938 to June 1948 and found that of a total of 81,000 post-partum women, 116 were admitted to a mental hospital with a puerperal mental disorder, a rate of 1·4 per 1000 deliveries. Among women delivered in a maternity hospital the admission rate was lower—1·0 per 1000 births—but short-lived mental reactions such as depression and delirium not requiring admission to a mental hospital occurred with a frequency of 0·7 per 1000 deliveries. Similar transitory illnesses among women delivered at home or at a nursing home generally led to admission to a mental hospital, so that in this group the admission rate was higher—1·8 per 1000 births.

Oltman and Friedman (1965) have suggested that the prevalence of post-partum mental disorder is declining. They reviewed all admissions of women aged 17 to 45 years to a mental hospital in Connecticut during the years 1942 to 1963 and noted that before 1956 puerperal mental illnesses represented 7·3 per cent of the total admissions, while after 1956 the proportion dropped

Table 9.11

PREVALENCE OF PUERPERAL PSYCHOSES

Authors	Place of study	Criterion for duration of puerperium	prevalence of puerperal psychosis (per 1000 deliveries)
Hemphill (1952)	Bristol (U.K.)	Not stated	1·4
Tetlow (1955)	Warwick (U.K.)	6 months	1·5
Pugh et al. (1963)	Massachusetts (U.S.A.)	6 weeks	3·3
Jansson (1964)	Göteborg (Sweden)	1 year	4·6
Paffenbarger (1964)	Ohio (U.S.A.)	6 months	1·9

to 3·7 per cent. Moreover, they observed that schizophrenic and manic-depressive reactions appeared to be decreasing in incidence. During 1942 to 1955, these illnesses accounted for 97 per cent of all the puerperal disorders, whereas during 1956 to 1963 they represented only 83 per cent. A similar decrease in prevalence was, however, not shown by Protheroe (1969) whose data on women admitted with puerperal psychoses to a mental hospital in Newcastle-upon-Tyne demonstrated no change in annual admission rates over the period 1927 to 1961.

Clinical Aspects of Post-Partum Psychosis

Diagnosis

In accordance with the generally accepted view that post-partum psychoses do not constitute an entity distinct from non-puerperal psychoses, the International Classification of Diseases (World Health Organization, 1967) allocates them to diagnostic categories which are independent of any relationship to childbirth, and most cases can be classified as schizophrenic, affective or organic. However, in the early stages of the illness the clinical picture is often not typical. There are very often non-specific prodromal symptoms, lasting a few days, of insomnia, restlessness, depression and irritability proceeding to euphoria, refusal of food and the expression of irrational ideas, and differentiation into schizophrenic, affective or organic types of mental reaction may occur only later in the course of the illness (Hamilton, 1962). Furthermore, clouding of consciousness, particularly early in the illness, occurs much more commonly than in non-puerperal functional psychoses. Thus, Arentsen (1968) noted disturbance of consciousness in 66 per cent of a series of 168 puerperal patients and in 42 per cent this disturbance dominated the clinical picture. Melges (1968) found evidence of confusion in 92 per cent of his patients, but this was generally mild and only 19 per cent were disorientated in time. In Protheroe's (1969) series, consciousness was clouded in 34 per cent of all cases, but was much more common among patients admitted before 1942. Confusional symptoms were seen in 30·3 per cent of cases by Jansson (1964) and in 34 per cent by Vislie (1956).

Within one or two weeks of the onset of a puerperal psychosis, it is usually possible to make a specific diagnosis. Ostwald and Regan (1957) reviewed nine studies published between 1911 and 1955 and noted that overall there was approximately equal representation of schizophrenic, manic-depressive and organic reactions. More recent studies (summarized in Table 9.12) show a much lower prevalence of organic mental reaction. This trend appears to be a definite one, and Protheroe (1969) has noted that at a hospital in Newcastle-upon-Tyne puerperal admissions during 1927 to 1941 had organic reactions in 10·4 per cent of cases, whereas during 1942 to 1961, the proportion had fallen to 1·2 per cent.

Table 9.12

PUERPERAL PSYCHOSIS. SPECIFIC DIAGNOSES.

Author	Number in series	Diagnosis (*per cent of series*)			
		Schizophrenia	Mania	Depression	Organic psychosis
		%	%	%	%
Hemphill (1952)	116	21	7	50	16
Fondeur *et al.* (1957)	100	50	5	25	0
Martin (1958)	75	59	1	36	3
Seager (1960)	42	36	0	52	0
Arentsen (1968)	168	11	5	19	2
Melges (1968)	100	51	31		0
Protheroe (1969)	134	28	14	54	4

Differential Diagnosis

The frequent occurrence of delirium, impairment of consciousness and confusion in puerperal mental disorders may occasionally mislead the clinician and cause him to overlook an intracranial or other lesion responsible for the mental disturbance. In young women, cerebral arterial thrombosis occurs more commonly in the puerperium than at other times and may be associated with disturbances of consciousness (Cross, Castro and Jennett, 1968), but puerperal cerebral thrombophlebitis is particularly common. Cerebral thrombophlebitis may cause drowsiness and confusion, as in 17 per cent of 181 cases reviewed by Carroll, Leak and Lee (1966), but there are usually other abnormalities present which allow the correct diagnosis to be made. Thus in Carroll's series, hemiparesis occurred in 45 per cent of cases, epileptic fits in 34 per cent, dysphasia in 24 per cent and severe headache in

34 per cent. The cerebrospinal fluid was abnormal, with raised protein level and increased numbers of red and white cells, in the majority of cases, and there was sometimes concomitant subarachnoid haemorrhage causing neck stiffness and a positive Kernig's sign; in more than one third of cases however the CSF was normal. Goldman, Eckerling and Gans (1964) have also pointed out that psychotic symptoms early in the puerperium may be due to cerebral thrombophlebitis and may lead to a mis-diagnosis of puerperal psychosis.

Time of Onset

Apart from the first few days after childbirth, the risk of developing a puerperal psychosis decreases markedly as the puerperium advances. Thus about 90 per cent of mental disturbances arising in the year following parturition start in the first six months (Jansson, 1964), while of cases arising in the first six months, the majority begin in the first four weeks (Table 9.13), and a number of investigators have shown that the risk of onset is greatest during the first week or ten days (Tetlow, 1955; Vislie, 1956; Seager, 1960; Melges, 1968; Protheroe, 1969).

Table 9.13

TIME OF ONSET OF PUERPERAL PSYCHOSIS

Time of onset after delivery	Jansson (1964) (117 patients) %	Paffenbarger (1964) (242 patients) %
0-1 month	53·9	67·8
1-2 months	16·2	11·2
2-3 months	14·5	8·7
3-6 months	15·3	12·4
	100	100

There is usually an interval of at least a few days between delivery and the onset of the psychotic disorder and Hamilton (1962) has stated that symptoms are almost never noted before the third day post partum. Paffenbarger (1964) observed such a lucid interval in every one of his 242 cases, but Melges (1968) noted that 16 of his 95 patients had symptoms on the first day of the puerperium.

Prognosis

Table 9.14 lists seven studies on a total of 702 patients with puerperal psychosis. Overall the recovery rate was 68·5 per cent but this varied in different series from a minimum of 34·0 per cent (Fondeur, Fixsen, Triebel and White, 1957) to a maximum of 80·7 per cent (Martin, 1958). The proportion of patients remaining permanently psychotic has been estimated by a number of investigators and ranges from 2·7 per cent (Martin, 1958) to 15·5 per cent (Hemphill, 1952); Vislie (1956) reported persistent chronic psychosis in 7·5 per cent of his cases and Arentsen (1968) in 12·5 per cent. The overall prognosis of post-partum psychosis is probably like that of similar non-puerperal illnesses and Fondeur *et al.* (1957) found no significant difference as regards condition at discharge, between 100 puerperal patients and 100 matched control patients with non-puerperal illnesses.

The consensus of opinion is that the prognosis is best in patients with affective disorders, even though Hamilton (1962) has suggested that manic-depressive psychosis occurring in the puerperium has a worse outcome than

Table 9.14

PROGNOSIS OF PUERPERAL PSYCHOSIS

	No. in series	Proportion showing complete recovery per cent
Hemphill (1952)	116	80·1
Vislie (1956)	67	58·2
Fondeur et al. (1957)	100	34·0
Martin (1958)	75	80·7
Seager (1960)	42	50·0
Arentsen (1968)	168	78·0
Protheroe (1969)	134	73·9
Total	702	68·5

similar non-puerperal illnesses. Of 66 patients with post-partum affective psychosis reported by Hemphill (1952), one committed suicide but all the others recovered, while Martin (1958) found that all her affectively disturbed patients made a good recovery. In a series of 91 patients with affective psychosis described by Protheroe (1969) the recovery rate was 89·0 per cent (Table 9.15).

Table 9.15

RECOVERY FROM PUERPERAL PSYCHOSIS
(Protheroe, 1969)

Type of psychosis	Proportion showing complete recovery among admissions during:		
	1927-41	1942-61	1927-61
	%	%	%
Affective	87·9	89·6	89·0
Schizophrenic	21·4	54·5	41·7
Organic	40·0	100·0	50·0
All types psychosis	65·4	80·2	74·4

The prognosis of post-partum schizophrenia has been assessed differently by different investigators. Martin (1958) has suggested that the outcome is very much better than that of non-puerperal schizophrenia in that all of her 15 schizophrenic patients and 24 of her 29 schizo-affective patients recovered. The opposite view has been expressed by Hemphill (1952) who found that puerperal schizophrenia had an extremely bad prognosis and was practically incurable, although he noted that all five patients with schizo-affective psychosis in his series made a very good recovery. Patients with puerperal organic mental reactions may die in the acute phase of the illness, but if they survive, the prognosis appears to be excellent (Hemphill, 1952; Protheroe, 1969).

Protheroe (1969) has noted that the outcome of puerperal psychosis, particularly of schizophrenia, has improved in recent years, as reflected in the proportion of patients recovering (Table 9.15) and in the duration of stay in hospital. He found that during the period 1927 to 1941 only a minority of affectively disturbed puerperal patients were discharged within six months of admission and that the majority of schizophrenics stayed in hospital for at least three years. In contrast, during the period 1942 to 1961 more than half the patients with affective psychosis were discharged within three months, and the majority of schizophrenics left within six months of admission. It seems likely that the improved prognosis is related to the introduction of physical methods of treatment, particularly of ECT and the phenothiazines.

A recent development in the treatment of patients with puerperal psychoses has been to admit the infant with the mother (Baker, Morison, Game and Thorpe, 1961; Grunebaum and Weiss, 1963; Fowler and Brandon, 1965; Bardon, Glaser, Prothero and Weston, 1968; Van der Walde, Meeks, Grunebaum and Weiss, 1968) while Albretsen (1968) favours the admission of the patient's husband as well. There seems to be general agreement that even seriously disturbed women can take some responsibility for their babies, that the presence of the infant does not place an undue burden on the nurses, doctors or other patients in the ward, and that the practice may have important advantages. Very careful supervision of the mother is of course necessary if there appears to be even the slightest risk of infanticide. Bardon et al. (1968) have suggested that joint admission is beneficial to the mother in that separation from the baby may confirm the mother's belief that she is harmful to it, while Baker et al. (1961) found that women admitted with their babies stayed in hospital for less time and were less mentally disturbed on discharge than similar patients whose infants were cared for elsewhere.

Risk of Further Puerperal Psychosis

After a puerperal psychosis, a proportion of women have further pregnancies and occasionally they become psychotic again after delivery. Table 9.16 lists six studies where the risk has been evaluated by careful follow-up of the patients and overall 17·7 per cent (i.e. approximately 1 in 5 or 1 in 6) of women who have had a post-partum psychosis will have a recurrence if they become pregnant again. The risk that any *particular* subsequent pregnancy will be associated with a puerperal psychosis is shown in Table 9.17 as 20·4 per cent. This risk is more than 100 times larger than that associated with pregnancies in the general population.

Relationship between Puerperal and Non-puerperal Psychoses

As has been pointed out earlier in this chapter, the consensus is that psychoses arising *postpartum* do not constitute an entity distinct from clinically similar non-puerperal psychoses. The evidence in favour of this is quite substantial. First, women with puerperal psychoses tend to come from

Table 9.16

PROGNOSIS OF PUERPERAL PSYCHOSIS. PROPORTION OF WOMEN HAVING
FURTHER POST-PARTUM PSYCHOSES.

	No. of women with subsequent pregnancies	Proportion of women with subsequent puerperal psychosis %
Fondeur *et al.* (1957)	22	13·6
Jansson (1964)	74	9·5
Vislie (1956)	15	20·0
Martin (1958)	63	23·9
Arentsen (1968)	72	15·4
Protheroe (1969)	53	26·4
All series	299	17·7

families where the incidence of mental disorder is as high as in the families of patients with non-puerperal psychoses (Tetlow, 1955; Martin, 1958; Seager, 1960; Jansson, 1964; Protheroe, 1969). Secondly, they tend to have other psychotic illnesses independent of pregnancy and the puerperium. Of 242 women with post-partum mental illness studied by Paffenbarger (1964), 10 per cent gave a past history of non-puerperal mental disorder whereas among 628 mentally normal puerperal women the incidence was one per cent. Hemphill (1952), Martin (1958), Arentsen (1968) and Protheroe (1969) have

Table 9.17

PROGNOSIS OF PUERPERAL PSYCHOSIS. RISK OF RECURRENCE IN
FURTHER PREGNANCIES.

	No. of subsequent pregnancies	Risk of recurrence per pregnancy %
Martin (1958)	80	18·7
Seager (1960)	8	37·5
Paffenbarger (1964)	102	34·3
Arentsen (1968)	114	14·0
Protheroe (1969)	121	14·9
All series	425	20·4

also noted a tendency for post-partum psychotics, particularly those with affective psychosis, to have had a previous non-puerperal psychosis. Following post-partum psychosis the risk of a woman having a non-puerperal psychosis has been estimated at 29·5 per cent by Jansson (1964), at 26·7 per cent by Arentsen (1968) and at 43·1 per cent by Protheroe (1969). These estimates suggest that after recovery from a puerperal psychosis the risk of further puerperal psychosis is less than the risk of non-puerperal psychosis.

The intimate connection between puerperal and non-puerperal psychosis has been further demonstrated by Bratfos and Haug (1966) who showed that among women diagnosed as suffering from manic-depressive disorder the incidence of puerperal depression was at least ten times higher than that in the general population. Winokur and Ruangtrakool (1966) also observed a well-marked increase in the incidence of puerperal breakdown in women with affective disorders, but they showed that this increase was not significantly greater than that at other times, and they conclude that the predisposition of such women to post-partum depression is entirely due to their predisposition to affective disorder in general.

The evidence cited so far supports the view that psychoses arising post partum do not form a distinct entity, but in the present state of knowledge it is not possible to dismiss an alternative theory that the puerperium has specific aetiological importance, and it may be that physical changes, perhaps hormonal or metabolic, or psychological changes, such as the activation of unconscious conflicts relating to pregnancy and childbirth, are responsible for psychosis when it occurs post partum. Various observations seem to support such a theory. First, there is some evidence that severe mental disturbance, particularly manic-depressive psychosis, is much more common during the puerperium than at other times. Pugh, Jerath, Schmidt and Reed (1963) showed that during the three-month period immediately after delivery, admission to a mental hospital with a psychotic illness is some five times more common than at other times. They also noted that during pregnancy there are far fewer admissions than expected and they point out that the post-partum excess is not due to the postponement of the admission of mentally ill pregnant women until after the delivery. Paffenbarger (1964) has also shown a similar disparity between the prevalence of mental disorder during pregnancy and that during the puerperium. Secondly, as has already been mentioned, puerperal illness tends to be recurrent, and in individual patients the mental disturbances tend to take the same form on each occasion (Martin, 1958; Paffenbarger, 1964; Protheroe, 1969). Thirdly, in apparently functional post-partum illness some of the clinical features, such as the frequent disturbance of consciousness and the symptom-free period immediately after the delivery, suggest an organic cause (Hamilton, 1962). However, even if post-partum psychoses were identical in form to non-puerperal illnesses the possibility of a physical basis cannot be excluded, because there is now good reason to believe that the symptoms of an illness do not necessarily indicate its cause. Thus, illnesses clinically indistinguishable from schizophrenia may be caused by temporal lobe epilepsy of long duration or by chronic amphetamine intoxication, while continued use of reserpine and other rauwolfia alkaloids may cause typical severe affective disorder. For these various reasons, the hypothesis that the puerperal psychoses are not a distinct entity is only likely to be proven or refuted when the aetiology of the functional psychoses they resemble is known with greater certainty than at present.

REFERENCES

ALBRETSEN, C. S. (1968). Hospitalization of post-partum psychotic patients, together with babies and husbands. *Acta psychiat. scand.* Supplement 203, pp. 179-182.

ARENTSEN, K. (1968). Postpartum psychoses, with particular reference to the prognosis. *Dan. med. Bull.* **15**, 97-100.

BAKER, A. A., MORISON, M., GAME, J. A. and THORPE, J. G. (1961). Admitting schizophrenic mothers with their babies. *Lancet*, **2**, 237-239

BARDON, D., GLASER, Y. I. M., PROTHERO, D. and WESTON, D. H. (1968). Mother and baby unit: psychiatric survey of 115 cases. *Brit. med. J.* **2**, 755-758.

BRATFOS, O. and HAUG, J. O. (1966). Puerperal mental disorders in manic-depressive females. *Acta psychiat. scand.* **42**, 285-294.

CARROLL, J. D., LEAK, D. and LEE, H. A. (1966). Cerebral thrombophlebitis in pregnancy and the puerperium. *Quart. J. Med.* **35**, 347-368.

CROSS, J. N., CASTRO, P. O. and JENNETT, W. B. (1968). Cerebral strokes associated with pregnancy and the puerperium. *Brit. med. J.* **3**, 214-218.

FONDEUR, M., FIXSEN, C., TRIEBEL, W. A. and WHITE, M. A. (1957). Postpartum mental illness. A controlled study. *Arch. Neurol. Psychiat.* (*Chic.*) **77**, 503-512.

FOWLER, D. B. and BRANDON, R. E. (1965). A psychiatric mother and baby unit. *Lancet*, **1**, 160-161.

GOLDMAN, J. A., ECKERLING, B. and GANS, B. (1964). Intracranial venous sinus thrombosis in pregnancy and puerperium. *J. Obstet. Gynaec. Brit. Cwlth.* **71**, 791-796.

GRUNEBAUM, H. U. and WEISS, J. L. (1963). Psychotic mothers and their children: joint admission to an adult psychiatric hospital. *Amer. J. Psychiat.* **119**, 927-933.

HAMILTON, J. A. (1962). *Postpartum Psychiatric Problems.* St Louis.

HEMPHILL, R. E., (1952). Incidence and nature of puerperal psychiatric illness. *Brit. med. J.* **2**, 1232-1235.

JANSSON, B. (1964). Psychic insufficiencies associated with childbearing. *Acta psychiat. scand.* Supplement 172.

MARTIN, M. E. (1958). Puerperal mental illness. A follow-up study of 75 cases. *Brit. med. J.* **2**, 773-777.

MELGES, F. T. (1968). Postpartum psychiatric syndromes. *Psychosom. Med.* **30**, 95-108.

OLTMAN, J. E. and FRIEDMAN, S. (1965). Trends in postpartum illnesses. *Amer. J. Psychiat.* **122**, 328-329.

OSTWALD, P. F. and REGAN, P. F. (1957). Psychiatric disorders associated with childbirth. *J. nerv. ment. Dis.* **125**, 153-165.

PAFFENBARGER, R. (1964). Epidemiological aspects of parapartum mental illness. *Brit. J. prev. soc. Med.* **18**, 189-195.

PROTHEROE, C. (1969). Puerperal psychoses: a long term study, 1927-1961. *Brit. J. Psychiat.* **115**, 9-30.

PUGH, T. F., JERATH, B. K., SCHMIDT, W. M. and REED, R. B. (1963). Rates of mental illness related to childbearing. *New Engl. J. Med.* **268**, 1224-1228.

SEAGER, C. P. (1960). A controlled study of post-partum mental illness. *J. ment. Sci.* **106**, 214-230.

TETLOW, C. (1955). Psychoses of childbearing. *J. ment. Sci.* **101**, 629-639.

VISLIE, H. (1956). Puerperal mental disorders. *Acta psychiat. scand.* Supplement 111.

VAN DER WALDE, P. H., MEEKS, D., GRUNEBAUM, H. U. and WEISS, J. L. (1968). Joint admission of mothers and children to a state hospital. *Arch. gen. Psychiat.* **18**, 706-711.

WINOKUR, G. and RUANGTRAKOOL, S. (1966). Postpartum impact on patients with independently diagnosed affective disorder. *J. Amer. med. Ass.* **197**, 242-246.

WORLD HEALTH ORGANIZATION (1967). *Manual of the International Statistical Classification of Diseases, Injuries and Causes of Death.* Eighth revision. Geneva.

Neurotic Post-partum Disorders

"Post-partum Blues"

About two-thirds of puerperal women have short-lived emotional disturbances early in the puerperium (Robin, 1962; Hamilton, 1962; Yalom, Lunde, Moos and Hamburg, 1968). Most commonly there is a tendency to weep either following some slight rebuff which would not normally produce an overt reaction, or occurring for no apparent reason, and the condition is therefore sometimes known as "maternity blues" or "post-partum blues". Intellectual disturbance has been reported and Kane, Harman, Keeler and Ewing (1968) found that of 137 women interviewed on the third day post partum, 51 complained of difficulty in thinking, concentrating or remembering. Psychological tests of neuroticism have shown a tendency for post-partum women to be more neurotic, more anxious and more depressed than non-puerperal women of childbearing age (Kear-Colwell, 1965). The condition appears to be quite benign and of 22 patients followed up by Yalom *et al.* (1968) only one was in need of psychiatric treatment eight months later.

Minor Mental Disorder in the Puerperium

During the puerperium there is an appreciable incidence of mental disturbance more severe and long-lasting than "post-partum blues" but generally not so disturbing as to require admission to hospital. Ryle (1961) studied the records of all the women in his general practice who had been confined on at least one occasion during a four-year period (1955 to 1959) and noted the development of puerperal endogenous depression after 2·6 per cent of all deliveries. He calculated that in his practice such depression was five times more common during the year after childbirth than at other times. Tod (1964) in a general practice survey found a similar incidence (2·9 per cent) of puerperal depression among 700 women and observed that it tended to be associated with pathological anxiety during pregnancy and with a previous history of depression. Pitt (1968) studied 305 women who had been confined six to eight weeks previously in hospital and found that only one patient had symptoms of "classical" depression with suicidal ideas, early morning wakening and with more severe symptoms early in the day. There were however 32 patients with "atypical" depression, where neurotic disturbances were prominent. The symptoms of these patients usually began in a mild form during the first few days post partum and became worse after discharge from hospital. Typically the complaints were of tearfulness, despondency, feelings of inadequacy, irritability, inability to cope (particularly with the baby) and moderately severe anxiety. Pitt (1968) followed up 28 of these depressive patients and noted that one year later only 16 had completely recovered, but that only a small proportion had had any psychiatric treatment.

REFERENCES

HAMILTON, J. A. (1962). *Postpartum Psychiatric Problems.* St Louis.

KANE, F. J., HARMAN, W. J., KEELER, M. H. and EWING, J. A. (1968). Emotional and cognitive disturbance in the early puerperium. *Brit. J. Psychiat.* **114**, 99-102.

KEAR-COLWELL, J. J. (1965). Neuroticism in the early puerperium. *Brit. J. Psychiat.* **111**, 1189-1192.

PITT, B. (1968). Atypical depression following childbirth. *Brit. J. Psychiat.* **114**, 1325-1335.

ROBIN, A. A. (1962). The psychological changes of normal parturition. *Psychiat. Quart.* **36**, 129-150.

RYLE, A. (1961). The psychological disturbances associated with 345 pregnancies in 137 women. *J. ment. Sci.* **107**, 279-286.

TOD, E. D. M. (1964). Puerperal depression. A prospective epidemiological study. *Lancet,* **2**, 1264-1266.

YALOM, I. D., LUNDE, D. T., MOOS, R. H. and HAMBURG, D. A. (1968). "Postpartum Blues" syndrome. A description and related variables. *Arch. gen. Psychiat.* **18**, 16-27.

CHAPTER 10

STATISTICS OF MENTAL DISORDER

The 1963 Census. Community Surveys. Psychiatric Morbidity in General Practice.

IN RECENT years much statistical information has been published concerning patients receiving treatment from psychiatrists in England and Wales, and in this chapter some of the statistics are discussed. The sources of these data are first, an important and comprehensive census on all in-patients in National Health Service hospitals in England and Wales, undertaken by the Ministry of Health on December 31st, 1963 (Brooke, 1967); second, surveys on the use of psychiatric services in circumscribed areas of the country and last, studies on psychiatric morbidity in general practice.

It should be emphasized that caution is required in drawing conclusions from these data, in particular those which might be applied to the planning of future services. These statistics, important as they are, merely state what was happening at the time they were collected and they are therefore determined by the psychiatric facilities available, by the health and welfare services in general and by the degree of social organization in the community as well as by the prevalence of psychiatric disorder. Indeed the number of psychiatric beds required in an area probably depends to a greater extent on the provision for out-patient and day-hospital treatment and on the amount of other accommodation for persons who cannot care for themselves, than on the actual numbers of patients or on the severity of their illnesses. Since information on these other facilities and factors is incomplete, no conclusions concerning the planning of psychiatric services are given in this chapter.

THE 1963 CENSUS

On the census date (31st December, 1963) there were 194,260 in-patients in psychiatric care in National Health Service hospitals in England and Wales, either physically present in these hospitals or on short-term leave. The total excludes the relatively small number of persons receiving treatment from psychiatrists in private hospitals and nursing homes. Of the total, 134,575 (69·3%) were in mental illness accommodation and 59,685 (30·7%) in that for subnormality (Table 10.1) and these two groups of patients will now be considered separately.

Mental Illness

The census showed that there were 132,895 patients in Regional Hospital Board (R.H.B.) hospitals for the mentally ill, representing 2·86 per 1000 of the total population of England and Wales; 93·1 per cent were in comprehensive hospitals, mainly large mental hospitals of the traditional type, and only 2·1 per cent were in psychiatric units in general hospitals (Table 10.1). There

Table 10.1

CENSUS OF PATIENTS IN NATIONAL HEALTH SERVICE PSYCHIATRIC BEDS
IN ENGLAND AND WALES, DECEMBER 31ST 1963
(Brooke, 1967)

Type of Hospital or Unit	Number of Patients Physically Present or on Short-term leave
Mental Illness	(Total 134,575)
Comprehensive mental illness	123,744
Units in non-psychiatric hospitals	2,781
Units in geriatric or chronic sick hospitals	1,312
*"Mixed" hospitals	4,933
Children's	125
Total Regional Hospital Board Hospitals	132,895
Teaching hospitals	849
Broadmoor	831
Subnormality and Severe Subnormality	(Total 59,685)
Regional Hospital Board Hospitals	58,373
Rampton and Moss Side	1,312
Total, all Psychiatric Beds	194,260

* Hospitals with beds for both mental illness and subnormality.

were a further 849 patients in Teaching Hospitals (mainly in London) and 831 patients in Broadmoor, the Ministry of Health special hospital for mentally ill and psychopathic patients with dangerous, violent or criminal tendencies, but these teaching hospital and Broadmoor patients will not be considered further here.

Table 10.2

CENSUS, 1963. AGE AND SEX DISTRIBUTION OF PATIENTS WITH MENTAL
ILLNESS IN R.H.B. HOSPITALS
(Brooke, 1967)

Age (years)	Males	Females	Total	Proportion of males per cent
0-14	215	143	358	60·0
15-24	1,982	1,662	3,644	54·4
25-44	14,379	10,678	25,057	57·4
45-64	25,214	27,006	52,220	48·3
65+	15,299	36,317	51,616	29·6
Total	57,089	75,806	132,895	43·0

Age and Sex

Table 10.2 gives the age and sex distribution of patients in R.H.B. hospitals for the mentally ill on the census date. Overall, 43·0 per cent were male and

57·0 per cent female, but these proportions were age dependent and over the age of 65 years, almost three-quarters of the patients were female.

The point prevalence of mental disorder requiring inpatient care in mental illness hospitals is 283 per 100,000 of the population, for England and Wales as a whole, but this varies from region to region. The rate is highest in the South-West Metropolitan region where it is 585 per 100,000 and lowest in the Oxford region where it is 209 per 100,000. It also varies with age and sex and Table 10.3 shows that it increases with age, particularly among women and is highest among women over the age of 75 years where about 1·4 per cent of the total female population in that age group were in mental hospital on the census date.

Table 10.3

CENSUS, 1963. NUMBER OF PATIENTS WITH MENTAL ILLNESS IN R.H.B. HOSPITALS. RATES PER 100,000 POPULATION BY AGE AND SEX
(Brooke, 1967)

Age (years)	Males	Females
0-4	1·3	1·5
5-14	4·9	3·6
15-19	34·7	33·0
20-24	89·9	71·7
25-34	149·3	120·3
35-44	308·8	225·3
45-54	389·4	338·5
55-64	512·1	550·7
65-74	652·6	812·5
75+	844·5	1,399·4
All ages	250·1	313·4

Legal Status

The vast majority (93·6 per cent) of patients had informal status; 3·1 per cent were detained for treatment under Section 26 of the Mental Health Act (1959) and 1·1 per cent by an order for observation under Sections 25 or 29 (Table 10.4). Sections 60, 71 and 72 of the Act provide for orders to be made

Table 10.4

CENSUS, 1963. LEGAL STATUS OF PATIENTS WITH MENTAL ILLNESS IN R.H.B. HOSPITALS
(Brooke, 1967)

Legal status	No. of patients	Per cent
Informal	124,378	93·6
Detained under section		
25	1,275	1·0
26	4,087	3·1
29	130	0·1
60, 71 and 72	822	0·6
Sixth Schedule	2,151	1·6
Other	52	0·0
Total	132,895	100·0

in respect of certain offenders or of certain other people brought before the Courts and accounted for 0·6 per cent of the total hospital population. Under the Sixth Schedule of the Act are detained patients who had been in hospital under compulsion before the Act came into operation, and on the census date 1·6 per cent of all in-patients were so detained.

Diagnosis and Length of Stay

Figure 10.1 shows the distribution of the 132,895 patients among seven diagnostic categories; the largest single category is schizophrenia which accounts for 46·6 per cent of the total.

N = 132 895

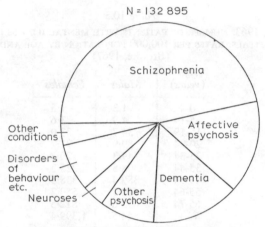

Figure 10.1 Census 1963. Distribution of in-patients in R.H.B. beds for mental illness in England and Wales, by diagnosis. (Data from Brooke, 1967)

On the census date there were 18,280 short-stay patients (i.e. those who had been admitted less than three months previously), 24,480 medium-stay patients (admitted between three months and two years previously) and 90,135 patients who had been in hospital for two years or more. Figure 10.2 shows that the distribution of patients among the various diagnoses varies according to length of stay; for example, the proportion of schizophrenics increases with length of stay, while that of neurotics decreases. Figure 10.3 shows the distribution of patients in four diagnostic categories (schizophrenia, affective psychosis, neurosis and dementia) by length of stay; it demonstrates that most schizophrenics had been in hospital for 11 years or more, that most neurotics had been admitted less than three months previously and that most patients with dementia had spent periods of between 3 months and 10 years in hospital. The data on which Figures 10.1 and 10.2 are based are given in Table 10.5.

That the variation in distribution of length of stay with diagnosis reflects differences in the prognosis of the conditions is demonstrated in Table 10.6 which shows that the rate of turnover of beds occupied by schizophrenics is

Short stay patients
(< 3months)
N = 18 280

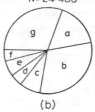

(a)

Medium stay patients
(3months- 2years)
N = 24 480

(b)

Figure 10.2 Census 1963. Distribution of in-patients in R.H.B. beds for mental illness in England and Wales by diagnosis and length of stay. (Data from Brooke, 1967)

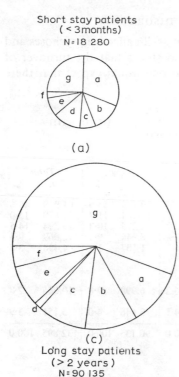

(c)
Long stay patients
(> 2 years)
N = 90 135

a · Affective psychosis
b - Dementia
c - Other psychosis
d - Neuroses
e - Disorders of behaviour etc.
f - Other conditions
g - Schizophrenia

Figure 10.3 Census 1963. Distribution of in-patients in R.H.B. beds for mental illness in England and Wales, by length of stay, for schizophrenia, affective psychosis, neuroses and dementia. (Data from Brooke, 1967)

Schizophrenia
N = 61 978

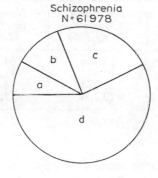

Affective psychosis
N = 19 879

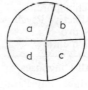

Neuroses
N = 4458

Dementia
N = 19 294

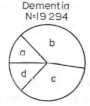

a - < 3months, b - 3mths - 2years, c - 2 - 10yrs, d - >11yrs

about one-fifth that of beds occupied by patients with affective psychoses and one-tenth that of places for neurotics. It also shows that the turnover of patients with dementia is relatively slow, and one would expect that there

Table 10.5

CENSUS 1963. DIAGNOSIS AND DURATION OF STAY OF PATIENTS WITH
MENTAL ILLNESS IN R.H.B. HOSPITALS
(Brooke, 1967)

Diagnosis	Duration of Stay							
	< 3m		3m-2 yr.		> 2 yr.		Total	
	No.	%	No.	%	No.	%	No.	%
Schizophrenia	4,563	25·0	7,356	30·0	50,059	55·5	61,978	46·6
Affective Psychoses	5,696	31·2	4,079	16·7	10,104	11·2	19,879	15·0
Dementia	2,458	13·4	7,561	30·9	9,275	10·3	19,294	14·5
Other Psychoses	1,217	6·7	1,906	7·8	8,946	9·9	12,069	9·1
Neuroses	2,298	12·6	1,053	4·3	1,107	1·2	4,458	3·3
Disorders of Behaviour, Character and Intelligence	1,549	8·5	1,519	6·2	6,998	7·8	10,066	7·8
Other Mental Disorders	499	2·7	1,006	4·1	3,646	4·0	5,151	3·9
Total	18,280	100·0	24,480	100·0	90,135	100·0	132,895	100·0

Table 10.6

ANNUAL RATE OF TURNOVER OF PATIENTS WITH MENTAL ILLNESS IN
R.H.B. HOSPITALS
(Data from Brooke, 1967 and Ministry of Health, 1969)

Diagnosis	Number of Admissions during 1964	Number of In-Patients 31.12.63	Annual Turnover Per 100 Beds
*Schizophrenia	35,226	64,496	54·6
Affective Psychoses	58,472	19,879	294·1
Neuroses	23,722	4,458	532·1
Dementia	12,706	17,374	73·1
All Diagnoses	158,861	132,895	119·6

* Including Paranoia

would be therefore a large number of very long stay demented patients in hospital at any given time. That the census figures do not indicate this is explained presumably by the high mortality rate of patients in this group.

Subnormality

The census count for in-patients in R.H.B. hospitals and units in England and Wales for the mentally subnormal was 58,373, of whom 94 per cent were in hospitals devoted solely to these patients; the remaining 6 per cent were either in hospitals which catered for mentally ill persons in addition, or in other types of unit. The figure of 58,373 represents a rate of 1·2/1000 of the total population of England and Wales, but there was wide variation between different parts of the country, ranging from 0·6/1000 in the Liverpool region to 2·1/1000 in the South-West Metropolitan region.

The census showed in addition that there were 1312 patients in Ministry of Health special hospitals (Rampton and Moss Side) for subnormal, severely subnormal and psychopathic patients of dangerous, violent or criminal propensities (Table 10.1) but these patients are not considered further here.

Age, Sex and Legal Status

Of the total number of patients in hospitals for the subnormal, 54·2 per cent were male. Table 10.7 shows that males outnumber females in every age group and that the highest rates are among young adults.

Table 10.7

CENSUS, 1963. NUMBER OF PATIENTS IN MENTAL SUBNORMALITY HOSPITALS.
RATES PER 100,000 POPULATION BY AGE AND SEX
(Brooke, 1967)

Age	Males	Females
<2	3·1	2·7
2-4	20·7	17·3
5-9	88·7	58·5
10-14	142·8	91·7
15-19	200·4	113·9
20-24	216·9	147·4
25-34	180·3	136·9
35-44	165·5	139·5
45-54	157·7	147·1
55 and over	102·7	98·2
All ages	138·6	110·4

The overwhelming majority (92·7 per cent) of patients were in hospital on an informal basis, and most of those who were not were detained under the Sixth Schedule of the Mental Health Act.

Diagnosis and Mental Category

Most patients in mental hospitals for the subnormal are suffering from various degrees of primary mental retardation (International Classification of Disease Code numbers 310-315) and relatively few from specific disorders such as mongolism, phenylketonuria, spastic paralysis or intracranial birth injury. A small proportion have mental illnesses or serious personality disorders which dominate the clinical picture (Table 10.8).

In categorizing patients in hospitals for the subnormal, a more useful classification than that based on diagnosis is the one described in Section 4 of the Mental Health Act (1959). This allocates mentally disordered subjects to four categories:

(*a*) mental illness.

(*b*) severe subnormality—"a state of arrested or incomplete development of mind which includes subnormality of intelligence and is of such a nature or degree that the patient is incapable of living an independent life or of guarding himself against serious exploitation, or will be so incapable when of an age to do so".

(c) subnormality—"a state of arrested or incomplete development of mind (not amounting to severe subnormality) which includes subnormality of

Table 10.8

CENSUS, 1963. PRIMARY DIAGNOSIS OF PATIENTS IN SUBNORMALITY
HOSPITALS AND UNITS
(Brooke, 1967)

Diagnostic Group	Number	Per cent
Schizophrenia	316	0·5
Other Psychoses	110	0·2
Neuroses	19	0·0
Antisocial Personality	73	0·1
Idiocy	8,463	14·5
Imbecility	26,018	44·6
Moron	14,992	25·7
Borderline Intelligence	887	1·5
Mongolism	3,167	5·4
Phenylketonuria	6	0·0
Mental Deficiency and Subnormality N.O.S.	2,597	4·4
Other Disorders of Behaviour, Character and Intelligence	95	0·2
Spastic Paralysis	334	0·6
Epilepsy	153	0·3
Congenital Malformations	161	0·3
Intracranial Birth Injury	96	0·2
Social Problem	8	0·0
Other Causes	878	1·5
All Causes	58,373	100·0

intelligence and is of a nature or degree which requires or is susceptible to medical treatment or other special care or training of the patient".

(d) psychopathic disorder—"a persistent disorder or disability of mind (whether or not including subnormality of intelligence) which results in abnormally aggressive or seriously irresponsible conduct on the part of the patient, and requires or is susceptible to medical treatment". (The General Register Office, 1968, in its *Glossary of Mental Disorders* has indicated that this mental category corresponds to a type of antisocial personality disorder in the International Classification of Disease.)

The 1963 census used the above classification to categorize patients in hospitals for the subnormal. The findings are set out in Table 10.9 which shows that more than three-quarters of the patients were severely subnormal.

Duration of Stay

Figure 10.4 gives the distribution of patients by length of stay. On the census date more than 80 per cent of patients had been admitted 2 years or

Table 10.9

CENSUS, 1963. MENTAL CATEGORY OF PATIENTS IN MENTAL
SUBNORMALITY HOSPITALS
(Brooke, 1967)

Category	No.	%
Severe subnormality	46,283	79·3
Subnormality	11,354	19·4
Psychopath	234	0·4
Mental Illness and other	502	0·9
Total	58,373	100·0

more previously and just under one-half had been in hospital continuously for more than 10 years. Consistent with this is the slow rate of turnover of beds in hospitals for the subnormal; during 1964 there were 10,364 admissions to these beds (Ministry of Health, 1969) and calculation from this figure and the census total gives an annual turnover rate in 1964 of only 17·8 per 100 beds.

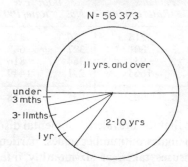

Figure 10.4 Census 1963. Distribution of patients in R.H.B. beds for mental subnormality in England and Wales, by length of stay. (Data from Brooke, 1967)

COMMUNITY SURVEYS

The Camberwell Register

In 1964, the Medical Research Council's Social Psychiatry Research Unit set up a cumulative psychiatric case register of Camberwell residents in contact with psychiatric services. Camberwell is an industrial working-class suburb of South-East London, with a population, in 1961 of 175,304. The main psychiatric services for adults in the area are provided by Cane Hill Hospital, an R.H.B. hospital which has over 2000 beds and which is responsible for a large catchment area in South-East London, of which Camberwell represents about one-third. In addition, the Camberwell population is served by two groups of teaching hospitals, the Bethlem-Maudsley group (post-graduate) and the King's College group (undergraduate). Services are also provided by the Local Authority Mental Health Department and by other agencies.

The register began on December 31st, 1964 with a census of all persons resident in Camberwell who were in contact, on that date, with a psychiatric service. Since then all new cases have been added to the register and further censuses have been undertaken at six-monthly intervals. Data concerning patients seen during the first three years (1965, 1966 and 1967) have now been published (Wing, Wing and Hailey, 1968) and some of the findings relating to mental disorder in adults (excluding subnormality) are presented here.

One-Day Prevalence

On December 31st, 1964 there were 1038 Camberwell residents aged 15 years or more in contact with psychiatric services (i.e. 758 per 100,000 of the population aged 15 years or more). Table 10.10 sets out the distribution of

Table 10.10

CAMBERWELL RESIDENTS IN CONTACT WITH PSYCHIATRIC SERVICES
ON 31.12.64, BY AGE AND SEX; ABSOLUTE NUMBERS AND AGE-SEX SPECIFIC
RATES/100,000 POPULATION
(Wing *et al.*, 1968)

Age (years)	Males No.	Males Rate/100,000	Females No.	Females Rate/100,000	Both sexes No.	Both sexes Rate/100,000
15-24	29	239	27	215	56	226
25-44	135	573	192	801	327	688
45-64	144	667	220	957	364	816
65+	72	1040	219	1663	291	1449
15+	380	592	658	905	1038	758

these patients by age and sex and shows that the prevalence of mental disorder increases with advancing age and that females outnumber males, particularly in the older age groups. Further censuses taken at six-monthly intervals showed similar findings (Table 10.11).

Table 10.11

ADULT CAMBERWELL PATIENTS IN CONTACT WITH PSYCHIATRIC SERVICES
ON 7 CENSUS DAYS (RATES/100,000 POPULATION AGED 15+)
(Wing *et al.*, 1968)

Census days	Males	Females	Both sexes
31.12.64	592	905	758
30. 6.65	643	1012	839
31.12.65	596	990	806
30. 6.66	629	930	789
31.12.66	582	953	799
30. 6.67	589	956	784
31.12.67	607	977	803

One-Year Prevalence and Rate of New Referrals

The one-year prevalence is the proportion of adults in contact with the psychiatric services at any time during the course of one year. During 1965 there were 2514 such patients (representing 1836 per 100,000 of the population aged 15 years or more), of whom 1038 were in contact at the beginning of the year while the remaining 1476 were those making new contacts during 1965. Table 10.12 gives the one-year prevalence rates, separately for the two sexes, and shows that they tended to increase during the three-year period.

Table 10.12

ONE YEAR PREVALENCE OF ADULT CAMBERWELL RESIDENTS IN CONTACT WITH PSYCHIATRIC SERVICES (RATES/100,000 POPULATION AGED 15+)
(Wing *et al.*, 1968)

Year	Males	Females	Both sexes
1965	1465	2164	1836
1966	1459	2194	1850
1967	1575	2364	1994

Table 10.13

CAMBERWELL RESIDENTS (NOT COUNTED IN TABLE 10.10) WHO BEGAN NEW EPISODES OF CONTACT WITH PSYCHIATRIC SERVICES DURING 1965, BY AGE AND SEX; ABSOLUTE NUMBERS AND AGE-SEX SPECIFIC RATES/100,000 POPULATION
(Wing *et al.*, 1968)

Age (years)	Males		Females		Both sexes	
	No.	Rate/100,000	No.	Rate/100,000	No.	Rate/100,000
15-24	121	996	173	1375	294	1189
25-44	235	998	400	1669	635	1336
45-64	164	759	231	1005	395	886
65+	41	592	111	843	152	757
15+	561	873	915	1259	1476	1078

Table 10.13 sets out the distribution, by age and sex, of patients who began new episodes of contact with psychiatric services during 1965; (a new episode is one which follows a period of at least three months during which the patient has made no contact with any psychiatric service). Table 10.13 demonstrates that there are many more new female patients than males, and that the rate of new contacts is greatest in the younger age groups. (In contrast, Table 10.10 shows that at a given point in time the prevalence of mental disorder is greatest among the elderly).

Table 10.14

ADULT CAMBERWELL RESIDENTS IN CONTACT WITH PSYCHIATRIC SERVICES ON DECEMBER 31ST 1964, BY TYPE OF SERVICE
(Wing *et al.*, 1968)

Type of service	Number	Rate/100,000 population aged 15+
In-patient		
Long stay	416	237
Medium stay	70	40
Short stay	81	46
Day-patient	14	8
Out-patient	457	261
Total	1038	592

Type of Service

Table 10.14 gives the distribution of patients who were in contact with a psychiatric service on December 31st, 1964 by type of service. In-patients were classified as *long stay* if they had been admitted one year or more previously, and as *short stay* if they had been admitted 60 days or less previously. Table 10.14 shows that, on the census date, 567 (54·6%) were in hospital and that of these in-patients most were long stay; more recent censuses have shown similar distributions.

Table 10.15

ADULT CAMBERWELL PSYCHIATRIC IN-PATIENTS ON DECEMBER 31ST, 1964.
DISTRIBUTION BY DIAGNOSIS AND LENGTH OF STAY
(Wing *et al.*, 1968)

Diagnosis	Length of stay			Total	
	Short stay	Medium stay	Long stay	No.	%
Schizophrenia	22	15	238	275	48·5
Severe depression	24	7	53	84	14·8
Organic conditions	9	23	48	80	14·1
Other diagnoses	26	25	77	128	22·6
All diagnoses	81	70	416	567	100·0

Diagnosis

The distribution by diagnosis of in-patients on December 31st, 1964 is given in Table 10.15 which shows that schizophrenics account for 48·5 per cent of the in-patient population and that the vast majority of schizophrenics in hospital are long stay.

Table 10.16

PROPORTIONS OF CAMBERWELL PATIENTS BEGINNING A NEW EPISODE OF
CONTACT DURING 1965, IN VARIOUS DIAGNOSTIC GROUPS
(Wing *et al.*, 1968)

Diagnostic category	Patients admitted %	Patients not admitted %	Total %
Schizophrenia	19	5	9
Endogenous depression	25	14	17
Organic conditions	11	1	4
Other diagnoses	45	81	69
Total	100	100	100
Number of persons	*471*	*1005*	*1476*

The actual numbers in each diagnostic category depend on the frequency with which the diagnoses are made, on the prognosis of each condition and on the proportion of patients in each diagnostic category that is admitted to hospital. Table 10.16 gives the distribution by diagnosis of the 1476 patients who began a new episode of contact with the psychiatric services during 1965. Schizophrenics accounted for 9 per cent of this total, but for 19 per cent of those admitted to hospital; hence a diagnosis of schizophrenia carries with it a much greater than average probability of admission. That eventually schizophrenics make up 48·5 per cent of the in-patient population (Table 10.15) is presumably due to the poor prognosis and to the tendency for schizophrenics to stay in hospital for longer than average. Severe depression accounts for 17 per cent of all new episodes, and for 25 per cent of all admissions (Table 10.16); here there is a probability of admission slightly above the average, but the prognosis seems to be good because these patients account for only 14·8 per cent of the hospital population (Table 10.15), i.e. there is no tendency for them to accumulate as in-patients.

Although only 4 per cent of new patients have organic conditions, Table 10.16 shows that these make up 11 per cent of the total admission. They tend to stay in hospital where they constitute 14·1 per cent of the population (Table 10.15). That the accumulation is not particularly great is presumably due to the high mortality associated with these conditions rather than to a good prognosis.

The Salford Register

Since 1959, a register of all adult patients from Salford, a city with a population of about 150,000 adjoining Manchester, has been maintained, and, like the Camberwell register, it records details of persons who come into contact with any of the psychiatric services. Adelstein, Downham, Stein and Susser (1968) have presented some of the statistics on Salford residents, who, for the first time in their lives, sought psychiatric care during the five-year period 1959-63, while Susser, Stein, Mountney and Freeman (1970a, b) have reported some of the findings concerning chronic disability associated with mental illness. (The Camberwell register has not published any data on either of these topics.) Figure 10.5 gives the age and sex specific rates for adults coming into contact with psychiatric services for the first time in their lives (these data, like others in this section, do not include mental subnormality). First illnesses are more common among women than men, although over the age of 60 the rate tends to be higher in men. Adelstein et al. (1968) also found that the risk of a first illness was greater among the divorced and widowed than among single persons and that it was least among the married.

From the Salford case register, Susser et al. (1970a) compiled a census of all adult persons who were on the register on September 30th, 1966 and who had been chronically disabled by mental illness for 12 months or more. The criteria of chronic disability were as follows:

1. For any patient: continuous residence in a mental hospital.
2. For any patient: for all practical purposes continuously confined to the home because of mental disorder.

3. For a man before retiring age or a single "working woman": continuously out of work (excluding brief unsuccessful attempts to work) because of mental illness.
4. For a man after retiring age: continuously unable, because of mental illness, to perform household or other duties previously carried out by him.
5. For a woman of any age: continuously unable, because of mental illness, to perform household duties previously carried out by her.

On the census date there were 685 persons chronically disabled because of mental illness on the Salford register, a one-day prevalence of 5·8 per 1000 of

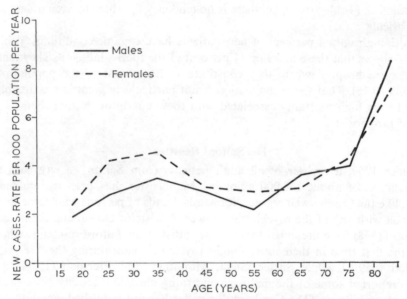

Figure 10.5 Salford residents coming into contact with psychiatric services for the first time in their lives during the period 1959-63. Age-sex specific annual rates per 1000 population. (Adelstein *et al.* 1968)

the population aged 15 years and over. Figure 10.6 shows the variation of the prevalence of chronic disability with age, separately for each sex. For both men and women the rate rises with age and with the exception of the over-70 age group it is higher in men than in women. Susser *et al.* (1970*b*) noted that, at the time of the census, 59·6 per cent of the chronically disabled were in hospital, the remainder living in the community. They also found that schizophrenia was the predominant diagnosis both in and out of hospital (Table 10.17). In the community, the chronically disabled tended to be younger than those in hospital, and this tendency was independent of diagnosis. Marital status also seemed to determine the location of these patients; most of those in hospital were single while the majority of those living in the community were or had been married.

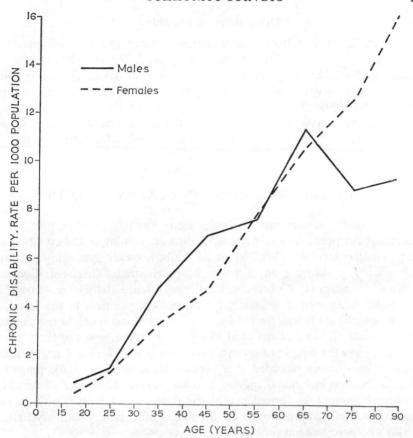

Figure 10.6 Point prevalence of chronic disability following mental illness in Salford on September 30th, 1966. Age-sex specific rates per 1000 population. (Susser *et al.*, 1970*a*)

Table 10.17

CHRONIC DISABILITY DUE TO MENTAL ILLNESS IN SALFORD,
SEPTEMBER 30TH, 1966. PER CENT DISTRIBUTION OF PATIENTS BY DIAGNOSIS,
SEX AND LOCATION OF PATIENT
(Susser *et al.*, 1970*b*)

	Men		Women		Both Sexes	
Diagnosis	*Community* (*N=125*)	*Hospital* (*N=192*)	*Community* (*N=152*)	*Hospital* (*N=216*)	*Community* (*N=277*)	*Hospital* (*N=408*)
Schizophrenia	52	70	30	51	41	60
Depressive psychosis	5	6	30	19	19	13
Senile dementia	3	2	9	12	7	7
Organic psychosis	4	3	3	3	3	3
Psychopathy	13	3	7	1	10	1
Psychoneurosis	8	1	11	1	10	1
Other	15	15	9	12	11	14
Total	100	100	100	100	100	100

Other Relevant Statistics

Most published data from official sources concerning psychiatric patients in England and Wales relate to those in hospital, but the Department of Health and Social Security (1970) has published statistics on the numbers of out-patients and day patients seen during 1967. A more detailed study of day patients who attended 15 selected psychiatric day hospitals during a twelve-month period in 1966-67 has been reported (Department of Health and Social Security, 1969) and this gives much useful information including diagnoses, duration of treatment and outcome.

PSYCHIATRIC MORBIDITY IN GENERAL PRACTICE

The in-patient census and the community surveys together give some estimate of the prevalence of psychiatric disorder coming to the attention of the psychiatric services. There seems no doubt however that many patients with psychiatric disorder are not seen by psychiatrists. Shepherd, Cooper, Brown and Kalton (1966) investigated the prevalence and nature of psychiatric disturbance seen in 46 fairly typical general practices in the London area. Before the study was started they constructed a one-in-eight representative sample of all the patients aged 15 and over on the books of these practices, and over the course of one year (beginning on October 1st, 1961) the participating doctors recorded every consultation involving these patients; the data obtained included diagnosis. Psychiatric conditions were allocated to two broad groups: (a) formal psychiatric illness and (b) psychiatric associated conditions (psychosomatic conditions, organic illness with psychiatric overlay and psychosocial problems).

Formal psychiatric illness was classified as follows:
1. psychosis (schizophrenia, manic-depressive psychosis, organic psychosis).
2. mental subnormality.
3. dementia (deterioration of mental powers in excess of normal ageing process).
4. neurosis (anxiety state, depressive, hysterical, phobic or asthenic reactions; others).
5. personality disorder.

Physical illnesses were allocated to one or other of eleven broad categories, e.g. cardiovascular, respiratory, gastrointestinal disorders etc.

The patient consulting rate for psychiatric morbidity (i.e. the one-year prevalence rate or the number of patients with a psychiatric condition who consulted the general practitioner on at least one occasion during the survey year per 1000 patients at risk) is shown in Table 10.18. Since some patients had more than one psychiatric diagnosis the total rates for formal psychiatric illness, psychiatric associated conditions and total psychiatric morbidity are less than the sum of the rates of the individual diagnoses.

The total psychiatric morbidity was 139·4 per 1000, that is to say during a single year about 14 per cent of the total population studied consulted their general practitioner with a psychiatric condition; formal psychiatric illness

Table 10.18

PSYCHIATRIC MORBIDITY IN GENERAL PRACTICE. CONSULTING RATES PER 1000
AT RISK, BY SEX AND DIAGNOSIS
(Shepherd et al., 1966)

Diagnostic Group	Male	Female	Both Sexes
Psychoses	2·7	8·6	5·9
Mental Subnormality	1·6	2·9	2·3
Dementia	1·2	1·6	1·4
Neuroses	55·7	116·6	88·5
Personality Disorder	7·2	4·0	5·5
Formal Psychiatric Illness	67·2	131·9	102·1
Psychosomatic Conditions	24·5	34·5	29·9
Organic Illness with Psychiatric Overlay	13·1	16·6	15·0
Psychosocial Problems	4·6	10·0	7·5
Psychiatric Associated Conditions	38·6	57·2	48·6
Total Psychiatric Morbidity	97·9	175·0	139·4
Number of Patients at Risk	6,783	7,914	14,697

accounted for just over two-thirds of this 14 per cent. Psychiatric prevalence varied with age and sex; it was higher among females than among males and was highest between the ages of 25 and 45 years. (Table 10.19).

Table 10.19

PSYCHIATRIC MORBIDITY IN GENERAL PRACTICE. CONSULTING RATES
PER 1000 AT RISK, BY AGE AND SEX.
(Shepherd et al., 1966)

Age (years)	Males	Females
15-24	62·0	125·4
25-44	104·8	194·6
45-64	110·8	208·1
65 and over	109·9	148·7
Not known	27·5	30·9
All ages	97·9	175·0

The records included data on "new" psychiatric illnesses (for which the patient had not previously consulted for at least one year) and on chronic illnesses (with a continuous duration of at least one year) and also the numbers referred to psychiatric specialists. New patients accounted for 37 per cent of all the patients with psychiatric disturbances, and of these only 3·5 per cent were referred during the survey year to a hospital for psychiatric assessment or treatment. Chronic patients accounted for 56 per cent of the total and of these 7·5 per cent received some specialist psychiatric supervision during the year. The referral rate was much higher among psychotic patients but even here only about one-quarter were referred for a psychiatric opinion.

Thus the vast majority of patients with psychiatric conditions seen in general practice were not referred to psychiatrists. Indeed of 100 chronic psychiatric cases in this investigation who were studied more intensively, only 32 had at any time been seen by a psychiatrist even though almost all of them had long histories of psychiatric disorder. Jones and Miles (1964), who undertook a survey of mental disorder in Anglesey (North Wales) during 1960 have also produced evidence suggesting this. They scrutinized the records both of the local psychiatric hospital (in-patients and out-patients) and of the general practitioners with patients on the island and found a total of 1966 cases of psychiatric illness (excluding mental subnormality). Of these cases, 1104 (56%) had never seen a psychiatrist and were known only to the general practitioner. Most were suffering from relatively mild conditions but there were 45 schizophrenics and 48 with organic mental disorders unknown to the psychiatric services. (Table 10.20).

There is some evidence that a proportion of psychiatric conditions may not be recognized by general practitioners. Goldberg and Blackwell (1970) investigated 553 consecutive patients attending a general practice surgery, of whom 200 were interviewed immediately afterwards by a psychiatrist. The general practitioner rated the patients on a five-point scale of severity of psychiatric disturbance as follows:

No psychiatric disturbance detected	66·7%
Mild subclinical emotional disturbance	13·0%
Psychiatric illness—mild	15·0%
Psychiatric illness—moderate	3·1%
Psychiatric illness—marked	1·4%

Thus the general practitioner noted an incidence of psychiatric illness in 19·5% of the patients, but the psychiatrist who spent half to one hour with each person he saw found that there were a number with mental disturbances whom the general practitioner had regarded as normal. These patients with "hidden" psychiatric illness presented with somatic symptoms and their emotional distress had been overlooked, and it was estimated that they accounted for about 10 per cent of all patients in the study. Follow-up showed that about two-thirds of patients with "hidden" illness were no longer mentally disturbed after six months, an outcome similar to that of patients whose psychiatric illnesses had been recognized by the general practitioner.

It is of course probable that there are some mentally disturbed persons who do not come to medical attention at all, but there is no indication as to their numbers.

REFERENCES

ADELSTEIN, A. M., DOWNHAM, D. Y., STEIN, Z. and SUSSER, M. W. (1968). The epidemiology of mental illness in an English city. Inceptions recognized by the Salford psychiatric services. *Soc. Psychiat.* (*Berl.*) 3, 47-59.

BROOKE, E. M. (1967). A census of patients in psychiatric beds, 1963. *Ministry of Health Reports on Public Health and Medical Subjects.* No. 116 H.M.S.O. London.

Table 10.20

ANGLESEY SURVEY OF MENTAL DISORDER. NUMBER OF PATIENTS, BY SEX, DIAGNOSIS AND TYPE OF TREATMENT
(Jones and Miles, 1964)

Type of treatment	Diagnosis										Total	
	Depression		Neurosis		Schizophrenia		Organic mental states		Psychopathy, alcoholism and epilepsy			
	M.	F.	M.	F.	M.	F.	M.	F.	M.	F.	No.	%
In Community												
Known to psychiatric services	165	271	57	72	45	43	11	11	41	14	730	37·1
Known only to G.P.	78	157	265	425	15	30	16	32	49	37	1104	56·2
In-patient or in care	8	16	–	–	53	30	9	5	9	2	132	6·7
Total	251	444	322	497	113	103	36	48	99	53	1966	100·0

DEPARTMENT OF HEALTH AND SOCIAL SECURITY (1969). A pilot survey of patients attending day hospitals. *Statistical Report Series* No. 7. H.M.S.O. London.

DEPARTMENT OF HEALTH AND SOCIAL SECURITY (1970). The facilities and services of psychiatric hospitals in England and Wales, 1967. *Statistical Report Series* No. 9. H.M.S.O. London.

GENERAL REGISTER OFFICE (1968). A glossary of mental disorders. *Studies on Medical and Population Subjects* No. 22. H.M.S.O. London.

GOLDBERG, D. P. and BLACKWELL, B. (1970). Psychiatric illness in general practice: a detailed study using a new method of case identification. *Brit. med. J.* **2**, 439-443.

JONES, D. A. and MILES, H. L. (1964). The Anglesey mental health survey. In *Problems and Progress in Medical Care.* (Editor McLachlan, G.) London.

MENTAL HEALTH ACT (1959). H.M.S.O. London.

MINISTRY OF HEALTH (1969). Psychiatric hospitals and units in England and Wales. Inpatient statistics from the Mental Health Enquiry for the years 1964, 1965 and 1966. *Statistical Report Series* No. 4. H.M.S.O. London.

SHEPHERD, M., COOPER, B., BROWN, A. C. and KALTON, G. W. (1966). *Psychiatric Illness in General Practice.* London.

SUSSER, M. W., STEIN, Z., MOUNTNEY, G. H. and FREEMAN, H. L. (1970*a*). Chronic disability following mental illness in an English city. Part I Total prevalence in and out of mental hospital. *Soc. Psychiat. (Berl.)* **5**, 63-69.

SUSSER, M. W., STEIN, Z., MOUNTNEY, G. H. and FREEMAN, H. L. (1970*b*). Chronic disability following mental illness in an English city. Part II The location of patients in hospital and community. *Soc. Psychiat. (Berl.)* **5**, 69-76.

WING, L., WING, J. K. and HAILEY, A. (1968). The Camberwell register. In *Triennial Statistical Report: Years 1964-1966.* (Editor Hare, E. H.) Bethlem Royal and Maudsley Hospital, London.

INDEX

Printed in Great Britain by T. & A. Constable Ltd., Edinburgh.